Sacred & Delicious

A Modern Ayurvedic Cookbook

Lisa Joy Mitchell

[swp]

SHE WRITES PRESS

Published October 16, 2018
Printed in Canada
Print ISBN: 978-1-63152-347-2
E-ISBN: 978-1-63152-348-9
Library of Congress Control Number: 2018939298

For information, address:
She Writes Press
1563 Solano Ave #546
Berkeley, CA 94707

Cover and interior design by Tabitha Lahr
Photographs by Roger Winstead, with a photo apiece by Ingrid Beckman (page 277), Jeanne Reinelt (page 71), and Ann Stratton (page 36)
Additional art and photographs © 123rf.com on pages 1, 3, 8, 14, 58, 73, 74, 81, 82, 83, 84, 101, 103, 105, 125, 137, 142, 153, 156, 159, 173, 177, 181, 191, 200, 212, 221, 236, 239, 241, 243, 248, 250, 254, 278; Shutterstock.com pages 16, 20, 23, 25
Front cover and Blessings lotus paintings © Karin Michele Anderson

A NOTE TO THE READER: This book is intended as an informational guide. The ideas and suggestions contained in this book are not intended as substitutes for medical care and treatment by a physician. For any medical condition, always consult a licensed health care professional.

She Writes Press is a division of SparkPoint Studio, LLC.

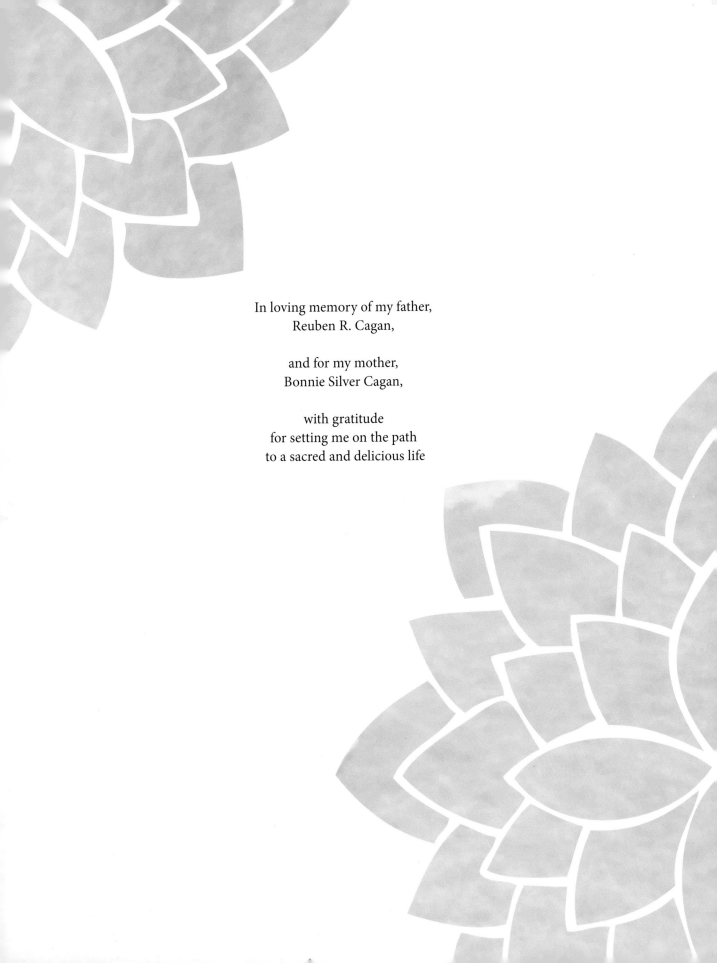

In loving memory of my father,
Reuben R. Cagan,

and for my mother,
Bonnie Silver Cagan,

with gratitude
for setting me on the path
to a sacred and delicious life

May all who explore *Sacred & Delicious* experience true nourishment
and delight through pure, delectable food.

May we awaken to the sacredness and joy of healthy eating.

May we learn to eat consciously so that we honor ourselves
and protect our Mother Earth.

May all who suffer find their perfect paths to healing.

And may all people everywhere have an abundance of healthy food.

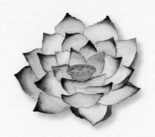

Contents

Part Two: The Recipes

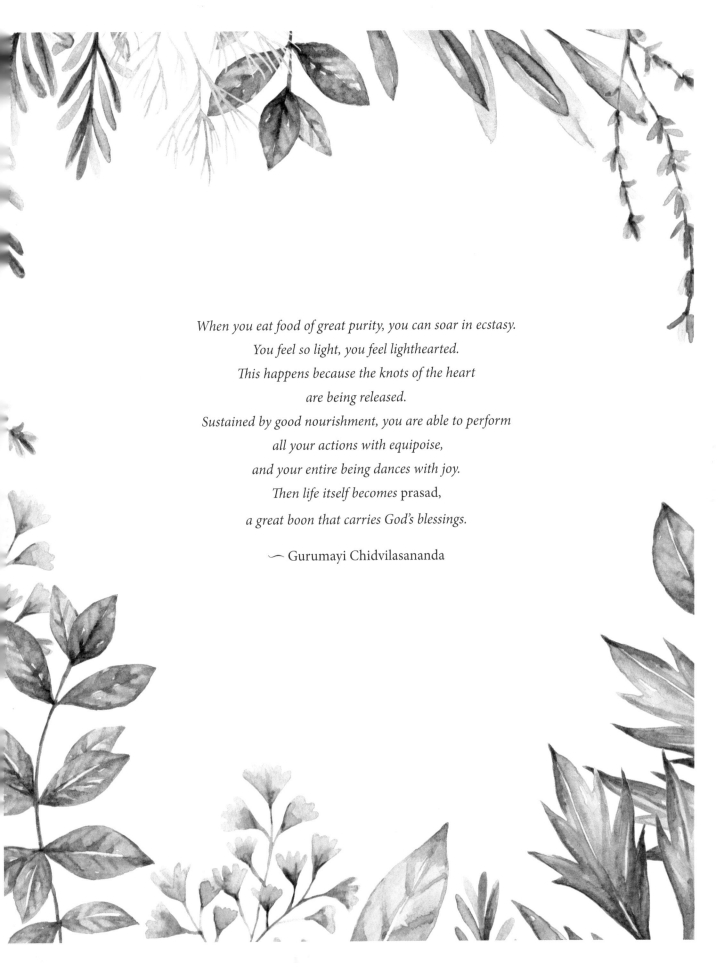

When you eat food of great purity, you can soar in ecstasy.
You feel so light, you feel lighthearted.
This happens because the knots of the heart
are being released.
Sustained by good nourishment, you are able to perform
all your actions with equipoise,
and your entire being dances with joy.
Then life itself becomes prasad,
a great boon that carries God's blessings.

⌒ Gurumayi Chidvilasananda

Introduction

*P*icture sitting around the table in your kitchen or dining room with those you love. As people take their first bites of a meal you have just prepared, for one brief moment no one speaks. Except for the faint sounds of forks clicking on plates, the room is silent. Then, as if on cue, comes a sweet chorus of murmurs: *Mmmmm . . . ooooo . . . aaaahhh!*

When we eat delicious food, we experience such deep satisfaction that most of us cannot refrain from vocalization. "Oh, my God!" someone will sigh, almost reverently, after sampling a particularly sumptuous dish. "This food is divine!" someone else will chime.

Moved by our passions as well as our fundamental need to eat, we build much of our lives, our relationships, and our most sacred occasions around the sharing of food. Whether we gather to commemorate life, give thanks for good fortune, or comfort the bereaved, we nourish and celebrate one another with meals that are intensely delicious and stoked in traditions both simple and elaborate. In my own life, food has been a primary source of celebration and comfort since I was very young. Many of my fondest childhood memories revolve around meals eaten with my family. For us, food was the sweet center of our existence.

I grew up in the 1950s and '60s in a Jewish home in Florence, South Carolina, where there were fewer than thirty Jewish families, a tiny percentage of the town's population. My mother invested great care in filling our family life with Jewish observances so we would love, and would never forget, our heritage. As Shabbat descended into our household each Friday evening at sunset, my father, brother, and I waited in anticipation for dinner while my mother sweetly sang a prayer over the Sabbath candles. The food remained untouched until we had said the final prayers over the wine and bread. Only then would we dive enthusiastically into our less-than-kosher Sabbath meal—roasted chicken or beef brisket smothered in tomatoes and onions, a vegetable side dish, dinner rolls with butter, and, of course, our favorite: the kugel. (For the uninitiated, kugel is a baked pudding. In our house, it was made with egg noodles, eggs, sour cream, and sugar. Just think of it: you're eating dessert, and it's still the main course!) It was heavenly.

Some of my happiest memories from childhood include the scent of food wafting through the house. Before our annual Yom Kippur fast and during the Passover seder, our family and friends would come together for a soul-satisfying meal. And how I loved that my mother always served whatever I requested for dinner on my birthday; I would mull this important menu over for weeks before announcing it to Mom—well in advance of my special day! After my brother and I became adults, I eagerly anticipated traveling to rural Virginia for the Thanksgiving dinners we would all cook together in his cabin in the woods. And I will never forget the jubilant stroke of the knife as my husband and I joined hands to make the first slice in our tiered and flower-bedecked wedding cake.

In my life much of what I find sacred is linked to something delicious. It was only recently, however, that I recognized this subtle connection. My first perception of it came when the name for this book appeared on the screen of my consciousness. I'd been considering various titles, waiting for something to click, and then one day the words "sacred and delicious" sprang forth from inside like a gift. I received this inspiration as an invitation to explore my own sacred relationship with food.

Delicious and Sacred

I must admit that long before I recognized the sacredness of food, I reveled in the many layers of "delicious." For a good part of my life, the word "delicious" conjured up typically American comfort foods. I craved potted meats simmering in their juices, casseroles rich with cream and cheese, dairy-laden desserts like cheesecake and ice cream—the real deal, please; no low-fat or soy substitutes for me! And of course I craved anything chocolate! For some readers, this may still be your ideal, and if so, your definition of the word "delicious" will echo mine during that period: sweet, rich in fat, high in calories. The more delicious the food, the more of it I ate. The concept of moderation did not have a seat at my family's table. Love was doled out in second and third servings.

By the time I reached my early forties, I was suffering from a number of acute and chronic health conditions: acid reflux, irritable bowel syndrome, osteoarthritis, chronic back pain, periodic bronchitis, insomnia, and more. At the urging of my husband, who is a healing practitioner, I became a patient and student of Ayurveda, the ancient medical science of India.

What first attracted me to Ayurveda was its promise to resolve the underlying imbalances in body, mind, and emotions—imbalances that Ayurveda defines as the primary cause of disease and discomfort. As I began to learn about Ayurveda, I recognized that my health problems stemmed, at least in part, from a lifetime of dysfunctional eating. When I embraced Ayurveda's approach to eating and living, I experienced gradual—yet noticeable—improvements. Almost twenty years later, I can happily report cumulative and significant physical improvements. For one thing, I can digest most foods, and this shift happened within weeks of changing the way I eat. I am pain-free much of the time. Also, my sleep is greatly improved, my emotions are steady, and my mind is clear. Most exciting of all, at the age of sixty-two, my energy level is better than it was two decades ago! Back then I could hardly swim one lap, and today I can swim a half mile (thirty-six laps!) with ease.

How did these changes come about? Through the Ayurvedic practices of detoxification, herbal supplementation, and a health-sustaining diet. One of the most fundamental principles of Ayurveda is this simple concept: food, when used correctly, sustains and heals us; food, when misused, will surely make us sick.

Putting it another way: how we prepare food and which foods we eat—basic considerations of Ayurveda—are essential tools in sustaining health and resolving illness. Indeed, Ayurveda was the earliest systematic approach to nutrition.

I started experimenting with Ayurvedic cooking in 1999. Over time, I gathered recipes from family and friends, and I adapted these for my own sensitive constitution according to Ayurvedic principles. As I became more adept with this style of cooking, I began to develop my own recipes. This book grew out of my desire to share what I've learned with those who enjoy delicious food yet may have delicate digestion, a chronic illness, or sustained pain that they would like to address, at least in part, through their diet.

Although healthy food seems to have had a rebirth in the urban American gastronomic scene, there are parts of the country where it's still considered to be boring. My guess is healthy food first got a bad name around the time of the misguided low-fat craze of the 1970s, when conscientious home cooks began to sacrifice their cheesy casseroles for plain, steamed vegetables as a daily regimen. About this time, people began to think of "healthy" and "delicious" as mutually exclusive notions.

Of course, nothing could be further from the truth! What I've happily discovered on my own journey back to health is that "healthy" and "delicious" are highly interdependent. According to Ayurveda, the more interesting and delicious a food becomes through the informed use of diverse spices, the more balanced and healthy that food is.

In my investigation of Ayurvedic cooking, I began using spices I'd never tried before, never even heard of! With these spices, I could intensify the flavor of simple soups and vegetable side dishes—really, just about everything! So, rather than experiencing sensory deprivation, I had a sensory awakening.

As I regained my health, I began to have surprising new cravings. I found that the healthier I became, the more I wanted healthy food! Now in times of stress, when I crave food for comfort, what I want on a cold day is a bowl of delicious vegetable soup—because when warm soup is going down, it feels exactly like love. In the summer, I long for a bowl of sweet ripe blackberries or a luscious papaya. "Delicious" remains my prerequisite for comfort, but my repertoire for "delicious" is no longer limited to foods that might actually make me feel worse.

Please don't misunderstand me: it's not that I now disdain all foods rich with cream and sugar. Heavens no! Nor do I subscribe to a puritan lifestyle. I do indulge sometimes for the simple pleasure of indulgence. What is summer without an occasional scoop of ice cream! And what would blowing out the birthday candles be without the cake! But as a rule, I have found delicious ways to stay in balance.

Early in my recovery process, I saw that I had to take responsibility for my own healing. Day in and day out, I have sole responsibility for protecting my health. I saw that my food choices really matter. It was more recently, however, as I began to examine the connection between food and sacredness, that I saw a deeper truth: only in feeling well can we walk lightly upon the earth and have the energy to serve others. As I've contemplated my relationship with food, I've come to recognize that not only is taking care of my body a sacred duty, it's also a subtle form of worship. "How so?" you may ask. To fully respect and nurture the body we have been given is the most direct way for each of us to honor this gift of life and to pay homage to the divinity that resides within us. The ultimate form of self-love is choosing food that is delicious *and* healthy.

Your Sacred Relationship with Food

Just as *Sacred & Delicious* was an invitation to me, it is also an invitation to you—an invitation to learn about the nurturing power of food and spices. I offer this book to all who wish to sustain or reclaim their health deliciously! Within these pages you will find directions for healthy eating, delicious eating, and conscious cooking—road maps that lead to the same sacred and delicious destination.

The heart of *Sacred & Delicious* is a collection of recipes that I've joyfully adapted or developed to support my own optimal health. These recipes come from various cuisines, yet each is accompanied by an analysis from the Ayurvedic perspective. By working with these recipes, you can learn to adapt recipes from other sources to your specific needs.

It is not necessary that you make a commitment to Ayurveda, or even understand Ayurveda, in order to enjoy these delicious dishes and to reap benefits to your health. I did find, however, in my own exploration of this form of traditional medicine that learning even a few of its concepts was helpful in supporting my quest for better health. So, for readers who are unfamiliar with this tradition, I have distilled the most fundamental Ayurvedic principles in part one. These principles provide a context for understanding the Ayurvedic approach to eating. As you go through *Sacred & Delicious*, you will discover the health benefits of engaging consciously with food. You will explore how to experience cooking and eating as joyful, sacred events in daily living.

I begin this book by sharing some of my spiritual discoveries about preparing and eating food. With the book title, I've already given one of Ayurveda's core teachings: the notion that food is sacred. On a physical level, Ayurveda recognizes that food is necessary not only to sustain life but also to maintain an optimal quality of life so that we can perform our *dharma*, our life's purpose. **Ayurveda recognizes food as energy—not just fuel, mind you, but as an expression of divine Consciousness, the living power of creation.** In other words, food does not only come *from* God; food is the energy *of* God. Food is part of God. This understanding of the true nature of food and all creation is articulated in every mystical spiritual tradition. As my friend Rabbi Raachel Jurovics says, "It's all Godstuff."

Once we acknowledge our sustenance as divine energy, we give ourselves an opportunity to engage in a new relationship with food. Rather than seeing it as a mere object in our lives, we see food as a form of God, as Consciousness itself. Recognizing this truth intellectually and knowing it experientially are, of course, two different things. But even the most elementary understanding adds a deeper level of meaning to the exclamation, "This food is divine!"

Let me tell you a story: When the title *Sacred & Delicious* came to me, I loved the sound of it, loved the feeling it gave me. Even so, I couldn't have explained what it actually meant to me. For years I'd heard the statement "Food is sacred" without examining it. When this book title took form, a longing for insight into this seminal concept was kindled. "Delicious" I could grok, but what did it mean to say that food is sacred? I wasn't going to be satisfied if I only pretended to know what it meant! No!

Over the next few years I prayed to understand the sacred nature of food. I prayed again and again—and again. One summer day when the question was far from my mind, an answer came.

I was working at home, and I stopped to prepare lunch for myself. There wasn't much in the refrigerator, but I did find some fresh mesclun greens, a ripe avocado, and a couple of eggs I could hard-boil. I chopped a handful of walnuts. I assembled this salad on a dinner-sized plate, and whipped up an easy vinaigrette with olive oil and lime juice. I sat down at the table, and before I began to eat, I took a moment to become present. I closed my eyes to bless my food and offer gratitude for what promised to be a luscious meal.

As I opened my eyes, my head still bowed, I looked intently at the fresh greens, which contrasted so vividly with the white and gold of the egg and the pale gold of the nuts. In that moment my mundane perception shifted, and I felt a wave of pure bliss bubble up from the food before me. It was almost effervescent, like bubbles rising in a flute of champagne. It seemed as if the food itself was giggling with delight. Feeling this salad's blissful energy as if it were my own, I laughed aloud and thanked the food for revealing its essence, its spark of divinity. For this, I knew, was what I'd perceived as this salad's irrepressible joy—the bliss of Consciousness that exists in all of creation.

I continue to contemplate this remarkable experience. It seems to me that what occurred was a sublime exchange of energy. While I was blessing my lunch, the Consciousness of the food was sending waves of blessing right back to me.

Each time we eat something delicious, there is the potential for bliss to bubble up inside us. The moment we taste an exquisite soup—or, yes, a morsel of perfect dark chocolate—we can tap into a natural wellspring of inner joy so pure that, in truth, it is nothing less than the bliss of the Divine. We may think that the food gave us that joy, but, in fact, a more subtle and mystical process has occurred. As we eat, the inherent divinity of pure food pulsates with a scintillating energy that explodes and merges with our own true Self. In that moment, when the blessedness of the food meets the purity of an open heart, we experience the bliss that—as the ancient sages say—was there, inside us, all along.

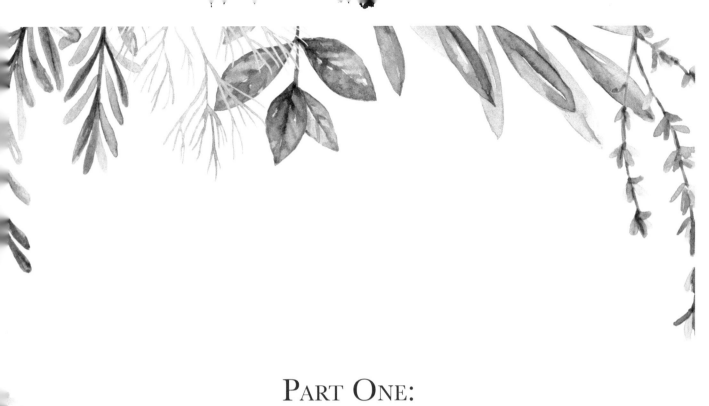

PART ONE:

The Fundamentals

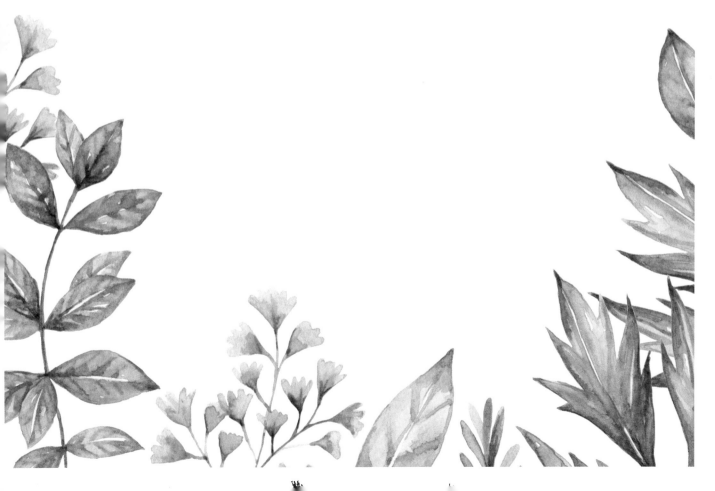

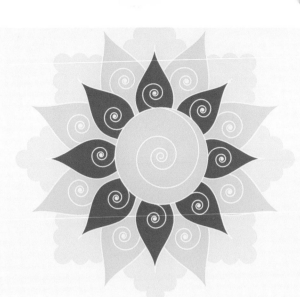

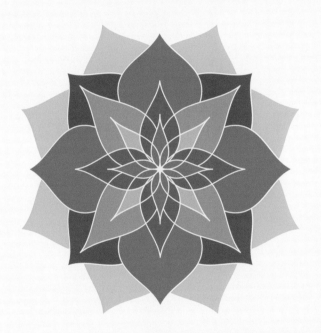

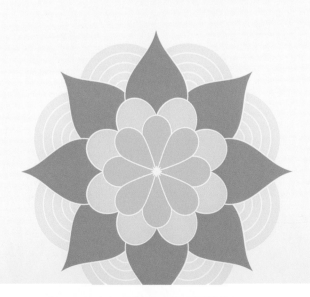

CHAPTER 1.

Principles of Ayurveda

When recommending food,
the most important question in Ayurveda is this:
Recommended for whom?

— Dr. Vasant Lad

The Body's "Organizing Intelligences"

The subtle wisdom of Indian medicine, Ayurveda, is said by most scholars to be at least five thousand years old. The Sanskrit term *ayurveda* means, literally, "knowledge of life." This broad body of knowledge seamlessly integrates science with the sacred by recognizing diseases of—and offering prescriptions for—body, mind, and spirit. Like the Vedas themselves, Ayurveda was passed orally from master to disciple for millennia before its tenets were first committed to writing, some time around 1500 BCE.

During the five hundred years of India's occupation, first by the Moguls and then by the British, Ayurvedic practitioners once again kept their knowledge alive through oral transmission while India's conquerors burned thousands of books of ancient writings. Today, Ayurveda thrives through the work of a number of respected colleges and physicians. Practiced widely in India and England, Ayurveda is now recognized by the World Health Organization as an effective form of traditional medicine.

In the United States, Ayurveda has grown in recognition and esteem as thousands of people have been introduced to its benefits by master practitioners and renowned teachers who have traveled in this country, such as Dr. Deepak Chopra and a number of others who have supported my own journey from sickness to health: Dr. Vasant Lad, Dr. Smita Naram, Dr. Pankaj Naram, and Ed Danaher.

Ayurveda is a vast branch of medical science that includes comprehensive dietary recommendations tailored to each individual. Please understand: Ayurveda is not a weight-loss diet. For one thing, the primary goal of Ayurveda is not weight loss—although one can certainly lose weight following the suggestions it sets forth—and for another,

Ayurvedic medicine involves more than just the way we eat. Ayurveda is a holistic approach to both conscious eating and conscious living that can manage and sometimes reverse disease, resolve acute health problems, and establish ongoing wellness. Ayurveda's core philosophy acknowledges the innate intelligence of the body to heal itself, and the most essential means of doing so is through nurturing food. As Dr. David Frawley and Dr. Subhash Ranade write in *Ayurveda, Nature's Medicine*, "All Ayurvedic therapies start with the right diet. Food builds up the physical body; the wrong foods cause disease." With this approach to food and the support of herbal remedies and detoxification treatments, Ayurveda has supported the health of millions of people over thousands of years. The guidelines are that supple, that universal, that accurate!

Although Ayurveda is inherently vegetarian, those who eat meat can follow the Ayurvedic approach to food and benefit greatly. Certainly, no one who eats meat eats *only* meat. And it's important to note that Ayurveda has a unique and useful perspective on the impact of different types of meat on the body, mind, and emotions. Thus, Ayurveda can help omnivores choose not only the vegetables and spices but also the meats that are most beneficial for their health and well-being.

As an empirical science, Ayurveda systematically addressed anatomy and disease—even surgery—thousands of years before the emergence of Western medicine, a fact that often surprises those who are new to the study of ancient healing arts. However, Ayurveda goes far beyond describing the physical body and its maladies. This was the original mind-body system of medicine, an approach that has gained credibility in recent decades as Western medical doctors have begun pursuing a more holistic approach to healing.

Ayurveda also describes the interplay between the various systems of the body. Dr. Sunil Joshi writes in *Ayurveda & Panchakarma*: "The strength of the Ayurvedic paradigm is that it not only gives us in-depth understanding of the physical substances that comprise the body but the organizing intelligences that create and govern their functions." **These "organizing intelligences" Dr. Joshi refers to are called the three *doshas*.** (The word is pronounced "DOE-shuh.")

Dr. Vasant Lad, founder of the Ayurvedic Institute in New Mexico and a prolific writer, describes the *doshas* as "dynamic principles that govern the body, mind, and consciousness." These principles, or biological humors as they are sometimes called, are identified as *vata*, *pitta*, and *kapha*. The *doshas* are derived from the five elements that, according to this system of traditional medicine, constitute everything in the universe: *vata dosha* is associated with air and space, *pitta* with fire and water, *kapha* with earth and water. "All the elements are present in each individual," Dr. Lad explains in his book *Ayurvedic Cooking for Self-Healing*, "but the proportions and combinations vary from person to person." Every living body, animal as well as human, is a unique collection of the three *doshas*—what Dr. Deepak Chopra refers to as our "unique blueprint" given by nature.

Right now you may be wondering why you're reading about something as esoteric as the *doshas* in a cookbook. The reason is that, according to Ayurveda, what we eat plays a primary role in keeping the *doshas* in balance, and keeping the *doshas* in balance is essential to good health. The *doshas* affect the way we move, think, feel, and—depending on whether or not they are in balance—the very health of our psychic and physical systems.

At any given time, one *dosha* is usually predominant in an individual. Each *dosha* has its own constellation of traits or qualities, affecting everything from metabolism to mental acuity, from complexion to emotional pitch. The *doshas* combine to manifest as the physical, mental, and emotional characteristics of each individual, or what Ayurveda would call that individual's constitution.

When the *doshas* are balanced, our constitution is strong, and we experience good health, vitality, ease, strength, flexibility, and emotional well-being. When the *doshas* are out of balance, we experience energy loss, discomfort, pain, mental or emotional instability, and, ultimately, disease. Sustaining or reclaiming our unique *doshic* balance is a primary focus of Ayurveda.

How do the *doshas* get out of balance? In his book *Ayurvedic Medicine,* Sebastian Pole explains, "The constitution is fixed at birth, but the traits have a tendency to accumulate." Imbalances come as we are drawn to expand what is already our dominant trait through lifestyle choices, as we experience the inevitable pressures of living and aging, and as we consume foods that are impure or are incompatible with our basic constitution. In all of these ways, the *doshas'* traits naturally "accumulate" within us.

The good news is that we have the power to correct these imbalances, and this we can do, in large part, through our daily meals. How does this occur? Ayurveda explains this rebalancing, in part, through the lens of a fundamental premise: **like increases like; opposites create balance.**

To state this less elliptically, foods and spices with qualities similar to a *dosha* typically increase or aggravate that *dosha;* foods and spices with qualities that are the opposite or at least different from a *dosha* typically decrease or pacify that *dosha.* It is this pacification, or balance, that is the goal of *Sacred & Delicious* recipes. Throughout the book, I will discuss qualities of the *doshas* as well as the qualities of specific foods and spices in some detail so that you can learn to harness their healing power. Let me underscore that each food or spice has a particular effect on each of the *doshas.* As you learn which foods support or antagonize the particular *doshas,* you will have unlocked one of the secrets to healing your body, mind, and emotions.

If you're blessed with a strong constitution and a cast-iron stomach—lucky you!—then you may see this information as unnecessary. If, however, you have any health issues at all, you may find it worth your time to take note. Some of the foods you have favored are likely, unbeknownst to you, to have played a role in the development of your condition. **Changing your diet to bring your *doshas* back into balance can be one step you take to restore yourself to good health.** Also, it's important to recognize that foods which may seem fine for you now could create problems for you later in life. This is not an unusual experience.

The three *doshas* are associated not only with an individual's tendencies but also with certain seasons of life. For instance, *kapha* is connected with the first stage of life—infancy, childhood, and the teen years. This is a time when the body is growing—a time of earth and water—and it's also when the physical system needs more sleep. The *pitta* stage of life is the twenties and thirties, when most people function at their highest energy, which is for some a truly fiery pitch. After forty, comes *vata*—air and space—and the inevitable aging process begins.

Again, the three *doshas* are part of every person's makeup and constantly interact with each other. The most skilled Ayurvedic physicians will make dietary and herbal recommendations only after checking a patient's pulse because the state of the *doshas*—their degree of balance or imbalance—can best be perceived through this refined and exacting form of diagnosis. Pulse diagnosis is invaluable in recognizing subtle and dramatic changes in the *doshas* even before health problems become apparent in the body. This can give you the opportunity to make dietary and lifestyle changes that can fend off illness. "Through the *doshic* model," Dr. Sunil Joshi says, "a physician can locate the seeds of disease long before clear clinical symptoms appear."

Unfortunately, true expertise in pulse diagnosis isn't always available in the West. Even without the help of a pulse master, however, you can begin to recognize your *doshic* imbalances by paying attention to your body. Just by reading the lists of conditions related to *dosha* imbalance in the discussions on each *dosha* that follow, you can get some strong hints about your body's constitution and current needs.

Because of its significance, both to life itself and to the movement of the other *doshas,* most discussions of the *doshas* begin with *vata.*

Understanding *Vata*

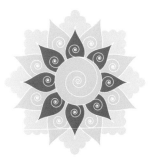

Vata, the *dosha* that is most challenging to keep in balance, is composed of air and space. The qualities of *vata* listed in Ayurvedic literature include these: cold, rough, dry, light, subtle, and mobile. *Vata* is necessary for all movement in the body, both gross and subtle—from blinking the eyes and expanding and contracting the lungs and heart to the more subtle movement of impulses throughout the nervous system. Since *vata* is the principle of air, it acts to dry out the moisture in both the skin and the internal organs, much as a brisk wind dries a puddle of water.

People with predominant *vata* tend to be thin. They often think, move, and speak quickly. They often have an irregular appetite and digestion; something they were able to digest easily one day may cause problems a week later. Because they like to stay in motion, they often accomplish a great deal. When *vata* is in balance, people have great enthusiasm and energy. Balanced *vata* is the foundation of joy, happiness, creativity, and imagination.

When *vata* is excessive, a person may experience an exaggeration of the qualities listed earlier—cold, rough, dry, light, subtle, and mobile—which manifests as one or several kinds of discomfort or disease. *Vata* imbalances include cold extremities, dry skin, constipation, intestinal gas, osteoarthritis, joint and muscular pain, insomnia, anxiety, and depression. For a more complete list of *vata*-related disorders, see the sidebar on page 22.

Looking over the list of *vata* imbalances, almost anyone over forty—and certainly over fifty—will likely recognize the connection between *vata* imbalance and aging. Even those of us who are in generally good health naturally experience some of the signs of increased *vata* as we grow older. Dry skin or cracking joints, for instance, are signs of excess catabolism, which is associated with an excess of *vata*.

It is especially helpful for people who suffer from chronic pain to understand that imbalanced *vata*—often coupled with toxins—is the source of much pain, according to Ayurveda. (A discussion about the role of toxins in disease begins on page 30.) This is not a connection recognized by Western medicine, yet from my own experience, I know it has validity. A decade ago, I experienced the excruciating nonstop pain of two frozen shoulders, known clinically as adhesive capsulitis. I declined a somewhat risky surgery proposed by an orthopedic specialist, and instead went to the Ayurvedic Institute for a week. My shoulders healed completely once I embarked on an Ayurvedic regimen to address the excess *vata* and toxicity problem. The remedy? A cleansing diet, Ayurvedic treatments (such as warm oil massage and colon cleansing), and Ayurvedic herbs. So, I can attest that keeping *vata* in balance is one of the great gifts we can all give ourselves to minimize the body's deterioration and sustain health into old age.

The experience of pain, particularly prolonged pain, creates anxiety, which exacerbates *vata* further, which causes more pain and contributes to many other related disorders—depression, insomnia, digestive problems, and so on. This debilitating cycle, known in Ayurveda as "deranged *vata*," must be broken to restore health.

There are a number of foods that will pacify or balance *vata*-related conditions, and anyone in good health who eats these foods regularly can slow the body's aging process. To choose wisely, remember the principle: like increases like, while opposites create balance. If you want to pacify *vata*, you need to return to the list of *vata*'s primary qualities—cold, rough, dry, light, and mobile—and then identify foods that are opposite in nature. Let me give you a few examples:

- Since cold is a quality of *vata dosha*, eating cold foods will increase *vata*, whereas warm foods pacify *vata* because their warmth acts in opposition to the cold.
- Because *vata dosha* is dry, staying hydrated with beverages is important. (Warm beverages are recommended since *vata* is also cold). Cooking with moderate amounts of oils, ghee (clarified butter),

or butter is also excellent for pacifying the dry nature of *vata* as is eating nut butters, which contain a lot of oil.

- ◉ Squash of any variety is easy to digest and particularly nourishing to *vata* because when cooked, squash becomes soft and moist—in opposition to rough and dry.
- ◉ Sweet potato, a heavy vegetable, balances *vata*'s light quality.

Although recognizing these qualities and their opposites may not seem intuitive at first, over time and with some observation, it becomes second nature. Then when you're feeling anxious, you can learn to recognize that your *vata* is high or on the rise. Instead of reaching for ice cream or chocolate, you can investigate what kind of food will balance your condition. Try a tablespoon of almond butter (because oily nut butter counters *vata*'s dryness). Or prepare sweet potatoes with a little ghee or butter (to counter dryness) and warming cinnamon (to counter the cold nature of *vata*). Or make a bowl of warm winter squash soup for dinner. Or do all of the above!

Vata is pacified by sweet, sour, and salty tastes. In the context of Ayurveda, "sweet" refers to cooked foods that are naturally sweet in taste or aftertaste, such as sweet potato, pumpkin, squash, carrots, and rice. "Sweet" also means unrefined sugar (like coconut sugar, Sucanat, or jaggery). Refined sugar (white table sugar) is not recommended by Ayurveda. When eaten in excess, pungent, bitter, and astringent tastes aggravate *vata*. (I address the concept of taste further on pages 27–28.)

Whole mung beans or split-mung dal, commonplace foods in India, are the ultimate sources of complete, digestible vegetarian protein for *vata* when combined with rice or millet. When soaked overnight, these legumes absorb water and become soft, making them ideal for *vata*. Although the pairing of dal with rice anchors traditional Ayurvedic meals, I prefer millet for pacifying *vata* because of the complication raised by the modern-day arsenic contamination of rice. (See "The Troubling Story of Modern Rice" on pages 157–158.)

All nuts (except dry roasted) are excellent for *vata*. Most vegetables that have been cooked until tender are good for *vata* (though there are exceptions), and most warm soups are *vata*'s best friends.

Vata types, or people with *vata* disorders, thrive when they eat foods with a variety of spices. Nearly all spices are fine for *vata* as most spices have a warming effect, which is especially helpful in pacifying cold *vata*. Try cooking with moderate amounts of garlic and fresh ginger as well as black mustard seeds, cumin, cinnamon, cardamom, and freshly ground pepper. The exceptions are pungent cayenne and chili peppers as well as Tabasco sauce, all of which should be used sparingly. Yes, these are heating, but too much heat in the diet can be drying, which also aggravates *vata*. (Think of a chili's high heat as a fire that dries out the body's moisture.)

Just as certain foods balance a *dosha*, other foods increase, intensify, or (to use an Ayurvedic term) "aggravate" that *dosha*, as noted above regarding a chili. Once again, you can take your cues from the *dosha*'s list of qualities. If you suffer from any of the numerous *vata* disorders, it is best to reduce your intake of foods that have a cold, dry,

Five Easy Ways to Balance *Vata*

1. Favor cooked rather than raw foods, especially during the fall and winter.
2. Learn to cook with warming spices.
3. Avoid or dramatically reduce your intake of sugar and caffeine, including coffee, caffeinated tea, and chocolate.
4. Avoid ice-cold drinks the year round. Switch to warm or hot beverages in the cold months and room-temperature drinks during the summer.
5. Avoid or reduce your intake of deep-fried foods and dry, crispy snacks such as chips and crackers.

Some Signs of *Vata* Imbalance

- Cold hands and feet
- Difficulty falling asleep, restless sleep, insomnia
- Constipation
- Hemorrhoids: dry, cracked; anal fissures
- Burping and hiccups
- Intestinal gas, colicky pain
- Dry skin, wrinkled skin, chapped lips, dryness in mouth
- Vaginal dryness
- Body and joint aches, pains, and stiffness
- Cracking joints
- Arthritic degeneration of joints and spine
- General pain, muscular pain, spasms, and cramping
- Low back pain, sciatica
- Hearing loss, tinnitus, weakened eyesight

- Stammering, tremors, convulsions
- Irregular heartbeat, palpitations
- Tremors, ticks
- Difficulty concentrating or maintaining focus
- Anxiety, insecurity, fear, phobias
- Depression, loneliness
- Lack of enthusiasm, motivation, vitality, and stamina
- Chronic fatigue
- Lack of mental clarity, sense of confusion or of being ungrounded
- Short-term memory loss
- Urinary incontinence
- Hypothyroidism, low endocrine system function
- Headaches in back of the head or left side

light, rough, or astringent quality. These include chilled foods or drinks, corn, popcorn, and the vegetables classified as nightshades: white potatoes, tomatoes, eggplants, and peppers of all kinds. Several modern food writers discuss nightshades in a way that concurs with the Ayurvedic paradigm. As Annemarie Colbin suggests in *Food and Healing,* "The no-nightshades diet, regardless of the disdain of official medicine, seems to be extremely effective for arthritic conditions, joint pains, and bursitis."

If I've just warned you to avoid all of your favorite foods, I urge you not to feel discouraged. Keep in mind that most of the foods listed in the paragraph above can be tolerated by many people with *vata* conditions if eaten just once or twice a month and if they are balanced with heating spices (such as ginger and garlic) and cooked in the proper fats (ghee, butter, olive oil, or coconut oil). It's also important to note that everyone responds differently to foods. For that reason, it's best to view these injunctions about what to eat and not to eat as general guidance rather than ironclad rules. There is, however, lots more guidance for *vata* disorders.

Other vegetables to be aware of in regard to *vata* are those that are naturally cooling to the metabolism: broccoli, cauliflower, cabbage, Brussels sprouts, chard, kale, rutabagas, and turnips. These cruciferous vegetables will increase *vata* but can also be eaten in moderation—say, about once or twice a week—when they are cooked with heating spices and with ghee, butter, or olive oil. The leafy greens mentioned above have a bitter taste, which in excess also increases *vata*, and this can be balanced with a drizzle of pure maple syrup or teaspoon of coconut sugar, making the greens better for a *vata* type, and also more delicious.

If you eat poultry, the dark meat is better for *vata*, while the white meat, because of its relative dryness, increases *vata*.

Beans are often the source of jokes precisely because they aggravate *vata*—the air element—causing flatulence. However, this problem can be lessened or avoided altogether when beans are cooked properly, which includes soaking them overnight so they are able to absorb enough water. In this way once they've been cooked, beans are transmuted from hard and dry to soft and moist. With the addition of appropriate heating spices, beans' natural *vata* quality can be countered so that most people can tolerate eating beans at least once a week. (See "Cooking Legumes" on pages 115–117.) If, however, you bring undercooked or unsoaked beans to your table, expect some comedy later on!

I'm sorry to report that raw foods, which are light and naturally cooling, increase *vata*, particularly when eaten in excess or during cold months. If you love salads with raw vegetables, it's best to save them for the summer months and to limit them to once or twice a week. When you do eat a salad, be generous with an oily dressing to bring about balance; a little balsamic vinegar, lemon, or lime can add some balancing heat with their sour taste. Even better, add some roasted vegetables to your salads so that you're not eating too much raw food.

Perhaps more than anything else, *vata* is aggravated by stress and overstimulation, so it's important for people with *vata* problems to avoid stimulating foods and beverages—that is, caffeine and white sugar. Have trouble getting to sleep at night? Your first and easiest remedy to this *vata* problem may be to kick the coffee habit! Cooking with small amounts of unrefined sugar or pure maple syrup is fine in moderation, if you have normal blood sugar. It's excessive white sugar that takes most people over the top.

Because *vata* is aggravated by cold, *vata* disorders are more prevalent in the fall and winter months, so it is especially important to avoid cold food and drinks during the cold seasons. Although taking the ice out of our iced tea is really an adjustment for Southerners, it will make a world of difference if you have *vata* disorders!

Finally, it is worth noting that the same balancing principle—like increases like; opposites create balance—is true in the body's relationship with the seasons. For instance, people with high *vata* tend to be cold all the time, and so they suffer more during a cold winter and they feel better in the warm summer months. As we move into a discussion of *pitta*, you'll learn that *pitta*'s primary quality is heat. Because of their hot nature, *pitta* types thrive during the cooler weather of fall and winter and often feel miserable at the height of summer.

Understanding *Pitta*

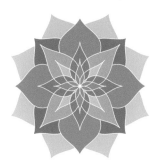

Pitta dosha comes from the elements of fire and water. Its predominant qualities include hot, sharp, sour, pungent, burning, oily, and spreading. "Spreading" refers to the propensity of *pitta* to erupt or break out. The *pitta dosha* is associated with digestion, absorption, and assimilation, including the digestive enzymes and amino acids that metabolize food into energy. This *dosha* also regulates body temperature and complexion. *Pitta* types have a medium build, and they often have oily skin. Their hair often grays prematurely, and they have a tendency toward baldness.

Healthy *pitta* produces a strong intellect and understanding. It generates ambition, courage, energy, and the motivation to achieve goals and overcome obstacles. *Pitta* types usually have great organizational skills and leadership capacity, and they are competitive in nature. When your *pitta dosha* is out of balance, you tend toward perfectionism and sharp criticism of yourself and others. The colors red and yellow are associated with *pitta*—for instance, red hair and ruddy cheeks are signs of a *pitta* constitution. The overproduction of bile that manifests in yellowing skin or stool signals an overabundance of *pitta*.

When *pitta* becomes too high, it erupts in a number of physical and emotional symptoms. Disorders related to imbalanced *pitta* include skin problems, such as acne, rashes, and itchiness. Hyperacidity and acid reflux, vomiting, diarrhea, inflammation, difficulty staying asleep, irritability, and aggression are all outcomes of disturbed *pitta*. Know anyone who is hot-tempered? You can bet that person's *pitta* is out of balance! For a more extensive list of *pitta*-related disorders, see the sidebar on page 24.

Some Signs of *Pitta* Imbalance

- Skin eruptions, including acne, rashes
- Rosacea, dermatitis, eczema
- Hyperacidity and acid reflux disease
- Vomiting, nausea
- Diarrhea or loose stools
- Hemorrhoids: bleeding, itching, burning
- Headaches at the temples and temporal area
- Sensitivity to heat, excessive perspiration
- Hot flashes

- Inflammation, itching
- Rheumatoid arthritis
- Yellow or green mucous formation
- Difficulty staying asleep, awakens at 3:00 or 4:00 a.m.
- Anger, jealousy, irritability, aggression
- Overly controlling, easily frustrated
- Tendency to criticize self and others

In eating to balance *pitta*, choose foods that are cooling to the metabolism rather than those that are too oily, sour, pungent, or hot (as in cayenne pepper). Eat foods cooked with cooling spices: coriander, fresh cilantro, and mint. Ghee and coconut oil in moderate amounts are also excellent for pacifying *pitta*. Milk, if your system can tolerate it, as well as coconut milk will benefit *pitta* for their cooling effect on the metabolism.

In general, favor sweet, astringent, and bitter vegetables. These include sweet and white potatoes, parsnips, asparagus, broccoli, cabbage, cauliflower, Brussels sprouts, green beans, okra, and leafy greens.

Whole mung beans or split-mung dal, traditional Indian fare, are excellent sources of digestible and complete vegetarian protein when served with rice or quinoa. All legumes tend to cool *pitta*'s hot nature. Nuts and nut butters can be eaten in *small* quantities by most *pitta* types; almonds are the least *pitta*-aggravating of all the nuts.

To lower *pitta*, it is best to avoid or greatly reduce pungent foods and hot spices, including raw onions, horseradish, chilies, cayenne, red pepper flakes, Tabasco, and other hot sauces. *Pitta* also may be aggravated by garlic, especially in excess. If a recipe calls for four to six cloves of garlic, I advise *pitta* types to use only one or two cloves. People with acid reflux disease are likely to feel best by eliminating garlic from their diets or by limiting its use to no more than once a week. Because *pitta* is aggravated by heat, it is especially important to avoid excessively hot spices during the hot summer months.

Women in perimenopause and beyond will probably relate to this: you eat Indian, Thai, or Mexican food with lots of chilies, and it seems that your night sweats get hotter and more intense. That's not your imagination! And chilies have other effects as well. I think it's no coincidence that over the past decade or two, as American chefs have introduced greater quantities of hot spices to our food, acid reflux disease has risen dramatically in the United States.

Although I've mentioned nightshades in the section about *vata*, it's also true that eggplants and tomatoes increase *pitta*.

Salty, fermented, and sour foods (particularly vinegar and tomatoes) are also harmful to *pitta*. This means that condiments such as mayonnaise, mustard, and ketchup, as well as relish and pickles, may wreak havoc when eaten in excess, as will too much salt. People with *pitta* problems often cannot tolerate the juice of lemons or sour oranges. Lime juice, however, is usually fine in moderation.

Likewise, red meat increases *pitta* and is best avoided by people with *pitta* problems. Dark-meat poultry will also disturb *pitta*, as will most seafood, especially salmon, tuna, shrimp, and oysters. If you have *pitta* problems and you enjoy beef, dark-meat poultry, and seafood, you may want to limit these items to once or twice a month.

Understanding *Kapha*

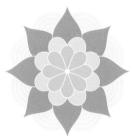

All of our cells, tissues, and organs are comprised of the *kapha* elements, water and earth. *Kapha dosha* gives solidity and structure to the body. It is the *dosha* of cohesion and also of lubrication and liquidity. *Kapha's* qualities include heavy, dense, cool, slow, oily, and damp. People with *kapha* constitutions usually have large bone structures and thick, shiny hair. They may have damp skin. They move slowly and tend to need a lot of sleep. They also tend to resist change or intense activity. Although they may be extremely intelligent, they are often slow to make decisions.

When this *dosha* is in balance, people with *kapha* constitutions are physically strong; they have great physical endurance and a strong immune function. Although they have the slowest metabolisms of all the types, their digestive capacity is regular and strong. People with predominant *kapha* are calm, steady, loyal, loving, and compassionate. When a loving relationship is absent, *kapha* types tend to replace love with food, and they are often attracted to sweets. Anyone with a *kapha* constitution has to be careful not to put on weight.

Other disorders related to *kapha* imbalance include weak kidney function; water retention; and a susceptibility to colds, sinus, chest congestion, and ear infections. For a more detailed list of *kapha*-related disorders, see the sidebar on page 26.

In general, people with *kapha* constitutions or disorders feel best when they eat warm, cooked foods with pungent, bitter, and astringent flavors. These include leafy green vegetables, green beans, beets, onions, garlic, peppers, and cruciferous vegetables (such as cabbage, bok choy, broccoli, Brussels sprouts, and cauliflower). Heating and pungent spices are good support for *kapha*. Vegetarian *kapha* types do well when getting most of their protein from legumes and pulses or dals. Light snacks such as popcorn (made without oil or butter) and pumpkin seeds or sunflower seeds also suit *kapha* well.

Of all the types, *kapha* can best tolerate caffeine, and since people with *kapha* constitutions tend to move slowly in the morning, a cup of tea or coffee can help them to get the day started.

To reduce *kapha* when it is in excess, it is helpful to reduce or eliminate the intake of cold and raw foods, wheat, red meat, dark-meat poultry, and dairy, especially cow's milk, and the cheeses that are made from cow's milk. A glass of cold milk is a double whammy for *kapha* types—both cold in temperature and cooling in its metabolic effect on the system. People with *kapha* problems should generally cook with modest amounts of vegetable oil, butter, and ghee, and they do best when they avoid olive and coconut oil altogether. Anything with a sweet taste will also increase *kapha*—particularly white sugar but also squash, sweet potatoes, and white rice. Sour and salty foods, in excess, also increase *kapha*, as do heavy foods such as bread, pasta, cooked oats, and rice (though brown rice is preferable to white). For someone addressing a *kapha* imbalance, it's best to eat these foods infrequently.

Some Signs of *Kapha* Imbalance

- Sluggish metabolism, digestion, and bowels
- Easy weight gain, difficult weight loss, obesity
- Lethargy, complacency, lack of motivation
- Excess sleep
- Weak kidney function, water retention, clammy skin
- Puffy skin
- Excess mucus, congestion, productive cough
- Susceptibility to colds and ear infections
- Seasonal allergies
- Headaches at the frontal and nasal areas of the head
- Increase in secretions: saliva, ear wax
- Growths such as fibroids, cysts
- Swelling
- White discoloration of eyes, skin, or stool
- Craving sweets
- Slow decision-making
- Excessive attachment to people, feelings, and possessions

Five Easy Ways to Balance *Kapha*

1. Keep your fat consumption low. Although everyone needs some fat in their diets, use only small amounts of butter, ghee, or cooking oil. Also eat nuts and nut butters in moderation.
2. Avoid or greatly reduce your intake of dairy products. If you drink milk, it's best to drink it warm or hot and with spices like ginger and cardamom, as in chai, the Indian-style spiced tea.
3. If you eat beef, do so infrequently and choose low-fat cuts; favor white-meat poultry.
4. Avoid or greatly reduce your intake of foods high in carbohydrates, including sugary desserts, wheat, all breads (even gluten-free but especially white), rice (especially white), and white potatoes.
5. Avoid or greatly reduce your intake of salty foods like pretzels and potato chips.

Working with the Three *Doshas*

As we've been exploring, the main medicine of Ayurveda is the foods we eat—and, often, the most striking quality of a food is the way it tastes to us.

Taste

Every food has a particular taste, and it is mainly this taste that makes eating a pleasure—or not! In the West we traditionally think of foods as being sweet, sour, salty, or bitter. This list was originally drawn in the fourth century BCE by the Greek philosopher Democritus, and it was expanded fairly recently to include savory (which is what most of us might call "spicy hot") by the American food scientist Harold McGee. Ayurveda identifies six tastes, or rasas, as they are known in Sanskrit: sweet, sour, salty, bitter, pungent (which is, again, that "spicy hot"), and astringent. The "astringent" refers to the slight sense of drawing or puckering you can get in the mouth or throat when you have a bite of pomegranate or a sip of red wine. As a taste, astringent is associated with foods such as quinoa, legumes, and sprouts.

According to Ayurveda, each taste has its own effects on the body or mind. When eaten in moderation, each taste contributes to optimal health. When eaten in excess—or taken into a system that already is leaning too much in that direction—the result can be adverse. (See "The Effects of Taste" on page 28.)

The Ayurvedic system of six *rasas* was first recorded in the third century BCE in the *Charaka Samhita*. Here, in one bite, is how each of the three *doshas* responds to each of the six flavors:

The *Doshas* and The Tastes

	Pacify	Aggravate
Vata	sweet, sour, salty	pungent, bitter, astringent
Pitta	sweet, astringent, bitter	sour, salty, pungent
Kapha	pungent, astringent, bitter	sweet, sour, salty

Since every living organism is seen as a combination of the three *doshas*, it follows that a balanced meal should include all six tastes. That way each *dosha* receives nourishment. We need be concerned about creating an imbalance only if we consistently overemphasize any one taste—which, of course, most of us do.

Most Western diets are rich in sweet, sour, and salty tastes, and in recent decades pungent chilies have been embraced by many. We rarely incorporate bitter and astringent tastes in our diets. The concern here is that the bitter and astringent tastes serve a purpose as they help keep *pitta* and *kapha* in balance. The solution to this problem, I'm happy to say, is delicious. We can simply expand our use of spices, particularly cumin, coriander, and turmeric.

I use a combination of cumin, coriander, and turmeric in at least one dish at every meal, and here's why: cumin's intrinsic taste is pungent and bitter; coriander is sweet and astringent; turmeric is a combination of bitter, pungent, and astringent. Add a dash of salt and a splash of lemon or lime and there you have it—all six tastes coming together deliciously (and sugar-free) in a minute or less. An aside: Ayurveda recommends using cumin and coriander together for another reason, as well—together they balance *agni*, the digestive fire. If *agni* is low, cumin elevates it; if it's too high, coriander subdues it.

Over time as you experiment in the kitchen, you will become attuned to each of the spices, its flavor, and its energetic qualities. With experience, you'll learn to select and combine spices that are appealing to your palate even as they help keep you and your loved ones healthy. In the meantime, you can cook with the recipes in *Sacred & Delicious*, as they balance the tastes as well as the intrinsic cooling and heating aspects of foods and spices.

The Effects of Taste

Taste	Eaten in Moderation	Overconsumption
Sweet	Good for plasma, blood, muscles, fat, bones, marrow, reproductive fluids. Promotes strength and healthy skin and hair. Heals emaciation.	Increased cough, congestion, loss of appetite, laziness, obesity, diabetes. Linked to lymphatic congestion, tumors, edema.
Sour	Stimulates appetite and improves digestion. Good for heart and mind.	Linked to tooth sensitivity, excessive thirst, hyperacidity, acnes, boils, dermatitis, eczema, edema, psoriasis, burning bladder
Salty	Laxative, lessens spasms, maintains electrolyte balance, aids digestion and absorption.	Thickens blood. Worsens skin conditions, hair loss, hyperacidity, hypertension.
Pungent	Clears sinuses, dries excess mucous. Good for circulation. Kills parasites and germs.	Drying for *vata*; contributes to cramping and insomnia as well as to diarrhea, heartburn, nausea, peptic ulcers, skin problems, and sexual dysfunction.
Bitter	Kills germs, moves toxins. Relieves burning and itching. Relieves intestinal gas and supports digestion. Reduces fever. Reduces fat.	Contributes to emaciation. Depletes plasma, blood, muscles, fat, bone marrow, and semen. Linked to fatigue and dizziness.
Astringent	Aids healing of ulcers. Promotes clotting and cleanses blood. Tones watery tissues.	May cause excess thirst, constipation, blood clotting, convulsion, sexual debility.

Balance

Now we come to balance. As we've discussed, Ayurveda categorizes every known food, spice, and condiment based on their qualities—in other words, their ability to increase or pacify the *doshas*. In the sections on *vata*, *pitta*, and *kapha*, I have promoted eating certain foods and discouraged others based on various health issues. Understand, however, that most people can eat almost anything on occasion—especially once they've learned the alchemy of cooking for balance.

How do you go about balancing a dish? The first step is that principle I've repeated many times now: *like increases like; opposites create balance.*

As you've read, among the *vata* qualities are light and dry, so when you eat, for example, some dry, light popcorn or a piece of dry, crispy toast, you're likely to be revving up *vata*. That doesn't mean, however, that a person with high *vata* should never eat popcorn or toast! Remember the second part of the principle: *opposites create balance.* If you drizzle melted ghee or butter over that popcorn or slather your toast with butter or olive oil, you will partially neutralize the *vata* quality of those foods. Following this principle, popcorn and toast become tolerable even for people afflicted with high *vata* when eaten in moderation. Let me repeat this: *when eaten in moderation!* Eat these foods every day, and my bet is you'll be constipated, a typical *vata* condition.

So, what is moderation? Since everyone is different, you're the best judge of what that means for you. To continue with our example, if you feel fine eating toast once a day or, say, twice a week, then it works for you. If you find you start having *vata* symptoms when you eat toast more often—or any bread, for that matter—this is your clue. You may find that you can digest one piece of bread and butter (or oil) with a meal perfectly well, but if you eat more than that, you feel bloated or gassy. Take notice. One piece is enough for your system.

The principle *like increases like* also holds true regarding the influence of nature. For instance, cold, windy weather will increase the *vata dosha* because *vata* is already cold and mobile. Therefore, eating cold or light foods during the winter season will have a greater negative impact on *vata*, just as eating hot, spicy foods is particularly hard on *pitta* during the warmest months of summer.

That said, you can balance most foods—for the *doshas* and for the seasons—once you've learned the Ayurvedic alchemy of cooking by which you play with the innate healing power of foods and spices. Cruciferous vegetables like broccoli and cauliflower, which are inherently cooling, can be balanced with a mildly heating spice such as fresh ginger or garlic. Or you can combine them in a dish with a heating food such as onion. Fats, particularly ghee, can be used to counterbalance the dryness or lightness of certain foods, as in the earlier example of popcorn or toast. As you learn to work this alchemy of cooking, you can eat almost any food in moderation and still maintain your health.

I find it fascinating how often national and regional cuisines intuitively combine opposites for balance. For instance, when Southerners eat corn on the cob (which aggravates *vata*), they pile on the butter, salt, and pepper (which all balance *vata*). Mexican salsa—basically, tomatoes and raw onions—uses cumin to balance the tomatoes' acidity and lots of fresh, cooling cilantro to balance the heat of tomatoes and onions.

With the right spices, the attributes of many foods can be mitigated if not reversed altogether. As I just mentioned, cumin is an antidote for the acidity of tomatoes, making tomatoes much easier to digest and, if they're eaten only on occasion, making them somewhat more acceptable for some *pitta* people. Cardamom pacifies *kapha*, making milk somewhat more acceptable for *kapha* types, who might otherwise not be able to tolerate milk. And cardamom is considered a partial antidote to caffeine.

The cooking method itself can also play a role in balancing foods. Although nightshades increase *vata*, they are less *vata*-aggravating when roasted. Roasting nightshades with ghee further modifies them, even making them tolerable for *vata* on occasion. Likewise, a pungent food such as a raw onion can cause havoc for people with *pitta* problems; however, when an onion is cooked until it browns, it no longer aggravates *pitta* because onions—pungent when raw—become sweet when caramelized.

For these reasons, I caution you not to be alarmed as you read Ayurvedic books, this one and others, listing foods to favor and avoid based on your *dosha*. Always keep in mind that with the right spices or in combination with other foods, most foods can be balanced. This is not the same as saying that you can eat just anything you crave on a daily basis. If the foods you habitually eat aggravate your *doshic* imbalance, you will pay the consequences! You can, however, maintain your health if you pay attention to food choices, eat in moderation, and favor those foods that are most healing for your body—and you can still enjoy, say once a week, some of your favorite foods that might be less than ideal for your constitution.

The recipes in *Sacred & Delicious* distill Ayurvedic cooking to its essential gift: how to balance the innate healing qualities of food with spices and other foods that have an opposite quality, bringing each dish or menu into perfect balance. If you don't have the time to learn about these principles today, or you're simply not interested, you don't need to go into this alchemy in detail. The recipes are already balanced for you.

When Balancing Is Complex

Typically, the *doshas* appear in combination, with one *dosha* being dominant and another being secondary—*pitta-vata*, for instance, or *vata-kapha*. The dominant *dosha* (the first named) will lead that person's tendencies, although the secondary *dosha* will be evident. Some people experience the *doshas* in equal measure, which is called a *dual dosha* or even *tridosha*.

Unfortunately, because of life's inherent challenges and our history of poor food choices, most of us have one or more *doshas* out of balance. Ayurveda recommends dietary changes to address a *doshic* imbalance, but since the foods that pacify one *dosha* often aggravate another, finding the right foods can be confusing. This challenge is compounded when you're cooking for a family in which family members have different constitutions and manifest a variety of maladies and imbalances.

What to do? In these cases, Ayurvedic experts suggest that you focus on eating for the season. By balancing the qualities that are predominant in the season, you will be counteracting the health difficulties that typically arise certain times of the year.

Let me explain this concept with a few examples. In the cold months of fall and winter, take care to eat warm foods and heating spices that are calming to *vata* and *kapha*, without increasing *pitta* problems. Essentially, this means enjoy all spices without overdoing cayenne pepper. Enjoy lots of fresh ginger and, if you wish, some garlic. Warm, wet dishes, such as soup, stew, and dal, are ideal centerpieces of any meal. Drink hot tea, especially ginger, if you feel a cold coming on.

In the spring when seasonal allergies peak, it's fine to eat all of the above but best to avoid all dairy products, which add to congestion. During late spring and certainly by early summer, you'll naturally gravitate toward cooling salads and side dishes instead of hot soups. Rather than eat a totally raw-food salad, which will increase *vata* and *kapha*, try topping salad greens with roasted vegetables. By summer add avocado to the mix. Lower the heat in your spices and add cooling ingredients to your meals: fresh cilantro, mint, and cucumbers. During summer, snack on cooling fruits such as melons and papaya.

Still sound complicated? Not to worry—just use the recipes in this book! Because I've experienced problems with all three *doshas*, I developed these recipes with the goal of keeping everything in balance. After you try any new dish, observe how you feel. The more you pay attention to how you feel after eating each meal, the more your inner barometer will recognize what works for you, both in terms of the season and your own *doshic* tendencies. When you monitor your experience of food, your self-awareness will naturally grow, and this will help you choose foods that allow you to feel good all the time.

We've spent a lot of time with the *doshas*, and now there are just a couple more of the fundamentals of Ayurveda to consider.

The Digestive Fire

Since ancient times, Ayurveda's primary tenet has remained the same: good digestion is the secret to sustaining good health. For this reason, it is helpful to understand the basis of good digestion and the result of poor digestion—*agni* and *ama*, respectively.

Agni and *Ama*

Agni means "fire" in Sanskrit, and in the context of Ayurveda it means "digestive fire." The term refers both to the digestive enzymes and to the metabolic process whereby food is chemically transformed into energy. With strong *agni*, we can digest most anything without suffering negative consequences. Even toxins, microorganisms, and foreign bacteria are destroyed by strong *agni*. When the digestive fire is strong, our energy is strong—we are healthy and we live longer.

When *agni* is weak, our health is likely to be more fragile, our energy decreases, and our immunity is compromised. People who suffer from allergies in the spring and fall tend to have weak *agni*; this is why their bodies are unable to eliminate the pollens to which they are exposed. If we have a low digestive fire, our bodies are unable to complete the chemical work of digestion, and this means that undigested food is trapped in the large intestine, where it ferments and decays. It is this undigested food that ultimately becomes the sticky and smelly mucus Ayurveda calls *ama* or *aam*. Simply put, *ama* is toxins.

Signs of Toxic Buildup—*Ama*

- White or yellow coating on tongue
- Bad breath
- Smelly stool
- Runny nose, especially while eating
- Aches and pains
- Joint inflammation
- Poor circulation
- Intestinal bloating and gas
- Diarrhea
- Swelling
- Acne
- Fever
- Indigestion
- Fatigue after eating
- Lack of mental clarity
- General weakness

These toxins are distributed throughout the body via the circulatory system. Deposits of *ama* can appear in the body in its joints, organs, or hollow channels—the veins, arteries, glands, lymph nodes, and nerves. Dr. Smita Naram explains in *Secrets of Natural Health* the significant consequences *ama* has for health:

> *If it blocks the circulatory system, it can lead to arteriosclerosis, thrombosis, or infarct in the brain or heart. If it blocks the respiratory channel, it results in asthma, bronchitis, or sinusitis. If it blocks the mental channels, it causes confusion, fear, excessive worrying, lack of focus, and irritability. Emotionally, it can cause sadness and oversensitivity.*

The consequential link between our digestive power, *agni*, and the toxins that accumulate in the body cannot be overstated. Although it may take months or even years for symptoms to appear, once toxins begin to accumulate, be assured you will experience their effects. "*Ama* is the starting point of any form of illness," Dr. Naram says. A weak digestive fire leads to the accumulation of toxins and, once the toxins begin to build, they further weaken the digestive fire.

Do you wonder whether or not you have toxins in your body? Then try this quick self-test. In the morning, before you drink or eat anything, take a toothbrush or tongue scraper and pull it down your tongue, starting at the back of the tongue near the throat and moving toward the front of your mouth. Do you find a thick, sticky substance coating your tongue? Bingo. This is *ama*. For a list of the telltale signs of toxin buildup in your body, see the sidebar above.

It is vital to understand the importance of the digestive power. To survive you need to eat every day, and to thrive you need to digest what you've eaten. You may be eating a diet of pristine foods that are just right for your constitution, but if you aren't digesting those foods well, your health will be compromised. Ultimately, as Dr. Naram indicates, even your emotions can become unstable. Toxins will accumulate in your body, and as toxins accumulate, the body's innate organizing intelligences—the *doshas*—go awry.

Ed Danaher, director of the Panchakarma Clinic at the Ayurvedic Institute in Albuquerque, New Mexico, explains it this way: "The balance or imbalance of the *doshas* is dependent upon *agni*. Therefore, anything that imbalances *agni* should ideally be given up."

Setting a Healthy Routine

The diet and lifestyle choices that either support or sabotage *agni* demonstrate a fundamental truth of Ayurveda: it is up to each individual to make daily lifestyle choices that strengthen digestion and lead toward the goal of optimal

Choices to Support or Sabotage Digestion

What Weakens Agni

- Excess *vata*
- Cold drinks and food
- Excessive raw food
- Heavy foods: deep-fried foods, red meat, hard cheeses, wheat
- Overeating
- Eating when not hungry
- Eating late at night and at irregular times
- Incompatible food combining (See page 43.)
- Refined sugar
- Refined and processed foods
- Eating when emotionally upset
- Anxiety, stress, negative emotions
- Sensory overload
- Lack of exercise
- Excessive sleeping during the day or lack of sleep

What Supports Agni

- Ghee in moderation
- Fresh lime
- Fresh ginger
- Warm or hot drinks, water or herbal tea, depending on the season
- Cumin, coriander, fennel, saffron, black pepper
- Eating at a regular time in a peaceful setting
- Finishing the last meal of the day no later than 7:00 p.m.
- Prayer and meditation
- Singing and chanting
- Hatha yoga, stretching exercises
- *Pranayama* (yogic breath)
- Walking, being in nature
- Thinking positive thoughts
- Keeping good company

health. Certainly, we don't always have control over what we eat. Yet even when we're traveling, eating in restaurants, or taking a meal in someone else's home, we can always make the healthiest food choice possible in that situation. And for the rest of the time—which, for most of us, is most of the time—we can set a healthy routine for our diet.

Although we may not be able to avoid stress as easily as we control our food intake, we can support ourselves with practices such as meditation (preferably daily) that reduce stress, calm the mind, and support digestion. If we focus on foods and lifestyle choices that enhance *agni*, the strength of our digestion will literally burn up the occasional toxins that are unavoidable in our diets.

One of the most significant lifestyle choices to support *agni* is what I call **the vital rule of digestion: eat only when you are hungry, and stop eating before you are full.** The first part of this equation is important because hunger is the signal that the inner digestive fire is kindled and the body is ready to ingest more food. Typically, it takes three to four hours to digest any meal, and for this reason, Ayurvedic experts caution us not to eat between meals. (The exception is for people with hypoglycemia, who may need to sustain their blood sugar with small protein snacks such as a few nuts every two or three hours.) By avoiding most between-meal snacking, we give the body time to complete the digestion process before we eat again. If you find that you're hungry an hour or so before mealtime, it's the ideal time to enjoy a light snack—a piece of fresh fruit, a handful of nuts, or a small glass of almond milk.

Just as it's vital to wait for the inner coals to get hot before throwing a meal on the fire, it is equally important that we stop eating before we're totally full—in other words, while there is still space in the stomach. Ayurvedic texts suggest that to sustain good health we need to eat only as much food as we can hold cupped in two hands. When we overeat, we overwhelm *agni*. When we habitually overeat, much of our food is never digested. Stuck in the colon for weeks and months at a time, this undigested food putrefies, becomes toxic, and then is absorbed into the body.

For many people, deciding to stop eating before they're full is easier said than done—especially when tantalizing

Healing Tips on Cooking with Spices

Garlic and Ginger: Cook almost any dish for four—vegetables, soups, dal or other lentils, or beans—with a clove of minced garlic and one teaspoon of freshly ground ginger. This will stimulate the digestive enzymes. If you suffer from acid reflux, double the ginger and skip the garlic or cook the whole clove in the pot without chopping or pressing it. Then remove the clove, just before serving. The taste of both garlic and ginger is pungent.

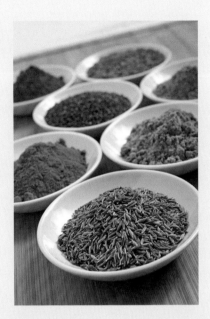

Asafetida: Add one pinch of asafetida per cup of dried legumes to avoid flatulence. Add two pinches asafetida per cup of dried hard beans such as black beans and chickpeas. Add a pinch of asafetida to the marinade for a 15-ounce block of tofu. Add a pinch or two of asafetida to a four-serving pot of any cruciferous vegetable. Asafetida has a pungent taste.

Cumin and Coriander: Sauté any green vegetable in a little oil or ghee with ½ to 1 teaspoon each of ground cumin and coriander. The combination is delicious and aids digestion by balancing agni. These spices are also essential to digesting legumes. Cumin is pungent and bitter. Coriander is sweet and astringent.

Turmeric: Add ½ to 1 teaspoon of ground turmeric, an antibacterial agent, to any soup stock, soup, stew, or bean or vegetable dish to keep it fresh longer. When you add turmeric to cumin and coriander, the trio creates a quick and yummy "gravy" flavor. Turmeric's added benefit is that it helps the body detoxify. Also, recent studies suggest that the consumption of turmeric as part of the daily diet in India may contribute to a low incidence of Alzheimer's disease there. Turmeric is bitter, pungent, and astringent. It pacifies all *doshas*.

food is left in the serving dish! Nonetheless, this advice is a critical part of sustaining good health. As I mentioned earlier, when I was growing up, my family always went for second and third helpings. In recent years, I've had to learn a new way of eating—paying attention while eating, noticing that I'm getting close to full, and then stopping. I don't succeed every day, but I'm getting much better at it. When I overeat, I feel lethargic or get indigestion. When I eat modest portions, I feel so much better.

Ayurveda and Vegetarianism

There are several reasons why Ayurvedic practitioners favor vegetarianism. First, a non-flesh diet is lighter and, so, easier to digest. This contributes greatly to supporting health because, as we've discussed, with good digestion, we're less likely to accumulate toxins. As well, fresh vegetarian food is more likely to have the subtle force known as *prana*—the life force or energy that distinguishes what is living from what is dead. For creatures, at the time of death all *prana* leaves the body. From the Ayurvedic perspective, this means that meat, poultry, and fish all lack *prana* and are seen as foods that cannot sustain good health—yet another reason that Ayurveda is an inherently vegetarian discipline.

The health benefits of a well-balanced vegetarian diet have been confirmed repeatedly in recent decades by Western medical science, which reports a lower risk of heart disease, cancer, and obesity for those on a vegetarian or restricted-meat diet. Interestingly, some research points to significant genetic changes that increase disease prevention and disable disease-promoting genes in those who switch to a vegetarian diet.

Ayurvedic texts suggest that the lighter vibration of a vegetarian diet enhances spiritual evolution, supporting seekers on the path to enlightenment. These authorities are not, however, universally opposed to eating meat and fish. Even India's most ancient medical texts recommend meat to those weakened or depleted by illness. Also, eating a little meat is sometimes prescribed to help ground *vata*.

Many feel better when they eat meat, and this may be an indicator that these individuals do need some flesh in their diet. (This happened to me for a few years, as I later discuss.) At the same time, this could also indicate that these people haven't eaten a sufficiently balanced or varied vegetarian diet. A vegetarian diet that includes a daily intake of legumes and grains, which form a complete protein, has the best chance of succeeding. Millions of Asians have good health and vitality eating a daily diet of vegetables, rice, a simple legume known as mung dal, and little or no dairy.

Vegetarian diets are often deficient in DHA and EPA, omega-3 fatty acids, as well as vitamin B₁₂, which can lead to anemia. I highly recommend that vegetarians take these nutritional supplements to ensure optimal health. Getting enough protein is another issue for many vegetarians—particularly for vegans. Although I'm passionate about eating fresh food, vegetarians may need to supplement their diets with pea or hemp protein powders. Some will also tolerate soy or whey protein.

Ayurveda advocates drinking raw milk (for *vata* and *pitta* types; not for *kapha* or people with *kapha* disorders) and cooking with ghee (which is clarified butter) because of the healing properties of these foods. Also, Ayurveda is not opposed to eggs for certain people. So even though Ayurveda generally suggests abstaining from meat and fish, it is not a vegan regimen. I would say, though, that vegans can benefit from Ayurveda's wisdom about balancing foods and still avoid the use of ghee.

There are more issues involved in vegetarianism than one's own health. My own decision to embrace a vegetarian diet—in my twenties for a few years and recently for a fifteen-year stretch—was a spiritual and ethical choice, reinforced by my study of Ayurveda. In an Ayurvedic cooking class I took, one of the students asked the teacher, Dr. Vasant Lad, why he subscribes to a vegetarian diet. I was struck by his simple answer: **"It's a way of practicing nonviolence."** *Ahimsa*, nonviolence, is one of the tenets of classical yoga and the heart of the philosophy put into practice by the Indian statesman Mohandas Gandhi. There are levels of nonviolence, and the most basic is to avoid causing needless harm. As Dr. Lad went on to say, "Most of us no longer have to eat meat to survive."

A vegetarian diet or reduced meat intake is also being advocated by many scientists worldwide as a way of practicing nonviolence in our relationship with planet Earth. The unintended byproducts of industrialized meat processing include the annual production of millions of tons of nitrous oxide and methane gas, which comprise 18 percent of all greenhouse gas emissions and have been shown to contribute significantly to global warming. If you are considering experimenting with a vegetarian lifestyle for yourself, you might want to read one of the many excellent books that address the ethical, environmental, and health concerns associated with eating meat.

Understand, however, that food choices are personal decisions. I feel that we should never impose on others our own decision about whether or not to eat meat. There was a period a few years ago when I experienced some debilitating health problems, and I was advised by several health-care practitioners—including my vigilant vegetarian husband—to eat foods derived from animals. Doing so was beneficial for my health, though I struggled mightily with this choice. My decision was complicated by the fact that I don't feel well if I eat eggs regularly; if not for this, I could have avoided eating animals and sidestepped an ethical dilemma (since I've never chosen a vegan lifestyle).

In retrospect, I'm grateful for the opportunity handed to me during this period: a chance to see myself more clearly. Although I had stopped eating meat for good reason, I came to recognize that I had enormous pride in identifying myself as a vegetarian. I put this book on hold for a few years so I could wrestle with the feeling of being a fraud. How could I publish a vegetarian cookbook while eating fish and poultry?

I've moved beyond that now. Though I continue to eat fish on occasion, I've been able to maintain my energy level by eating a vegetarian diet most of the time. I do accept that, in eating fish, I am taking conscious life forms as food for my body so that I can sustain my energy for a busy life of service. This goal, I feel, is congruent with Ayurveda. Before eating a once-conscious life form, I offer a prayer I have borrowed from the Native American tradition: I pause to thank this individual being for its sacrifice, to honor its divinity, and to offer that being my blessing.

Of course, there are millions of people who do live long, healthy, vital lives as vegetarians. I don't want my health issues to dissuade anyone from experimenting with becoming a vegetarian. What I do intend is to be in integrity about publishing a vegetarian cookbook. I also want to share a very important message: if you've adopted a vegetarian lifestyle for ethical or spiritual reasons and then find it's not working for your health, it's appropriate to rethink your choice.

Even the Dalai Lama, who says he would prefer a vegetarian diet, acknowledges that he eats some meat. I've learned the hard way that if you've grown up as an omnivore and switch to a vegetarian diet, it can be challenging to sustain good health for the long-term. This is especially true if you are anemic or have blood-sugar issues. People who suffer from anemia, hypoglycemia, or insulin resistance may need some animal protein for a time or long-term to maintain healthy blood sugar levels—though it's possible that supplementing your daily diet with protein powder and B vitamins will be enough support for optimal health.

If you want to live as a vegetarian but struggle with health issues, my advice is to be gentle with yourself. Listen to your body, work with a trusted health-care practitioner, and decide what is best for you at this particular time.

Because I've had to renew my commitment to a vegetarian lifestyle more than once, I chafe when someone is self-righteous about being a vegetarian. For readers who are vegetarians and are concerned about the eating habits of omnivorous friends and family, my advice is to not pressure them. A gentle invitation is good—and even better when it is accompanied by delicious vegetarian food! Ultimately, people choose a vegetarian or vegan lifestyle only when they are physically and emotionally ready to take that stand.

It's my hope that the recipes in *Sacred & Delicious* will support all readers—vegetarian and omnivore alike—in your search for delicious, healthy food, whether vegetables are your mainstay or side dishes on your table.

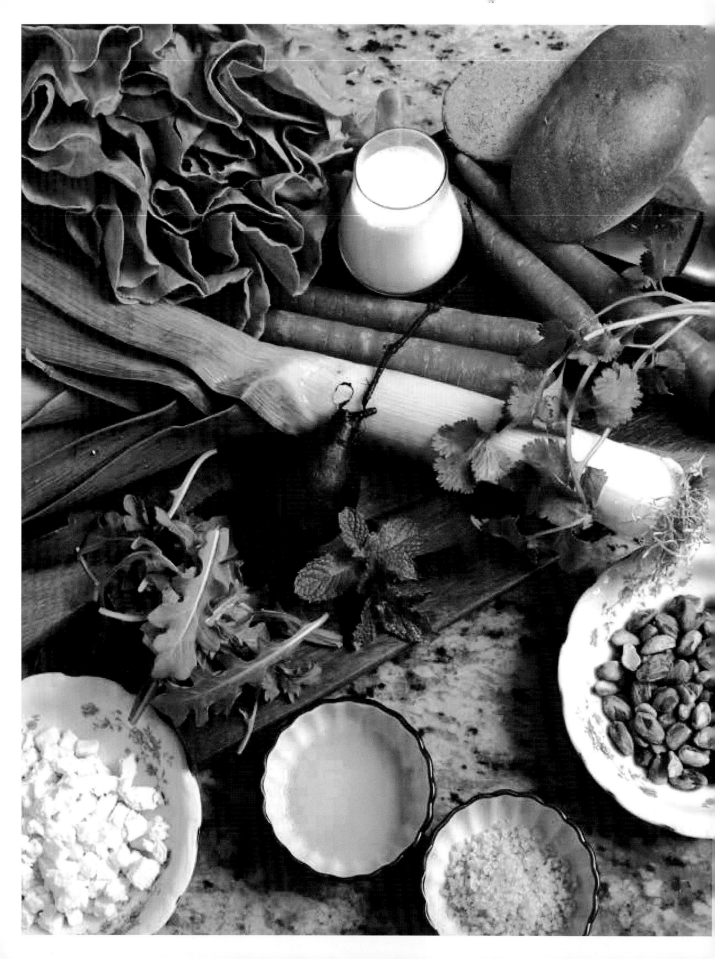

CHAPTER 2.

Eating Well in the Modern World

Ayurveda teaches what kind of food will support your health,
calm your mind, and increase your energy.
Eat food that is nourishing and easy to digest.
Then you will have great enthusiasm for life,
and you can be of service to others.

⁓ Dr. Smita Naram

What to Eat: Eight Guidelines

After all this information, you may be asking, "So, what *do* I eat?" Good question!

When I began learning about Ayurveda, I found myself obsessing about which foods had been recommended and which had been discouraged for each *dosha*. I studied lists of foods to favor and to avoid, given my various conditions, and although these lists can be extremely useful, I found that for the first time in my life I was worrying about food—particularly when I found myself "cheating."

Looking for guidance, I often quizzed my mentor, Ed Danaher at the Ayurvedic Institute, about whether or not I could eat specific foods. On several occasions he offered me the same wise counsel: *It's what you eat day in and day out, day after day, that has a significant, long-term impact on your health.*

As a recovering perfectionist, I've taken his words to heart. A statement that bears repeating is that most people can sustain good health eating almost anything, as long as it's fresh, whole food, and they eat it in moderation. This is especially true for people with strong constitutions who are in generally good health—signs of strong *agni*. Worrying about food choices creates anxiety, and that never contributes to good health.

Ideally, each of us would only eat the foods that support our *doshic* balance, but there are bigger issues to tackle in the twenty-first century. If we're mostly eating processed food on the run, then the first choices we must make revolve around eating real food. For this reason, I've purposefully taken a general and gentle approach with dietary recommendations in *Sacred & Delicious*. My goal is to offer what I think of as Ayurvedic common sense: traditional nutritional wisdom applied to food in modern times. If you suffer from an acute or chronic condition, you may want to learn more of the particulars on what foods support or aggravate the *doshas* so that your diet can more fully support your healing process. For that I recommend *Ayurvedic Cooking for Self-Healing* by Usha Lad & Dr. Vasant Lad. You'll find additional details about my food plan at sacredanddelicious.com.

As stated earlier, after we reach middle age, the accumulation of *ama* and aggravated *vata* are the ultimate sources of disease, physical degeneration, and pain. It's also important to note that aggravated *vata* also pushes the other *doshas* out of whack. For these reasons, I have come up with eight recommendations to address some of the present-day eating practices that contribute to creating *ama* and disturbing *vata*.

Here are the guidelines we'll be discussing in this section, which will help you assess your current diet:

1. Eat fresh, organic produce.
2. Eat whole foods rather than refined foods.
3. Avoid "junk," fast, frozen, and microwaved foods.
4. Eat mostly cooked food rather than raw food.
5. Reduce or avoid fermented foods in your diet.
6. Avoid cold food and drinks.
7. Avoid combining fruit with other types of food.
8. Determine if you have food sensitivities, and avoid those foods.

1. Eat fresh, organic produce.

Let me begin by adding ". . . whenever you can."

The first issue of "fresh" is when the food was harvested. Through the lens of Ayurveda, the longer food has been away from its sacred source—the earth—the less vital is that food's life force. If we could pick our vegetables fresh from the earth just before cooking, that would be ideal. But a working urbanite is lucky to have a tomato plant on the patio, so in the modern world, we do the best we can.

If you live near a farmers' market, the veggies sold there are likely to have been picked in the past day or two, at most. In many areas of the United States you can pay a fee to a local farm and receive a weekly box of fresh produce throughout the growing season. This movement is aptly named Community Supported Agriculture (CSA).

If your food source is a supermarket, try to shop a couple of times a week, so your vegetables are as fresh as possible when you cook them. Look for produce with bright, vivid color and firm texture.

"Fresh" also involves when the food was cooked. Ayurveda suggests that we eat food on the same day it is cooked and, ideally, within four hours. "Leftovers" are considered to be, energetically speaking, old or dead food—food that lacks *prana*, life force. Eating old food regularly can bring feelings of lethargy and a buildup of toxins. I have made a compromise with this guidance: I prepare enough food every night to have leftovers for lunch the next day.

Now we come to processed foods—the packaged, ready-made food products that line supermarket shelves, including the dinner-in-a-box to which you just add water. These have been engineered to sit in their packages for years and still appear fresh when eaten. In truth, this is dead food. If you feel your schedule requires you to supplement your weekly menus with processed food, try to make it the exception rather than the rule.

"Organic" is another consideration. Much research conducted in the United States points to organic food having higher nutrient content and less toxic residue, and so modern Ayurvedic practitioners universally advocate eating organic foods. Unfortunately, organic foods are more expensive than others—and may seem cost-prohibitive for anyone struggling financially.

If you are able to make this choice, I suggest restructuring your food budget to allow for organic foods. This shift would be particularly beneficial for anyone with chronic pain, which is often related to toxins stored in the body. Also, anyone whose family medical history involves cancer would be wise to go organic and avoid exposure to the chemicals that treat standard produce. The way I see it, buying organic food is a long-term value proposition, worth considering for the sake of your health.

You can compensate for the high cost of organic food by reducing meat consumption or even becoming a vegetarian. You could also stop buying junk food—the cookies, crackers, chips, and soft drinks, organic or otherwise. You would be amazed at the savings! And if you can't afford to go *all* organic, become familiar with the Dirty Dozen and Clean Fifteen lists developed by the Environmental Working Group and posted online with regular updates. These will help you make informed choices.

Certainly, there are millions of people who live in poverty and struggle to get any kind of food to eat, but for many of us, buying organic foods is a choice we *could* make.

The Dirtiest and the Cleanest Foods

The Environmental Working Group (EWG), a nonprofit organization based in Washington, DC, analyzes pesticide residue testing data annually from the US Department of Agriculture and the Federal Drug Administration for forty-eight foods. The EWG ranks those foods based on pesticide residue and publishes two annual lists: the Dirty Dozen and the Clean Fifteen. These lists identify the safest and most dangerous produce to eat, if you're not buying organic. The group estimates that individuals can reduce their exposure to pesticides by 80 percent if they switch to organic when buying those foods identified on the Dirty Dozen list. They started with twelve and fifteen foods on these respective lists, but they've been adding or deleting foods as agricultural processes change and new data is available. Sign up for information at ewg.org.

2. Eat whole foods rather than refined foods.

"Whole foods" are most easily defined by their opposite—fruits, vegetables, and grains that have not been refined, processed, or polished. These are foods that are closest to their natural forms. According to Ayurveda, foods that have been stripped of their natural identity have less life force, are more likely to create toxins, and contribute to disease.

Eat whole grains instead of white flour; eat unrefined sugar instead of refined sugar; and eat regular oatmeal instead of instant. Once I would have told you to eat brown rice instead of white, but now you might consider giving up rice altogether (see page 157). Whole foods are rich in micronutrient vitamins, minerals, antioxidants, enzymes, phytochemicals, and fibers, which are, at least in part, removed by the process of refining. Eating whole grains also helps to keep the colon moving, an essential component of health.

Many refined foods, on the other hand, are highly acidifying, which contributes greatly to inflammation in the body. In recent years, there has been a rise in inflammatory diseases, including allergies, asthma, arthritis, lupus, and Crohn's disease. Recent studies have also linked inflammation with heart disease, Alzheimer's, and certain types of cancer.

3. Avoid "junk," fast, frozen, and microwaved foods.

As Alfred E. Neuman, the fictional mascot of *Mad* magazine, once said, "We are living in a world today where lemonade is made from artificial flavors and furniture polish is made from real lemons." With a wary eye toward synthetic foods, additives, "natural flavors" that aren't found in nature, and the like, I'm lumping junk foods with fast foods, frozen foods, and microwaved foods for this discussion. From the Ayurvedic perspective, these have a similar impact on the body. They all contribute to the buildup of toxins. In other words, they are not worth eating. They don't support life.

JUNK FOODS: What nutritionists call "junk" are heavily processed foods with a nutritional value that is low relative to their calories, even if they are labeled "organic" or "all natural." Most chips, crackers, cookies, cakes, packaged pastries, processed cheeses, protein bars, and hybrid foods like chicken nuggets are often loaded with refined sugar and chemical additives. Some of these are suspected carcinogens; basically, I'm suspicious of any ingredient I can't pronounce. Even homemade cookies are junk when they are created with white flour, white sugar, and processed shortening. They don't suddenly become nutritious simply because you popped them into the oven yourself!

I understand that for many people, junk foods are comfort foods. Most people—and I am one—savor dessert at least once in a while. I live by "the special occasions rule" because to my mind special occasions do call for sweet celebration. The desserts in *Sacred & Delicious* (starting on page 223) are for people seeking sweets at the intersection of delicious and healthy.

When I'm out in a restaurant celebrating my birthday or wedding anniversary, I eat the dark chocolate dessert! I'm not willing to give it up absolutely and forever. Giving it up most of the time, however, has made a huge difference in how I feel. If you love junk foods, try limiting them to small quantities, eaten no more often than a few times a month—or less, if you're willing. Call it a treat.

A discussion about junk food is not complete without addressing the topic of carbonated drinks. The addition of carbon dioxide (the fizzy stuff) to sodas increases *vata* dramatically. And in colas, the refined sugar or sugar substitute isn't helpful either. In 2007 a study reported that drinking just one 12-ounce can of soda a day, either regular or diet,

About Sugar and Other Sweeteners

One of the greatest things you can do for your health is to dramatically reduce your intake of refined sugar—and if you can quit sugar altogether, that's even better. From an Ayurvedic perspective, white sugar aggravates all the *doshas* and creates *ama*, contributing greatly to chronic pain and disease. From the perspective of Western science, any amount of refined sugar—or too much of any other kind of sugar—contributes to inflammatory diseases, creates brain fog, suppresses the immune system, and weakens the kidneys and liver.

Vegetarians may be surprised to learn that, with the exception of 100 percent pure beet sugar, no white table sugar is vegetarian. The raw cane is whitened through a char derived from cow bones.

There are, of course, a number of alternative sweeteners available. Ayurveda suggests that *small* amounts of unrefined cane sugar, coconut sugar, date sugar, and maple syrup are fine and that both maple and date sugar are strengthening to the constitution. Unfortunately, most sweeteners will aggravate *kapha,* the exceptions being stevia and honey. Raw honey has many health benefits, but it can aggravate *pitta*, so anyone with a *pitta* imbalance may want to use honey in moderation. And cooking with honey is a problem. (See page 42.)

In my midfifties, I discovered that I was insulin resistant, which is the underlying cause of diabetes. Insulin resistance is a largely invisible health problem that affects perhaps 75 percent of Americans. When insulin resistance occurs, the body cannot efficiently absorb glucose, the digested carbohydrates that are used for energy. I dealt with my condition by avoiding sweets except on rare occasions. I switched from baking with Sucanat to using coconut palm sugar because of its low glycemic index (GI). This is the rate of how fast blood sugar levels rise after eating a particular type of food. Happily, I can now report that my blood sugar levels are normal again.

is associated with a 48 percent increased risk of "metabolic syndrome," a predecessor of heart disease and diabetes. Soft drinks are also extremely acidic because of their phosphoric acid content and contribute to acid indigestion, acid reflux disease, gastritis, inflammation, and osteoporosis.

The best beverage for the body is simple, filtered water. Most of the caffeine-free herbal teas are good for all *doshas*, but take note that all herbs have a *doshic* consequence.

FAST FOODS: Practitioners of Ayurveda call fast foods a fast track to disease. These are the prepared foods that you can purchase in minutes from drive-through and chain restaurants serving processed fare that is high in trans fats (the bad kind), full of calories, and light on nutrition. Most fast foods are the opposite of fresh. Those French fries were real potatoes once upon a time, but they've been sitting in a freezer for a while, maybe even months, awaiting their dip in hot fat. The sandwich meats come from animals that were routinely fed antibiotics. Chicken nuggets or other chicken-based finger foods sold at many fast-food restaurants and grocery stores are typically filled with lots of carbs: corn flour, cornstarch, and wheat. What's worse, these imitation foods are sometimes laced with unpronounceable chemical additives and preservatives such as dimethylpolysiloxane, "a suspected carcinogen," according to food journalist Michael Pollan. In any case, they're processed foods, not the real thing. Best bet: give them up.

FROZEN FOODS: Modern Ayurvedic masters say that freezing kills the life force that is in fresh foods. As Dr. Joshi writes:

> *To illustrate this point, notice what happens when you defrost food and set it beside the same food in fresh form. The defrosted food decomposes much more quickly, taking on a dried, colorless look, and starts to give off a putrid odor after a short time.*

This is true whether the frozen food is something you cooked and froze yourself or something you bought frozen at the store. The packaged frozen foods often have the additional problem of being laced with numerous chemical additives and preservatives to add color, enhance flavor, and sustain shelf life. These chemicals, Dr. Joshi says, "deplete *agni* and poison the body."

I'm sure some household cooks feel they have to freeze leftovers to save time. Freeze half of tonight's dinner, and you have a ready-made meal for another night. Nonetheless, if you suffer from chronic pain or illness, you may want to reconsider this modern convenience. Make a commitment to fresh food for a time, and see if you start to feel better.

MICROWAVED FOODS: Although there are conflicting opinions about the safety of foods that are heated or cooked in a microwave oven, modern Ayurvedic practitioners join those health experts who advise against them. Microwaving is known to alter food's molecular structure, and while the effects of eating such food are not conclusive, some scientists have expressed their concerns about the long-term impact of microwaving.

I do own a microwave, but I never cook with it. I use a microwave only to reheat leftovers when time is very important. It seems in our best interest to avoid this path to *ama*, even if we may not have clear evidence one way or another for some decades to come.

4. Eat mostly cooked food rather than raw foods.

In the Ayurvedic paradigm, cooking is recognized as the prerequisite to proper digestion. Just as crude oil must be prepared before it is a fuel an engine can use efficiently, we must prepare the fuel we give our bodies. According to

About Honey

There is one significant exception to Ayurveda's mandate to eat cooked food, and that is in regard to honey. Honey should not be cooked or even heated to more than 100°F. At this temperature, honey destabilizes and becomes toxic. As Dr. Lad explains:

> *According to ancient Ayurvedic literature, honey should never be cooked. If it is cooked, the molecules become a non-homogenized glue that adheres to mucous membranes and clogs subtle channels, producing toxins. Uncooked honey is nectar. Cooked honey is poison.*

Unfortunately, honey has been promoted as a health food by marketers who do not understand this principle, and today it is a common ingredient in breads, cookies, and other pastries as well as in baked granola.

When adding honey to tea, it is also best to wait until the tea has cooled to lukewarm.

Food combining is an issue for honey as well. Ayurveda recommends that honey not be eaten with milk, ghee, meat, or fish. The combination of honey with any of these foods produces *ama*.

classic Ayurveda, breaking the foods down for assimilation is begun during the cooking process. Heat breaks down the cell walls of foods, making their nutrients more accessible. Cooking also makes food easier to digest. The exceptions are lettuce and seeded cucumbers, which can be digested by most people when eaten raw.

This approach belies the basic premise of the raw-foods movement. Many people share their stories about recovering from cancer through a raw-foods diet, and some say they experience having more energy once they start eating raw foods. Nonetheless, I know people who report that after their initial success with a raw-foods diet, they found they needed to return to cooked foods; raw foods became debilitating over time.

Ayurveda's explanation for this reversal is simple. A diet of only raw foods can certainly help the body detoxify because in embracing raw foods, a person is typically renouncing meat, cheese, heavy grains, and—most importantly—processed foods, all of which contribute to the accumulation of toxins. A long-term diet of raw foods will, however, increase the *vata dosha*, particularly if you undertake that diet after the age of forty, which is the *vata* stage of life. An increase in *vata* is associated with many health problems, from constipation to insomnia. (See page 22.) Over time an exclusively raw-foods diet can also weaken the digestive fire. Raw foods can also increase *kapha*.

Why, then, do some people thrive on a sustained raw-foods diet? My guess is that they have very strong digestion and little constitutional tendency to develop *vata* problems.

5. *Reduce or avoid fermented foods in your diet.*

Today many Western nutritionists and naturopaths extol the virtues of naturally fermented foods because they are enzyme rich and are said to aid digestion. Ayurvedic practitioners see these foods from another perspective.

Ayurveda would agree that a limited amount of fermented foods, condiments, and drinks can be beneficial for certain people. This is true for those with high *vata* because fermented foods are naturally heating for the metabolism and therefore can help balance *vata*. Small amounts of balsamic or rice vinegar as well as good wine can be helpful in the diet, as these can kindle the digestive power if it is weak. For this purpose, Ayurvedic physicians sometimes give their patients a fermented tonic called *draksha*.

Eating fermented foods on a daily basis, however, is not advised for anyone. According to Dr. Smita Naram fermented foods can combine with any toxins lodged in the colon and increase the cycle of toxin formation. As well, fermented foods are likely to increase *pitta* and can lead to *pitta* maladies. (See page 24.) A steady diet of fermented

foods will also increase gases in the body, a *vata* condition. Systemic yeast infections such as candida thrive on a diet of fermented foods.

Although *kapha* can tolerate dry wines, beer, and tempeh, *kapha* will likely be aggravated by other fermented foods, including yogurt, hard cheeses, vinegar, and vinegar products. *Kapha* as well as *pitta* are aggravated by soy sauce and tamari, which are both fermented. (Instead, try Bragg Liquid Aminos, a nonfermented, gluten-free soy sauce.)

So, how does Ayurveda advise keeping enzyme function in proper working order? You can do this, according to Ayurvedic practitioner Ed Danaher, by keeping the *doshas* balanced, your digestive fire robust, and the toxins in your body minimal with pure foods and a healthy lifestyle. In addition, using spices properly (see page 33) will help sustain your body's naturally occurring enzymes.

6. Avoid cold food and drinks.

The average temperature in the stomach is 110°F, the temperature required for digestive enzymes to work effectively. Sending cold beverages or ice-cold foods into that warm environment is shocking to the body and weakens the digestive fire. In the summer, it's fine to drink liquids at room temperature or slightly cooler (such as filtered water from a tap). In the fall, winter, and early spring, it's better to drink warm or hot beverages unless you're suffering from hot flashes, ladies, in which case lukewarm will do!

7. Avoid combining fruit with other types of food.

Ayurveda has many suggestions about food combining—so many that I will not summarize them here. I am focusing on fruit because this is an easy dietary change that can be made without learning a list of food-combining recommendations.

Because fruit is digested much more quickly than other foods, eating fruit at the same time as grains, vegetables, dairy, fish, or meat can lead to indigestion, fermentation, and putrefaction in the digestive tract. These unwanted side effects of food combining can result in toxemia and disease, and this is particularly true for people who have weak digestion to begin with. Some Ayurvedic traditions advise that fruit be eaten by itself, at least thirty minutes to an hour before or after other foods are eaten. Using this time frame as a guideline, you can eat fruit as a between-meal snack or as a fruit-only meal. And because of the specific properties of melons, it's best not to combine them with anything else, even with other fruit.

This caution extends to some favorite American foods such as pancakes, cobblers, cake, and pies, which typically combine fruit with grains and dairy. No need to despair! If you have strong digestion, then an occasional blueberry pancake brunch or peach cobbler dessert will probably be fine. If, however, you experience chronic indigestion or illness, you may want to take a closer look at the Ayurvedic literature that explains the numerous considerations in food combining to avoid discomfort and disease.

8. Determine if you have food sensitivities, and avoid those foods.

At least some indicators of compromised health may be caused by invisible food sensitivities. Sinus problems, headaches, joint pain, skin eruptions, indigestion, irritable bowel disease, and many other disorders are often signals that some food or another is causing inflammation and excess mucous. Common culprits are gluten, dairy, eggs, sesame, corn, and other grains.

If you have any of these issues or other unresolved health problems, find a health-care practitioner who can check you for food sensitivities or support you in doing an elimination diet, where you eliminate all the foods listed above for at least three weeks. Take note of how you feel. After three weeks, begin to add these foods back to your diet, one by one, every few days. Typically, if you have an intolerance to a particular food, you will have obvious symptoms within hours or a couple of days after eating it again.

One of the most common food sensitivities in the United States today is to gluten. Many who are not allergic to gluten (celiac disease) still suffer from gluten sensitivity or "intolerance." This inflammatory response produces a broad range of symptoms, including abdominal pain, diarrhea, bloating, irritability, depression, anemia, joint pain, and mouth sores. If you decide to go gluten-free, it's important to recognize that gluten is ubiquitous and often an unseen ingredient in packaged foods or restaurant meals. It's not only in bread, cookies, and cakes but also in salad dressings and sauces, in gravy and soups. It's often the hidden ingredient on the label that says "natural flavoring." Giving up gluten requires constant vigilance unless you cook 100 percent of your food.

Also, some food sensitivities are triggered by low *agni*, weak digestion. When this is the case, people can improve dramatically—actually eradicate their food sensitivities!—through protocols and lifestyle changes that increase *agni*.

How to Eat: One Guideline

If I could invite you to make just one lifestyle change to improve your health, it would be this: **slow down; take the time to truly eat**. The pace at which you eat is crucial to your digestion, which is itself essential to your health. These days many of us have become habituated to eating on the run. If this is true for you, I have a few suggestions to help you slow down at mealtime. Although this looks like yet another list, if you go through it, I think you'll see that every single item has to do with the kind of time you give to eating.

- Make it a practice to plan enough time to eat, every meal, every day.
- Sit down when you eat. Avoid eating while you're standing, driving a car, or engaging in any activity other than eating.
- Pause, for at least a moment, before beginning to eat.
- Practice being present with your food. Notice what you're eating. Observe the food's colors and textures. Relish the various tastes.
- Chew each bite at least twenty times—as many as fifty is even better—until the food is completely masticated. When you swallow food that isn't adequately chewed, it's much more difficult to digest.
- If you're in the habit of eating quickly, practice putting the fork down between bites so that you consciously add space in your meals.
- After you've finished eating, savor what you've eaten. Pause for five or ten minutes after each meal. Don't immediately jump up to do dishes or run out the door. Instead of *doing*, take a *being* break! Have a pleasant conversation, invite a purring kitty to your lap (my favorite digestive aid), read a book, or just be still.

Simple Changes: A Step at a Time

When I first discovered the Ayurvedic approach to eating, I was, to put it mildly, a bit annoyed. I had already given up meat and was limiting my intake of white sugar, which felt at the time like huge sacrifices. I wasn't the tiniest bit interested in making *more* changes to my diet. And when I saw vegetables like tomatoes and eggplant—vegetables I enjoyed eating!—listed in the "best to avoid" category, I was shocked.

It took chronic pain and illness to motivate me to make the dietary shift away from the nightshades. In the process, I learned how to select foods that specifically support my health. I was fascinated to learn that certain foods I'd always seen as neutral, or even beneficial, were actually contributing to my health problems. It became exciting and empowering to discover that other foods and spices had the potential to heal me. As I began to absorb this ancient wisdom and make positive choices, I felt less victimized by my genetic tendencies.

And then, of course, as I've already mentioned, recently I've found that I occasionally need to include some *tamasic* food in my diet: I need to eat some animal protein. Many yogis have given themselves the dictum to eat only the purest foods, but this isn't advisable for every person. Your physical system may need the energetic boost of *rajas* or the grounding of *tamas*—in which case, you would do well to eat some of those foods, making the most discerning choices you can. This isn't an invitation to eat junk food, but it does open the door to eat eggs as needed or a little garlic or onions (cooked!) a few times a week. For many, garlic is a digestive aid as it increases *agni*. When onions are cooked until they start to brown and caramelize, they become sweet.

In any event, changing your diet is a step-by-step process.

Whatever your situation, I encourage you to try these recommendations one or two at a time to tackle any problems and pave the way for a comfortable old age. Even if you introduce a few very simple changes, they can make a positive impact on your digestion and your overall health. For instance, if you haven't already, you can move gradually toward a whole and fresh food diet. Try forgoing ice-cold drinks; in restaurants you can order water without ice. Rather than eating a piece of fruit with a meal, try saving it for a midmorning or afternoon snack. These steps wouldn't require any investment of your time or money, and even just this much can retard the aging process and the development of chronic disease.

One inherently practical rule of Ayurveda is this: **In dealing with dietary changes, moderation is always the key.** As my mentor said to me, it's all right to eat almost anything from time to time; it's what we eat day after day that has a real impact on our overall health. My approach is to cook well at home and sometimes cheat (so to speak) when I eat out. This gives me an opportunity to eat the food that's offered or available to me when someone else is feeding me, even though I might not consider eating the same thing every day.

If you are just now asking yourself whether or not Ayurveda might work for you, I suggest that you try these recommendations for a period of time—say for six months or a year—and then observe the changes in how you feel.

In the beginning, my advice is that you try one new guideline every week. Either add a new discipline to your daily regimen or subtract something from your diet that may be creating problems for your body. If you want to take one step at a time, you could undertake one of the following each week:

- Start with "How to Eat" on page 44. Pick one of the guidelines and practice it faithfully. You might begin with sitting down to eat every meal. This alone will support digestion and calm *vata* and *pitta*.
- Practice the guideline to stop eating before you feel completely full. This helps slow the buildup of toxins in the body.
- Give up snacking between meals, unless you're truly hungry. Then opt for a healthy snack: a piece of fresh fruit or a small handful of nuts.
- Stop eating junk food or at least give up eating junk food snacks on a regular basis. If you must have chips or ice cream, begin by limiting them to once a week. When you can, cut back further to see if you feel better without those snacks. Once you stop eating them regularly, the addiction will be easier to kick. Avoiding junk foods will become easier—and in time, second nature. Really! This is also the very easiest way to lose weight.
- If you don't already eat a lot of fresh vegetables, experiment with one new vegetable recipe each week.
- When you're ready to dive in more fully, read through the list of characteristics and symptoms associated with each *dosha* to determine which of your *doshas* seems most out of balance. Then go to the end of the section on that *dosha*, and practice one of the "Five Easy Ways to Balance."

- If you have chronic health problems, consider kick-starting your program with the help of a skilled Ayurvedic practitioner. It's extremely beneficial to have the assistance of a knowledgeable practitioner who can understand your problems, support you with herbal remedies, and help you to detoxify safely while you rebuild your digestion and overall health.

While you may be able to see some results immediately, understand that no one can undo a lifetime of unhealthy eating in just a few weeks. This will take time—and it's worth it. If you begin to eat by Ayurvedic principles and recognize the great difference this can make in your energy level, your digestion, your moods, and so on, I suspect that you will become as eager as I am to embrace more of what Ayurveda has to offer.

CHAPTER 3.

The Essential Ingredient

When you eat, have the feeling you are offering.
Offer every breath, so every action becomes an offering to the Divine.
That is love.

⁓ Sri Sri Ravi Shankar

The Cook's Inner State

I want to return to the reasons I love to eat and the reasons why so many of us are passionate about cooking. As imperative as it is to understand how foods affect health, it's equally important that every meal be delicious! The great pleasure of food has the power to connect us to our sublime inner joy. As well, food is a primal connection to family and community.

The phrase may sound clichéd to us, but food *is* love, and instinctively we know this to be true. From the moment we were born and took in our first mouthful of mother's milk or life-sustaining formula, our sense of safety and connection to the world was established through food. Our needs provided for, we joined the circle of life, the sacred cycle of giving and receiving that is essential to our existence as human beings.

When you bring dinner to the table, whether you're cooking for your partner, for your family, or simply for yourself, the act of cooking is your *dharma*, your sacred duty. You have cooked that food not only to quell hunger but also to sustain life, which is sacred. When you consider your body to be a temple of the Divine, then the food you cook becomes a pure offering to the divine presence within yourself and within others.

You may question whether it's practical to bring such a lofty perspective to the sometimes rushed and labor-intensive work of cooking. Such a perspective, however, requires only one extra ingredient: love.

There is a particularly delightful scene in the film *Like Water for Chocolate*, in which a dinner guest asks the cook, a Mexican woman, what makes her mole so remarkably delicious. The cook's answer? *"El secreto es hacerlos con mucho amor."*

The secret is to make it with lots of love.

Throughout the ages this truth has been espoused by saints and ordinary cooks alike. In cooking, love is the essential ingredient. It's love that transforms even the simplest dish into something quite wonderful. And I don't mean this metaphorically at all. When a dish is cooked with love, you can taste it—absolutely!

Not only does the cook's love enter the food as it's being prepared, so does any other feeling the cook may have: joy or sadness, serenity or agitation, resentment, or forgiveness. Whatever the cook is feeling—your inner state—goes straight into that food in the form of palpable energy. This is the ancient wisdom of Ayurveda and my own experience. Think about this! Whoever eats at your table will encounter the state of *your* mind while you were cooking! So, as you cook, isn't it worth asking yourself what you want to offer your family or guests?

I observed this one day when I overindulged my National Public Radio habit. I listened to upsetting news and political analysis for a few hours while preparing dinner for company. The news made me anxious, and what I'd hoped would be a special meal was disappointing. The food wasn't as tasty or as satisfying as I'd expected. Later I realized the difference came because of my own state of agitation as I cooked.

I have also experienced that when the cook's mind and emotions are peaceful or even exalted, then the cook's inner state itself becomes a blessing for the food and for everyone who eats it. Let me tell you this story.

In 1996 my husband and I had the privilege of hosting his meditation master, Sri Sri Ravi Shankar, in our home. Between Guruji's public events, some fifty or so people gathered at our house to visit with this spiritual master, and we were feeding everyone who came. One volunteer did all the cooking, and after a few days, we felt she needed a break. We decided to order the final day's lunch from a local Indian restaurant. A few hours later, Guruji asked how things were going in the kitchen. Hearing about our plans for the final meal, he shook his head in that uniquely Indian way, not from side to side but subtly from shoulder to shoulder. This expression is open to interpretation—yes or no?—and Guruji let us know what he meant by saying, "I'll cook lunch."

The next day, Guruji rolled up his sleeves and went to work in my kitchen with the woman who had been cooking for all of us. When I went to offer my help, I was captivated by what I saw. The bearded saint, small in stature, moved with fluid grace from stove to counter and back again, stirring the pots and adding the spices so easefully that it was apparent he knew exactly how much was needed in each dish. But even more evident was his delight in cooking. His eyes sparkled and a smile played on his lips. Despite the hot stove and the hungry crowd awaiting lunch, Guruji was cooking in a state of perfect equanimity and love.

After he had finished cooking and we'd set the food out on a table, he came into the dining room and helped serve each guest. As I watched these people file by holding out plates to receive food from their teacher, I, too, was filled with the pure joy of giving. When I finally sat down to eat, I was astounded by the food! The flavor was exquisite, unlike anything I had ever tasted—even though I was no stranger to Indian cuisine. With each savory bite, I could feel the sweet blessing of the master's enlightened state. People ate that meal quietly, their faces beaming, their hearts full.

And in that space of shared contentment, for at least a moment, we tasted divinity.

Setting a Sacred Intention

How can we transform cooking daily into a joyful and sacred experience? The answer is simple: by bringing awareness and love to our kitchen activities. And how we do this is a topic worth exploring.

Although I usually love cooking, I occasionally lose my enthusiasm for retesting recipes, delicious as they are! I typically cook an evening meal "from scratch" five or six days a week. If I'm particularly tired or feeling out of sorts that day, I'll sometimes notice that my heart just isn't into cooking. Once when I was in this kind of a slump, I decided to make a simple effort to shift my attitude. I turned to the teachings of Ayurveda and yoga that have become my life support. I wrote a statement of intention, imbedded with a prayer, and taped it to the hood above my stove:

I embrace my dharma *of cooking as an act of selfless service and self-love.*
O Lord, please come cook with me today, that I may experience your delight in all actions.

Each time I read these words, my heart soars! Once again I'm reminded to renew my intention to stay present while I cook, to bless the act of cooking, and to open myself to the experience of divine bliss that is available in every moment—even while performing mundane tasks like chopping vegetables. With this simple yet profound intention, I have been able to re-engage joyfully with cooking.

And something else magical happened when I took the time to contemplate my resistance to daily cooking. I had long seen cooking for others as an honorable form of service to *them*. What hadn't occurred to me was the possibility of cooking to expand my own consciousness, cooking to serve myself as well as others.

Another way that I reconnect to my intention is to practice a brief ritual before I start to cook. I borrow from the Indian tradition of performing *arati*—waving a lighted candle at a small altar in my kitchen, while I listen to a sacred chant. This takes only a few minutes. No matter how tired or harried I may feel at the end of the day, when I start my practice of cooking with *arati*, I am re-energized, refocused, and reconnected to grace.

Cooking as Spiritual Practice

Making a sacred intention is one thing; holding it and keeping it alive is something else altogether. It is the holding of a sacred intention and the coming back to it again and again that makes any activity a spiritual practice. Cooking provides an ideal opportunity for this effort. While we're washing vegetables, chopping, and stirring, we have ample time for the mind to wander and think positive thoughts or to get lost in a negative spiral. Each time we choose the higher path, we reinforce both our intention and spiritual understanding.

Thankfully, cooking as spiritual practice doesn't take any extra time. It takes only a shift in consciousness. As we cook, we can use that time to actively observe our inner state. In the yogic tradition this practice is called "witnessing." Sometimes while cooking I'll observe that my mind has launched a negative diatribe toward an unsuspecting character in my personal life! When I notice what I'm doing, I practice letting go of negativity and realigning my inner state with my essential Self in a lighthearted way.

"Well, that's a familiar record," I might say to myself good-humoredly, "but it doesn't feel so useful today!" I may take a moment to reframe whatever I was thinking in a more positive light; then I pivot the mind back to cooking and reabsorb myself in the task at hand. Sometimes when my inner witness kicks in, I notice that I'm begrudging my time at the stove. I do a quick attitude adjustment and remember my intention to make this meal an offering of love, a practice in generosity.

What's important is to notice your thoughts and feelings without getting too caught up in them or even believing them to be true! It's also important not to beat up on yourself. Just notice and return your focus to the work at hand. In the Buddhist tradition, this practice is called "mindfulness." As you focus your attention and enter deeply into the experience of any activity, you allow yourself to become one with whatever you're doing. In the kitchen, this can be as simple as focusing your attention on the food and the activities of cooking. Notice the colors, the textures, the smells. This is cooking with awareness. When you enter deeply into the experience of cooking (or any activity), the chatter of the mind naturally begins to quiet down. If you practice mantra repetition, as I do, cooking provides the perfect opportunity to become absorbed in the divine name. With either practice, mantra repetition or witnessing, you can move beyond the mind toward the space of the heart.

It's not uncommon for me to catch myself in an intense *rush-rush* pace, trying to get everything on the table by the promised dinnertime. In those moments, I notice that I'm feeling tense as I try to push through. When I find myself in this inner posture, I take a second to breathe consciously, smile at my old habit, and shift my awareness

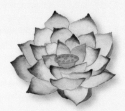
back to the mantra and the rhythm of cooking easefully—moving *with* time instead of against it. When I return to that calm flow, I feel the tender hand of grace guiding each move, and I start to resonate with joy once again.

The Power of Prayer and Blessing

Following Indian tradition, before anyone begins to eat a meal, the first morsels of food are offered back to God. This offering may be made to a deity on the family altar, or it may be made metaphorically, through prayer. Whenever we inwardly offer our food to the divine source, we link ourselves to universal love. In diverse cultures throughout the world, offering food to God before eating is seen as a way to give back to the divine source of all. Feeding other people is often another way of offering back because in many cultures this is considered a service the host performs on behalf of God.

For those readers who are not spiritually inclined or not drawn to rituals or prayer, I want to point out that the act of merely pausing for a moment before beginning to eat—the act of taking the time to recall that you're about to nourish your body—can transform your inner state from *rush-rush-rush* to inner quiet. Before I start to eat, I make it a practice to take a deep cleansing breath, stop all activity, and just be. This is only for a moment, but in this time my heart rate slows down, I reconnect to my center, and from that state I can then be truly present for my meal. This, in itself, can make eating a sacred experience.

And for readers who do embrace prayer, or who wish to renew or begin prayer as a mealtime practice, I've sprinkled a few of my favorite prayers and blessings from various cultures throughout this book. It is my hope that these prayers will serve as a sweet inspiration for your own creative blessings.

Although I grew up in a household in which a blessing was offered before every meal, my own offering of such prayers as a child was a bit perfunctory, and so it was many years before I recognized the value of invoking divine love before eating. The understanding came during an uncomfortable period in my early twenties when everything I ate made me sick. Some friends suggested that I speak with a healing practitioner who was visiting Columbia, South Carolina, where I lived at that time. It was this healer who introduced me to the true power of prayer before meals.

He explained that while I was eating, the state of my mind could affect the power of my digestion either positively or negatively. I took the healer's advice and renewed the ritual of praying before meals, a practice I had left at home when I departed for college. I then recovered quickly from that phase of chronic indigestion. At the time, I likened this recovery to a miracle, and in a certain sense it was. In any event, it was surely grace that pointed me toward the power of prayer.

When I turned to mealtime prayer in earnest, I no longer felt satisfied with the habitual prayers of my youth. Instead, I instinctively turned within to reestablish my connection with divine love. I began searching for words that had personal meaning for me. Words that attuned my heart to the divine pulsation of love and summoned my sincere appreciation of a delicious meal. Today, as I integrate my religious background with my evolving spirituality, the formal prayers I first learned as a child offer me comfort and inspiration as I also listen to the inner voice of gratitude.

For me, offering a prayer before eating is far more than asking for a blessing from the Creator because, in truth, grace has already been received in the form of the abundant food on my plate! I've come to recognize that when I summon my heart to the moment, I am offering my loving thoughts—my own blessing—to the food as well as to others around the table. A meal that might have been something mundane suddenly becomes a sacred event. Charles Poindexter, my friend and author of *Sacred Healing*, offers this observation:

The community meal when shared together with love is a sacred reflection of the divinity that lives within and among all beings. The blessing of that meal is an act of remembering the love that sustains and unifies us. When we choose to remember, each portion of food becomes saturated with the vibration of that love and becomes a vehicle for sharing the brilliance of divinity. When we regularly share our meals with such sacred intention we nourish, not only the gathered few, but also the collective consciousness of all creation.

The Sacred Principle of Food

As we practice cooking and eating with awareness and as we pause to bless our meals, we are able to connect with the sacred principle of food. With awareness, we notice how delicious the food really is, and suddenly, the table swells with those universal sounds of epicurean contentment:

Aaaah . . . oooooo . . . uummmm . . .

These are not just sighs of pleasure; they are some of our truest expressions of joyful living. They may even be our unconscious murmurs of gratitude to God. I once heard Dr. Lad say that when we utter the sound *uummm*, we are instinctively repeating the name Uma, one of the names of the Divine Mother in India. And *a-u-m* is the esoteric spelling of *Om*, the primordial syllable that the Indian traditions identify as the first sound to emerge from the cosmic silence, the syllable of creation from which all the universe is said to have sprung.

Ultimately, *uummm* means satisfaction. It means comfort. It says that the cook's efforts were well spent. It affirms, "This food is divine!"

The next time you taste something truly delicious and you start to feel that irrepressible joy bubble up, you may want to try this experiment. Become very still and see if you can trace the joy you're feeling back to its source. Take a long, full moment to pause and savor the taste of the food. Become totally present to the wonder of this delicious morsel in your mouth. Experience the food with every cell of your being. Sense the food's divine pulsations. Now follow the feeling of joy and sense the space from where that joy emanates inside yourself. Let go into the bliss!

Through contemplation and spiritual practice we can begin to understand that food is more than a path to sensory satisfaction. Eating can serve us as a portal to the Divine. As we bless our meals, thanking the food for offering itself to us, the very food that sustains us also can offer us an experience of our own true nature, which is boundless love.

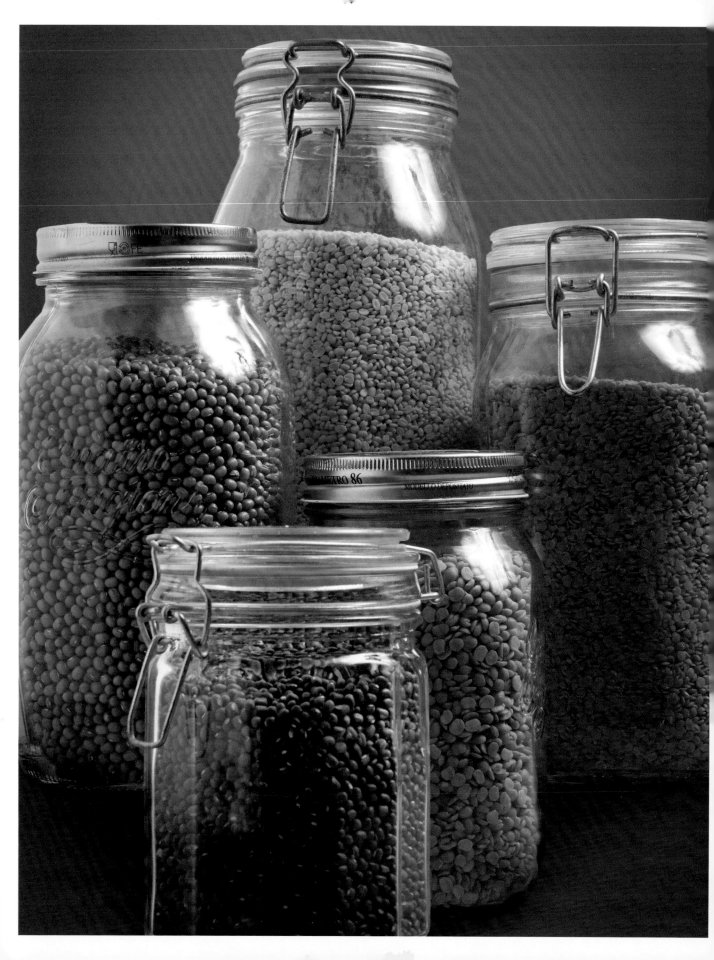

Chapter 4.

Getting Started

Be grateful for nature's unending gift of food,
and respect it as you do yourself.

⁓ Dr. Deepak Chopra

Notice How You Feel

If *Sacred & Delicious* is your introduction to Ayurveda, you have probably just taken on a new vocabulary and some new ways of approaching food. You may be asking yourself, "Is this for me?" This is not just a valid question; it's the right question.

It seems that every few months new research is announced extolling the benefits of one food or another. Within weeks, armies of marketers assault us with packaged foods containing the new magic bullet. We discover that X food has X nutritional components, and the word goes out: eat more X! This is the reductionist logic common to modern food research. It fails to take into account that while X may be great for some people—even most people—it can lead to imbalance for others. When your own experience of X differs with the advice of the "experts," it's easy to become confused.

I once heard the Ayurvedic master Dr. Lad say that when a food is recommended by researchers, most Western nutritionists and dietary approaches forget to ask what in Ayurveda is the most important question: **Recommended for whom?**

How could every person possibly benefit from every new discovery that food science unveils! Take tomatoes, which are lauded by many American nutritionists for their antioxidants but are among the foods that most aggravate *pitta*. If you suffer from acid reflux, acne, or inflammatory conditions such as rheumatoid arthritis, the antioxidant benefits of tomatoes are more than countered by their acidity, a *pitta*-aggravating quality that increases inflammation. Coconut oil has also received great press in recent years with research pointing to, among other health benefits, the antibacterial and antiviral properties of its lauric acid. While I recommend coconut oil for many people, I do so with one caveat: coconut oil greatly increases *kapha* conditions—colds, coughs, asthma, and allergies—and all coconut products are problematic for people with these maladies. These are just two examples; there are many more.

ꕥ 53

My advice is this: pay attention to your own body. Notice how you feel after you eat certain kinds of foods. Favor those that support your body in feeling light and energized. You can become the best arbiter of what food is right for you.

If you would like to explore Ayurveda and you have a chronic ailment for which you need professional support, try to do a consultation with an Ayurvedic practitioner. (For those who do not find a local practitioner, many qualified Ayurvedic consultants can be found online and offer telephone consultations.) As already stated, the science of Ayurveda categorizes every food, spice, and beverage according to how it impacts each *dosha*, and this is particularly helpful to study and learn if you have any chronic health problems. Once you've received advice about the specific foods to eat and to avoid for your constitution or condition, do your best to follow that advice for at least three and preferably six months to determine whether or not your new regime makes a difference for you.

In the short run, you can look at the list of chronic conditions by *dosha* in *Sacred & Delicious*, on pages 22, 24, and 26, and you can avoid or eat less of the foods that most aggravate the conditions you have.

"But"—I can hear you saying—"I don't want to have to figure this out! It's too complicated to even think about. Please, just give me a food list!"

OK. For you, I will! You can find the *Sacred & Delicious* Food List at my website: sacredanddelicious.com. By posting this list on the web, I can update it regularly based on any new food research and trends I discover.

About the Recipes

In the following pages you will find more than 108 recipes, all but two of them gluten-free, organized in traditional sections. They begin at dawn with "Breakfast, Breads, and Beverages," followed by an assortment of vegetable and legume-based soups that can star as the main course for any lunch or dinner. Most of the entrées can serve as a whole meal. I've provided a broad selection of vegetable side dishes and salads, offering options that will support each of the *doshas* so you can mix and match them at your table to bring overall balance to any meal. And I supply a number of gluten-free desserts that are not overly sweet but seem to satisfy even the most dedicated devotees of cakes, cookies, and other pleasures.

Ayurveda in the West

Sacred & Delicious endeavors to bring the principles of Ayurveda to a Western audience, catering to the varied tastes and adventuresome palates that seem to increase in sophistication year by year. I suspect that only a handful of these recipes will fit your idea of traditional foods of India, the motherland of Ayurveda. As I've mentioned, most of my recipes are modeled after traditional cuisines, sometimes with a different spice than you might expect to bring the dish into greater *doshic* balance. For instance, I hide some cumin in a tomato sauce to balance its acidity.

Most of the recipes in *Sacred & Delicious* are inspired by Ayurveda, whether or not the dish itself resembles traditional Ayurvedic cooking. This means that I strive in my own daily cooking to balance the various qualities of the food so that each dish is easy to digest and nourishing for the *doshas*.

I do use onions and garlic in a number of recipes to aid digestion, which is taboo to some Hindus and spiritual aspirants. From a Hindu scriptural perspective, eating onions and garlic is considered *rajasic*—overstimulating to the body, mind, and emotions. This prohibition is often characterized as an Ayurvedic dictate, but experts do not agree on this point. In fact, garlic and onions are often used medicinally in Ayurveda. Onions are recommended for convulsions, fainting, fever, sexual debility, rapid heartbeat, and high cholesterol. Garlic is prescribed for chronic indigestion, enlarged spleen, obesity, arthritis, high cholesterol, and chronic cough.

I do avoid raw onion in these recipes. Raw onion is highly aggravating to *pitta* and is also truly *rajasic* in its effect on the system. I heard Dr. Lad say that onions are no longer *rajasic*, however, when they are well cooked—especially when they become caramelized and sweet. Caramelized onion can add a depth of flavor to vegetarian dishes that spices alone cannot replace. I often use leeks instead of onions because of their milder flavor.

While I'm on the topic of breaking with Ayurvedic tradition, let me point to *Sacred & Delicious* recipes for breads, breakfast foods—pancakes!—and desserts that have absolutely no resemblance to traditional Ayurvedic cooking. All the more proof that I prefer flexibility over a rigid adherence to any model. When I want an occasional treat outside the Ayurvedic model, I look for ways to keep the recipes as healthy as possible. These recipes are based on Southern comfort foods, but are updated and reconstructed without white sugar and with gluten-free and vegan options.

As mentioned earlier, it could seem daunting at first to follow an Ayurvedic paradigm when cooking for a family since each individual has a unique *doshic* profile. However, families tend to have *doshic* patterns—the fruit doesn't fall far from the tree—so the children are likely to mirror their parents. Despite a family's differences, the cook supports everyone at the table by preparing foods that nourish all the *doshas*, taking the season into account. (For more information on *doshas* and the seasons, see page 30.) You will find recipes in *Sacred & Delicious* that support all of these differences and serve my main goal of managing *vata* and *ama* to support optimal health.

Finally, please don't be alarmed by the number of ingredients in many of the soups, entrées, and side dishes. Most are spices, and once you pull spices out of the cupboard, it takes only seconds to add them. I hope you won't let the length of the recipe or any unfamiliarity using spices keep you from trying something that could completely dazzle your senses! Once you learn some of these spice combinations, they will become as natural as salt and pepper.

Key to Reading the Recipes

Each recipe is set up with an estimated cooking time and number of servings followed by a brief introduction about its origins. Cooking time will vary by individual based on your familiarity with the recipe and ingredients, your skill with a knife or food processor, and your efficiency in the kitchen.

The number of servings is an estimate and will often be listed as a range. These numbers and ranges vary based on whether you are using a recipe as a one-course meal or as a centerpiece among other dishes on a menu when the portion size will naturally be smaller. It also depends on the appetites at your table.

This preamble is followed by a list of ingredients and cooking directions. You'll find ideas about advanced preparation in occasional notes called "Time-Saver."

Novice cooks or those new to Ayurveda can gain extra information about handling the ingredients, recipe variations, or the tools for a particular recipe in the notes called "Cook's Tip" or "Baker's Tip."

And at the end of most recipes in soups, entrées, and a few side dishes, you'll find a "Menu Suggestion" to suggest food pairings that work well together.

Ayurvedic Note

After each recipe you will find an "Ayurvedic Note." This explains how the ingredients combine to create a balanced offering to the *doshas* and maintain or improve health. In many recipes, these notes also describe how each of the individual ingredients affects the *doshas* so that you can begin to learn more about your favorite foods. I've developed these notes after almost two decades of studying Dr. Vasant Lad's guide, *Qualities of Food Substances*, and discerning from my own experiences how each food impacts my body and *doshic* tendencies and vulnerabilities—which many other Americans also have.

The notes also give you some tips on seasonal suitability and health conditions when it's best to favor or avoid a particular dish. For example, a recipe with cooling properties is ideal for the summer months, when *pitta* is most aggravated, but you may want to avoid or eat it less routinely during the winter. Dairy dishes aggravate *kapha* conditions, especially a cold or cough, which is when you may want to avoid eating dairy.

If you're not interested in learning about Ayurveda, skip over the notes and special instructions. Most people will benefit from most of these recipes most of the time. If you do suffer from chronic health problems, please accept this invitation to read a little bit at a time as you begin to explore how an Ayurvedic approach to eating can help you reach optimal health.

Icon Legend

(V) = *vata*   (S) = *summer*

(P) = *pitta*   (W) = *winter*

(K) = *kapha*   (G) = *includes gluten*

Following the "Ayurvedic Notes" I suggest an alternative way of cooking the dish if you have a health problem or are aware of (or suspect) a *doshic* imbalance. This may be an acute problem, such as a cold, or a chronic problem, such as acid reflux disease or difficulty maintaining a healthy weight. These recommendations are marked with a (V), (P), or (K) (short for *vata*, *pitta*, or *kapha*) and (S) or (W) (for summer or winter) to signify a change you can make— for instance, more or less of a certain spice—to increase the benefits to whichever *dosha* has been indicated. For example, the note may say: " (V) Add an additional clove of garlic." This means that if you have a *vata* imbalance, you may wish to add the additional garlic to the recipe.

There are no such suggestions in the "Desserts" section. These recipes are cleaner than typical American favorites as written, but they will increase the *doshas* to some degree. Creamy (even coconut oil), sugary (even unrefined sugar) frostings always increase *kapha*. Chocolate aggravates all *doshas*. Butter and eggs are not part of an Ayurvedic regime. There's no free dessert! But, as I often say, it's fine to treat yourself every now and again, and no dessert will trash your health if eaten in a modest quantity and only on occasion.

So, use your common sense and creativity. Always give highest priority to your own known health issues when following a recipe. If you are hypoglycemic or diabetic, then avoid added sugars that may be called for. If you don't eat high-glycemic white potatoes, experiment with other ingredients in a recipe, such as cauliflower or zucchini. And so on.

Finally, two recipes are made with spelt and, so, include gluten. Those recipes are noted with a bold (G) icon. All the rest are gluten-free.

It's Time to Start Cooking!

My hope is that you will find within these pages many new ways to make every mealtime a sweet occasion. If you are new to Ayurveda, I invite you to take your first steps on this journey to health by exploring the recipes that follow. If you've already been following an Ayurvedic lifestyle, I hope that you will find some interesting new menu options and perhaps even a few ideas that will help you deepen your commitment to taking care of your health and the health of your family in a meaningful way.

People who have eaten in our home and have cooked with my recipes will often say, "Mine didn't taste as good as yours." I'll mention four possible reasons why:

1. If a recipe calls for soup stock and you use a boxed or canned stock, it will have a noticeably different taste, including an unpleasant aftertaste that I notice because of the preservatives even in "natural" and organic products.

2. Salt can make a huge difference. I find that typical refined table salt cannot compare in taste to Celtic Sea Salt, Himalayan salts, and many fine artisan salts. For this reason, I always cook with unrefined salt. Unless otherwise specified, the measurement for salt in these recipes is always based on Celtic Sea Salt®-Light Grey. The light grey crystals are closer in size to kosher salt than to standard table salt. **If you use a finer grain of salt, I suggest that you start by adding half of what is called for in these recipes.** Then taste and add more to your liking. In fact, salt in food is such a personal and variable preference that I encourage you to experiment and add more or less, to satisfy your own taste.

3. One of the secrets to my cooking is that I spend more time caramelizing onions than my recipes dictate—I feared that many cooks would rebel if I told them to spend 30 minutes sautéing onions! But I do this routinely! The recipe may call for 10 to 15 minutes for sautéing onions until they turn "uniformly golden." But truth be told, I will cook onions for 25 to 30 minutes before adding other ingredients. I organize my cooking by starting the onions before preparing anything else. I sauté the onions on medium heat until they turn golden and just start to brown. Then I reduce the heat to medium-low for another 10, 15, or even 20 minutes, depending on how many I'm using, until they begin to caramelize and sweeten—without burning. This one step takes many recipes from good to delicious! And it does not always necessitate more time. Just let the onions cook as you're preparing other dishes.

4. My cooking always tastes better when I cook with joyful and uplifting music that opens my heart, anything from James Taylor to Sting to *The Sound of Music*! (Yes, my age is showing!) And I haven't even mentioned my true favorite for many years, sacred chants. You'd be surprised what a difference it makes in the final flavor of your food when you fill it with the music of love!

My wish for each reader is that you experience greater energy and well-being as a result of eating healthy, well-balanced, and as important, *delicious* food. I encourage you to experiment so that every dish turns out delicious for you. If a particular spice or food combination doesn't intrigue you, then adjust the recipe so that you and your family look forward to eating each and every meal that you cook. OR, consider giving the recipe a try as it is written—just once!—to see if you can expand your palate.

Perhaps most important of all, I hope that you'll have fun finding new ways to refresh your cooking experience so that preparing meals brings joy both to you and to those you feed.

And, finally, Dear Reader, may your life be filled with all that is sacred and delicious!

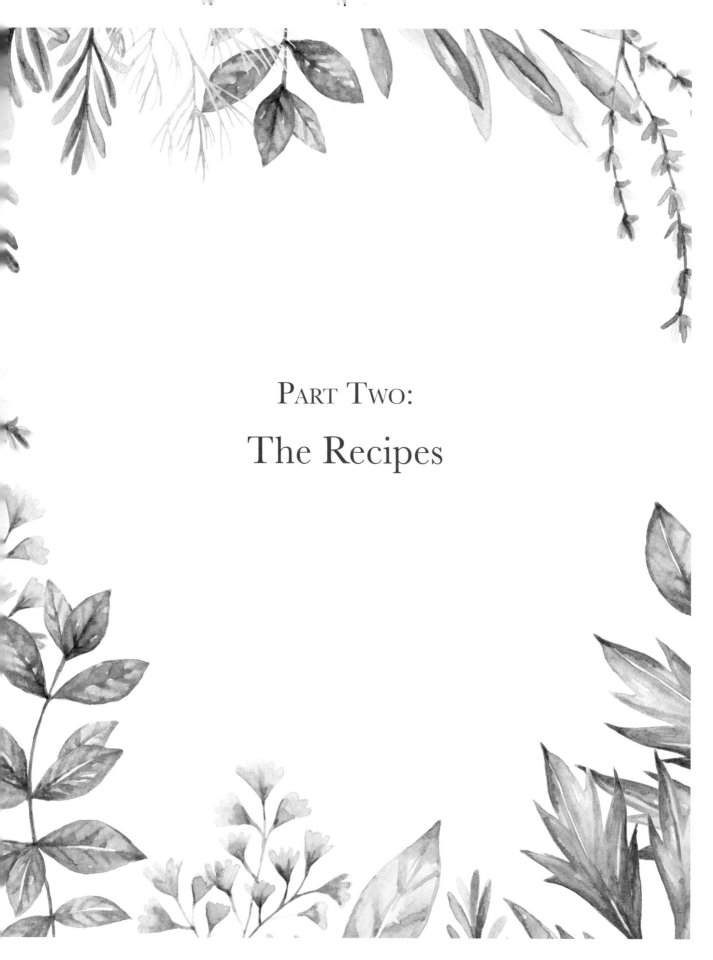

PART TWO:

The Recipes

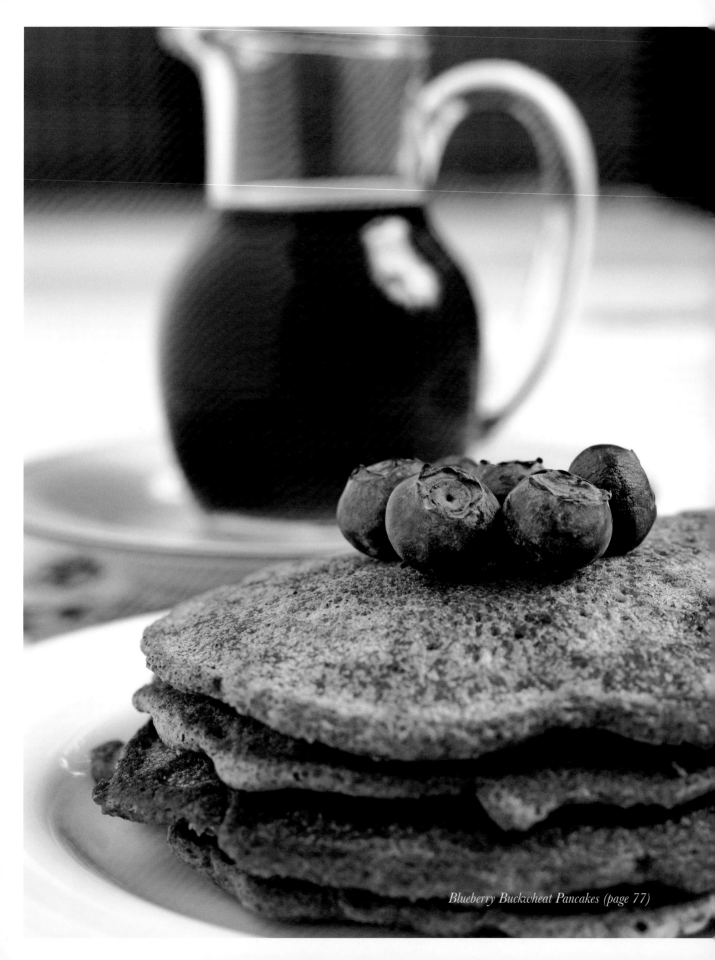

Blueberry Buckwheat Pancakes (page 77)

CHAPTER 5

Breakfast, Breads, and Beverages

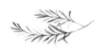

The wise see the Lord of love in all food.

⌐ Prashna Upanishad

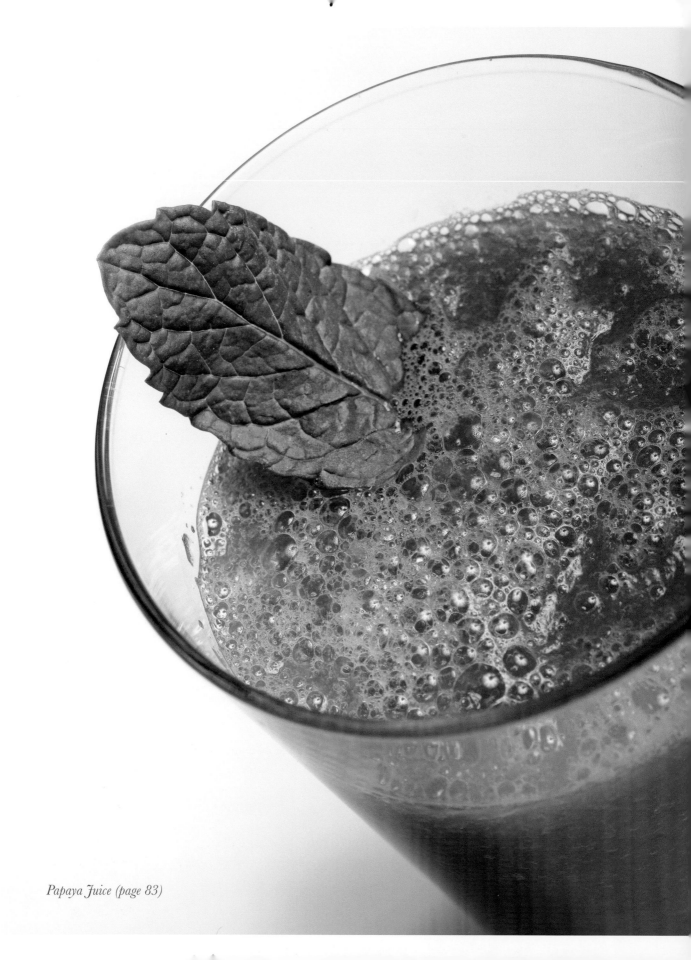

Papaya Juice (page 83)

Ayurvedic Breakfast Primer

Ayurveda generally recommends that you eat lightly in the morning and save your heaviest meal for midday, when your digestive power is strongest. Everyone's needs are not the same, of course, and Ayurveda has some tips for you based on your constitution.

- *Vata* loves warm, moist foods such as oatmeal with warming spices: cinnamon, cardamom, and fresh ginger in cold months.
- Nut butters and seeds are especially good for *vata*.
- Cooked quinoa with spices is good for *pitta* and especially *kapha*, because it is so light.
- Eggs are OK in moderation, as long as your digestion is strong. Egg whites are best for *pitta*.
- If you like a savory breakfast, all *doshas* benefit from mung soup, and *kitchari* is fine for *vata* and *pitta*.
- Smoothies are fine for all *doshas*, but only if they are room temperature!
- Dry cereals and granola are good for *pitta* and *kapha* and acceptable for *vata* on occasion, especially with a dollop or two of homemade yogurt.
- Commercial yogurt, eaten by the cup or two, is not recommended.
- Toasted bread is not recommended on a daily basis but can be eaten on occasion, especially with ghee or nut butter, to offset the dryness of toast.
- Pancakes are best saved for special occasion brunches. The sweet pancake recipes in *Sacred & Delicious* are provided as healthier versions of this favorite comfort food!

The Ayurvedic Perspective on Bread

One of the most standard additions to breakfast in the United States is toasted bread. However, the leavened bread we know so well in the Western world is not a part of Ayurvedic fare, which originated in India. There the norm is hand-rolled flatbreads called *chapati* or *roti,* which are similar to the flatbreads served for centuries throughout Africa, the Middle East, and Latin America. Utilitarian as well as filling, soft flatbreads are used to scoop up moist food and sauce.

Flatbreads offer a health advantage because they are made without yeast or baking powder. This is healthier because both yeast and baking powder release carbon dioxide when they interact with the liquid used to make a dough, and excess air is a quality that increases *vata*. The fermentation process of baking with yeast also increases *pitta*.

Regardless of a flatbread's health benefits, I have to tell you that they require a particular skill to make. With a little practice, though, it's easy! I've watched in fascination as my Indian friends roll out chapatis by hand, perfectly round, in just seconds. The cook forms thin circles of dough with a narrow rolling pin. She then folds each round and rolls it out again twice, refolding it to add air. The thin, flattened disc of dough is placed into a hot skillet. The heat combined with the air makes the chapati puff up momentarily, and when it's served immediately, this flatbread is as light as a feather. If you're game and want to try your hand at it, you'll find a gluten-free Indian-style chapati recipe in this section.

Because *Sacred & Delicious* takes a modern approach to Ayurveda, I do include three yeast bread recipes and corn bread made with baking powder to serve those readers who can't imagine life without bread from time to time.

Although Ayurvedic physicians have traditionally favored whole wheat for *vata* and *pitta* types, modern practitioners are aware of the many complications associated with the high-gluten wheat grown in the United States. When I first started moving away from gluten, I began by replacing wheat with spelt, an ancient grain with a lower gluten content. Happily, spelt tastes similar to wheat and can easily be used to replace wheat in most recipes. As I say in the chapter "Eating Well in the Modern World" (pages 43–44), anyone diagnosed as having a gluten sensitivity is wise to avoid it altogether—which ultimately was the choice I made. Although bread isn't required to complete a meal, it can be a lovely addition, and it's certainly helpful when you're traveling and want to take a sandwich on the road. So, I created a gluten-free loaf for my readers who miss baking bread and want a healthy gluten-free recipe.

Whether you approach eating bread from an Ayurvedic perspective or through the lens of contemporary nutrition, all breads are best eaten in moderation, say once or twice a week at most, and if you struggle with weight, you'll be served by saving bread for an occasional treat!

SPELT BREAD WITH FIGS AND WALNUTS

Preparation Time: 5½ hours (30 minutes active)
Makes 1 large loaf or 2 small loaves

In the early years of developing Sacred & Delicious—before I was diagnosed as gluten intolerant—I had a great time baking with spelt, which is a delicious wheat alternative with lower gluten content. Flash back to my senior year in college: I roomed with Ellen Brock, an incredibly bright woman who was as adept in the kitchen as she was in academia, and later medicine. It was Ellen who first taught me to bake bread, and I immediately welcomed that intoxicating scent of yeast rising in the oven. Talk about uuummm! Ellen created this recipe, and she offers the following commentary: "This is a dense bread with a fine crumb. It is vegan as it sits but is best slathered with butter or a nice goat cheese." To that I add, amen!

2 cups warmed water (100°F to 110°F)
3 teaspoons active dry yeast (1½ packages)
¼ cup coconut sugar, divided
2 tablespoons olive oil, plus 1 teaspoon
2 tablespoons walnut or almond oil
2 teaspoons Fine Ground Celtic Sea Salt
5½ cups whole spelt flour, plus 2 tablespoons for the
    surface if kneading by hand
¾ cup chopped toasted walnuts
1 cup chopped dried figs (optional)
1 to 2 tablespoons cornmeal (optional)

BAKER'S TIP: 1. For a savory loaf, mix 1½ teaspoons finely chopped fresh rosemary with the spelt flour in a food processor fitted with a steel blade, prior to assembling the recipe. Process until the rosemary is very fine. **2.** Instead of nuts and figs, try ½ cup kalamata olives, pitted and chopped.

AYURVEDIC NOTE

Because spelt is light, it may increase *vata*, as will yeast. The crispier the crust, the more *vata* will increase. The oils are balancing for *vata*. Ayurveda suggests that fruits be eaten separately from other foods; however, foods that are cooked together take on each other's qualities, making this recipe with figs fine for most people.

V Serve with a copious quantity of ghee, butter, olive oil, or nut butter to decrease dryness. Do not toast the walnuts prior to baking. Do not spray the loaf with water, which makes for a crispier crust and therefore increases *vata*.

P If using olives, reduce by half.

K Eat rarely. Serve toasted; avoid added ghee, butter, or oil.

1. Pour the yeast and 1 tablespoon of coconut sugar into a large mixing bowl. Stir in ½ cup water. Proof for 5 to 10 minutes until the yeast starts to bubble slightly (to ensure that the yeast is active).

2. Add to the yeast mixture the remaining water and coconut sugar plus the olive oil, walnut (or almond) oil, and salt.

3. Stir in 5½ cups spelt flour one cup at a time, until the dough reaches a texture that you can knead. Sticky dough is preferable, so add just enough flour to facilitate kneading.

4. Knead the dough for several minutes, unless making the dough in a food processor, in which case the dough will be ready once it forms a ball in the bowl of the processor. Place the dough ball in a large bowl greased with about a teaspoon of olive oil. Turn the dough to coat. Let the dough rise until it doubles in bulk, 1½ to 2 hours.

5. Chop the figs and walnuts. Punch the dough down and knead in figs and walnuts. Shape into two small loaves and place on a parchment-covered baking sheet dusted with cornmeal. Or shape into one large loaf. Make three diagonal slashes about ½ inch deep in each loaf. Let the dough rise until it doubles in bulk, 1½ to 2 hours. If using a loaf pan, transfer the dough to a greased 5x10-inch pan, and let the dough rise just to the top of the pan, about 45 minutes.

6. Preheat the oven to 400°F. Bake at 400°F for 10 minutes, then at 375°F for 35 to 40 minutes more. If you wish, spray water onto loaves with a spray bottle about 10 minutes before they are done to develop a crispier crust. When the bread is finished, cool the loaf on a rack for 15 to 30 minutes before slicing.

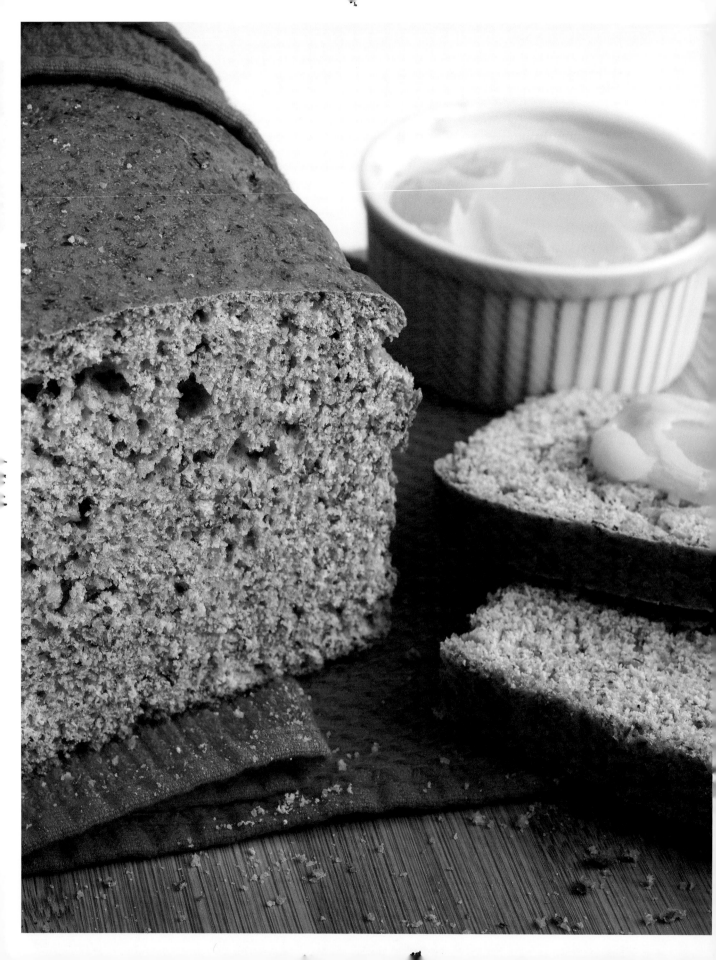

OUR DAILY BREAD (G)

Preparation Time: About 5 hours (20 minutes active)
Makes 1 loaf

This bread uses less whole grain for easier slicing when making sandwiches.

3 teaspoons (1½ packages) active dry yeast
¼ cup coconut sugar, divided
2 cups warmed water (100°F to 110°F), divided
2 teaspoons Fine Ground Celtic Sea Salt
½ cup rolled oats
½ cup oat bran
3 cups whole spelt flour
1 cup unbleached spelt flour
½ cup flaxseed meal
2 tablespoons olive oil, plus 1 teaspoon
2 tablespoons walnut or almond oil

BAKER'S TIP: These directions are based on making the dough in a food processor. The advantages of using the processor are speed and quality; you won't be tempted to add too much flour to the mixture because of dough sticking to your hands. Sticky dough makes perfect bread; too much flour can lead to a dry loaf. If you prefer kneading by hand, follow steps on page 65.

AYURVEDIC NOTE
Spelt and flaxseeds may increase *vata* for some people. Yeast also increases *vata*, as will a crispy crust. The oils are balancing for *vata*.

(V) Slather each slice with ghee, butter, olive oil, or nut butter to minimize dryness.

(K) Eat rarely. Serve toasted; avoid added ghee, butter, or oil.

1. Pour the yeast and 1 tablespoon of coconut sugar into a large measuring cup. Stir in ½ cup water. Proof for 5 to 10 minutes until the yeast starts to bubble slightly (to ensure that the yeast is active).

2. While waiting on the yeast to proof, measure and place the rest of the dry ingredients in the bowl of the food processor. Pulse a few times to mix. Add olive oil and walnut (or almond) oil and the rest of the sugar. Pulse a few times. When the yeast mixture is ready, pour it into the food processor with the processor on; then slowly add the remaining 1½ cups water. Process for about 1 minute until the dough forms a ball in the processor.

3. Place the ball in a large bowl greased with 1 teaspoon olive oil. Turn the dough to coat. Let it rise until doubled in bulk, about 1½ hours. Grease a large loaf pan (5 x 10 inches) with olive oil. Punch the dough down and knead briefly. Shape into one large loaf and place in the pan. Make three diagonal slashes about ½ inch deep in the loaf. Let rise until doubled in bulk, 1 to 1½ hours.

4. Preheat oven to 400°F. Bake at 400°F for 10 minutes, then at 375°F for 35 to 40 minutes more—less if you're using 2 pans. When the bread is finished, cool it on a rack for at least 30 minutes before slicing.

Jewish Blessing

This is a traditional blessing before eating bread.

בָּרוּךְ אַתָּה יְיָ, אֱלֹהֵינוּ מֶלֶךְ הָעוֹלָם, הַמּוֹצִיא לֶחֶם מִן הָאָרֶץ.

Baruch atah Adonai, Eloheinu melech ha'olam,
hamotzi lechem min ha'aretz.

Our praise to You, Adonai our God, sovereign of the universe, who brings forth bread from the earth.

GLUTEN-FREE WHOLE GRAIN BREAD

Preparation Time: About 3 hours (30 minutes active)
Makes 1 loaf

Yes! It is possible to bake a delicious gluten-free loaf of bread! This loaf strives to offer more protein and less carbs per loaf than most commercially available brands, and it holds up well as sandwich bread. This bread may not always rise to a perfect dome, but it is perfectly delicious!

1 cup millet flour

1 cup garbanzo (chickpea) flour

1 cup teff flour

1 cup oat flour

¾ cup ground flaxseeds

3 tablespoons psyllium husks (whole flakes)

1½ teaspoons Fine Ground Celtic Sea Salt

1 tablespoon baking powder

2¼ teaspoons rapid-rise yeast

2 tablespoons coconut sugar, divided

1¼ cups warm water (100°F to 110°F)

3 large eggs, room temperature

2 tablespoons olive oil

2 tablespoons walnut oil

1 cup coconut cream or whole coconut milk

BAKER'S TIP: If you don't want to invest in walnut oil, use more olive oil. If you prefer sweet bread, add 1 more tablespoon sugar.

AYURVEDIC NOTE

Millet flour is fine for all *doshas,* when eaten in moderation. Garbanzo and teff flours will increase *vata,* but this effect is somewhat balanced by the oat flour, eggs, oils, psyllium, flaxseeds, and coconut cream. Yeast also increases *vata,* and the crispier the crust, the more *vata* will increase. For these reasons, it's best for anyone with *vata* problems to eat yeasted breads only occasionally. The oils, coconut cream or milk, sugar, and oat flour will increase *kapha.*

V Eat occasionally. Serve with generous amounts of ghee, butter, oil, or nut butter to minimize dryness.

K Eat occasionally. Serve toasted and with no butter or oil.

1. Grease a large loaf pan (5 x 10 inches) with olive oil. Create a double-layer aluminum foil collar for the loaf pan by wrapping foil around the outside of the pan, about 1 inch higher than the pan height, and stapling the layers together.

2. Combine the flours in a medium-sized mixing bowl with flaxseeds, psyllium husk, salt, and baking powder. Stir with a whisk and set aside. Preheat the oven to 200°F. Then turn the oven off immediately.

3. Pour the yeast and 1 tablespoon of coconut sugar into a second mixing bowl or a 4-cup spouted measuring cup. Stir in ½ cup of warm water. Proof for 5 minutes or so until the yeast starts to bubble slightly, which ensures the yeast is active. Once it is proofed, stir in the remainder of the water and coconut sugar.

4. Whisk the eggs and add them to the yeast-water mixture, followed by the oil and coconut cream. Place the liquid in a stand mixer fitted with a paddle and set at a low speed or use a large food processor bowl fitted with a dough paddle and turned to the dough setting. Slowly add the flour mixture one cup at a time until you're able to combine all of it with the wet ingredients. Increase the speed to medium (in a food processor switch from pulse mode to "on") and mix the dough until it becomes sticky, another 4 to 5 minutes.

5. Using a spatula, transfer the dough to the prepared pan and gently press the edges of the dough around the entire pan. Move the pan to the warm oven for 10 minutes; then remove the pan from the oven and let the dough continue to rise until the loaf reaches the rim of the pan, another 20 to 30 minutes, depending on your kitchen's warmth.

6. Preheat your oven to 350°F. Let the loaf rise until doubled in bulk. Transfer the pan to the oven and bake for 45 to 50 minutes. When the bread is done, the top will be well browned, and the loaf will sound hollow when tapped. Remove the bread from the oven and let it cool in the pan on a rack for another 10 minutes. You can remove the loaf from the pan then, but let it finish cooling on the rack about 2 hours before slicing.

7. After 10 minutes, remove the bread from the oven and let it cool in the pan on a rack for another 10 minutes. You can remove the loaf from the pan then, but let it finish cooling on the rack about 2 hours before slicing.

Baking Gluten-Free Bread

Truth be told, I renounced bread in my midfifties, when I gained forty pounds because of a thyroid condition. I did lose most of that extra weight, but it was a slow process, and cutting back on unnecessary carbs was one key to reaching my goal.

Even so, as I was wrapping up *Sacred & Delicious*, I felt a sense of urgency about developing a gluten-free bread that meets my high standards for healthy and delicious food! Most gluten-free breads on the market and many online recipes are filled with highly refined starches—white rice flour, potato starch, and tapioca flour—and others have dairy. I wanted to avoid both. I'm excited to say that I believe I succeeded!

It helps to know that baking gluten-free bread is even more specialized than, say, cooking a gluten-free cake. If you've been baking breads for years, as I had, you'll have to push some of your most prized skills and knowledge aside. Here are the key differences:

- You won't be kneading a gluten-free dough. Say a sad farewell to that quaint pleasure. You'll combine the ingredients by using a stand mixer fitted with a dough paddle, or you can combine it by hand with a rubber spatula. You can also use a bread machine, if you own one, though the loaf may not turn out as pleasing to your perfectionist eye.

- You also won't be using traditional yeast. Rapid-rise yeast is required. Slow is not better with gluten-free breads. You can read about the science of gluten-free cooking in one of the excellent *The How Can It Be Gluten-Free Cookbooks* by America's Test Kitchen.

- America's Test Kitchen recommends using psyllium husk as a binder. Excellent idea! Psyllium husk is used in Ayurvedic medicine as a bulking agent to relieve constipation or diarrhea. Using psyllium in a bread recipe has health benefits as well as structural benefits when baking with gluten-free flours.

- It's tough, though perhaps not impossible, to make a gluten-free bread without eggs. My recipe includes eggs.

- Vegans may want to explore a new approach to egg replacers called aquafaba. Check out aquafaba. com or *Aquafaba*, the cookbook, by Zsu Dever.

CHAPATIS

Preparation Time: 1½ hours (30 minutes active)
Makes 8 small chapatis

A chapati is an Indian flatbread, which is typically made with wheat flour. This gluten-free recipe works best with a bit of xanthan gum, which gives gluten-free flours more stretch than they naturally have and makes it easier to roll the dough. I have had gluten-free, xanthan-free chapatis in India, made by Rosy in a village in Maharashtra state. Like many Indian women, Rosy is a wizard with a rolling pin! If you're similarly skilled, you may want to try the recipe without xanthan gum.

Special thanks to Usha Lad for her guidance on the chapati in her cookbook, Ayurvedic Cooking for Self-Healing, *which informed this recipe.*

1 cup chickpea flour
1 cup sweet sorghum flour, plus ½ cup more for
   rolling and dipping
¾ teaspoon xanthan gum
½ teaspoon Fine Ground Celtic Sea Salt
¼ cup plus 2 tablespoons melted ghee, sunflower oil,
   or olive oil for the dough and 2 tablespoons for brushing
⅔ cups plus up to 3 tablespoons more warmed water

COOK'S TIP: 1. The dough can also be made in a food processor. **2.** A cast-iron or nonstick ceramic pan is ideal for this recipe. **3.** It is also helpful to have a small rolling pin made for tortillas and small flatbreads. **4.** Well-chilled dough is the key to a successful chapati! **5.** You may enjoy these variations: Add 1 teaspoon of cumin seeds to the flour when preparing the dough. Or try adding favorite herbs, such as thyme or rosemary.

AYURVEDIC NOTE

Chickpea flour is somewhat aggravating to *vata*, but I added it to the recipe for some protein to balance the rice flour, which is fine for *vata*. It is possible to make chapatis using just rice flour. All breads and ghee or oil will increase *kapha*.

(K) Add ½ teaspoon of black pepper or a pinch of cayenne to the flour mixture.

1. Whisk together the flours with xanthan gum and salt in a medium mixing bowl. Stir in the ghee or oil and mix well with your hands or a rubber spatula. Add water a little at a time starting with ⅔ cup until it is mixed well. Add more water until the dough is moist and smooth. Cover the bowl and refrigerate the dough for 30 minutes to an hour. After the dough is chilled, it will bounce back if you press a finger in it.

2. When you're ready to make the chapatis, heat a nonstick pan on medium heat. Spread a few tablespoons of sorghum flour onto the surface where you'll do the rolling—a counter or large cutting board. Take a small handful of dough (about 2 tablespoons), roll it into a ball in your hands, and then place it on the floured surface. Next, flatten the ball with your hand and, using a rolling pin, roll it into a disc, 5 or 6 inches in diameter. When rolling a chapati, always roll outward from the dough's center.

3. Brush one side with a little ghee or oil, avoiding the edges. Dip the oiled side into flour. Fold the dough in half, covering the oiled side, and fold it in half again. Pinch the edges together and return the folded dough to the floured surface. Lightly flour the top (to keep the rolling pin from sticking) and again roll the chapati into the same size disc as before. Between rolls, gently lift the disc of dough and turn it. This turning is what helps to produce the perfect (or almost perfect) round shape. When you touch the dough, if it feels sticky, add a little more rice flour, both to the counter and to the top of the chapati. The size you're going for is 5 to 6 inches in diameter, as thin as you can make it without the disc tearing. It takes supreme skill to make a chapati thinner than ⅛ inch.

4. Add some ghee or oil to the pan, and cook 1 chapati at a time. In a minute or 2, the chapati will bubble up and the bottom will begin to show brown spots. Dab with ghee or oil, flip it over, and cook the second side until it is lightly brown on the bottom. Place the cooked chapatis on a paper towel to absorb any excess oil. Cover to keep warm until ready to serve. As you cook additional chapatis and the pan is getting hotter, reduce the heat just a little so the oil isn't smoking and the chapatis don't burn.

CORN BREAD

Preparation Time: 45 minutes (15 minutes active)
Makes 9 large muffins or squares

If you like having bread with a meal, a quick and easy option is corn bread. This recipe uses Bob's Red Mill Gluten Free Cornmeal, a particularly fine meal that requires more fat and liquid than some grinds of cornmeal.

9 tablespoons melted ghee, butter, or coconut oil, plus 1 teaspoon for baking dish
3 cups Bob's Red Mill Gluten Free Cornmeal
1 tablespoon baking powder
1½ teaspoons Fine Ground Celtic Sea Salt
1 to 2 tablespoons coconut sugar, to taste (optional)
1 tablespoon psyllium husk
2½ cups unsweetened almond milk

COOK'S TIP: 1. Bulk corn meal is not certifiably gluten-free, as it is often ground in facilities that process wheat flour. **2.** If you're making this as the base for Holiday Dressing (page 164), skip the sugar. **3.** If you wish, use 2 eggs, omit psyllium husk, and use 2¼ cups of almond milk.

AYURVEDIC NOTE
Cornmeal is an excellent grain for *kapha* and is ok for *vata* and *pitta*, on occasion.

V Use generous amounts of ghee, butter, or oil when serving to minimize dryness.

K Omit or reduce coconut sugar by half. Eat in moderation.

1. Preheat the oven to 375°F and lightly grease a 9 x 9 baking dish or muffin tin.

2. Melt fat in a saucepan. Let cool for a few minutes.

3. Combine dry ingredients in a mixing bowl.

4. Add almond milk and the cooled ghee to the dry ingredients, and stir well with a spatula.

5. Pour the batter into a muffin tin or 9 x 9 baking dish. Bake 30 minutes until firm in the middle and golden brown on top. Serve with ghee or olive oil.

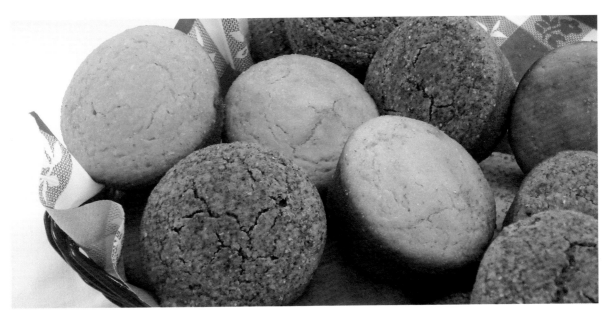

GHEE (Clarified Butter)

Preparation Time: Less than 1 hour
Makes two 13-ounce jars or one 1-quart jar

Ghee is a superlative spread on most breads, an ingredient in many of the Sacred & Delicious recipes, and an essential component of the Ayurvedic healing model. You can buy organic ghee in upscale grocery stores and online, but it is less expensive to make your own, if you have the time.

2 pounds unsalted organic butter

COOK'S TIP: Use a pure, organic, unsalted butter. Be sure to check the label since some butters contain lactic acid, which is not helpful

1. Place butter in a heavy medium-sized saucepan (preferably spouted) on medium-low heat, uncovered, until the butter melts. Reduce the heat to low and continue to cook uncovered. Let the butter come slowly to a boil, 20 to 30 minutes (on my slow electric stove). Periodically check the pot to make sure it is not cooking to a boil too quickly, in which case it will start to burn.

2. As foam begins to form on the top of the pan, reduce the heat to low. Skim the foam off with a clean, dry spoon. (Liquids and even a speck of food will spoil the ghee.) The milk solids or curds will fall to the bottom of the pan. Once the ghee comes to a boil the curds will turn from white to tan and the ghee will start to smell like popcorn—your signal that the ghee is ready. Remove the pan from heat immediately so it does not burn. Let the ghee cool for at least 30 minutes to an hour.

3. Cut a piece of cheesecloth to fit inside an 8-inch metal strainer, and place the strainer over a glass jar. When the ghee has cooled down, carefully pour the liquid through the strainer, making sure that none of the curds at the bottom of the pot fall into the jar, as they will cause the ghee to spoil. Let the ghee continue to cool completely before putting a top on the jar. If the ghee is not tainted with food or liquid, it will last six to eight months unrefrigerated.

The Many Essential Benefits of Ghee

Ghee (clarified butter) is the preeminent ingredient of Ayurvedic cooking, extolled and glorified by Ayurvedic texts and practitioners in both ancient and modern times. Ghee is often used in preparations of Ayurvedic medicine and has been an element of spiritual rituals in India for millennia.

Ghee is prepared by slowly heating butter and allowing the milk solids (casein, whey, and lactose) to settle to the bottom of the pot or be skimmed off the top. What remains is luscious, healthy fat. Once butter has been clarified in this way, all the milk solids are removed, making it much easier to digest.

The *Bhavaprakasha*, an Ayurvedic text from the sixteenth century, speaks about the benefits of ghee in these terms:

Ghee is sweet in taste and cooling in energy, rejuvenating, good for the eyes and vision, enkindles digestion, bestows luster and beauty, enhances memory and stamina, increases the intellect, promotes longevity, is an aphrodisiac, and protects the body from various diseases.

Since ancient times Ayurvedic doctors have recognized ghee as an aid to digestion. As noted, ghee is said to kindle *agni*, the digestive enzymes, improving the absorption and assimilation of food. Ghee also sustains *ojas*, the subtle essence gleaned from pure foods that sustains the body and increases vigor, immunity, and luster.

Among its many benefits, ghee operates as a vehicle to transport the medicinal qualities of foods, spices, and medicinal herbs, delivering their essential nourishment where needed in the body. Dr. Vasant Lad describes this process, saying that ghee "carries the medicinal properties of herbs to bodily tissues," which is how we gain the most benefit from cooking with ghee and spices.

Because ghee pacifies *vata* and *pitta*, it is grounding, calming to the nervous system, and cooling to the temper. For *kapha* types too much of any fat is problematic, but everyone needs some good fat for physical energy and brain function. Ayurvedic practitioners prescribe ghee for *kapha* in moderation.

Ghee is a highly stable fat and can sustain high temperatures without burning, a big plus when you compare it with regular butter. Also, unless it has been tainted by another food or by water, ghee almost never goes rancid.

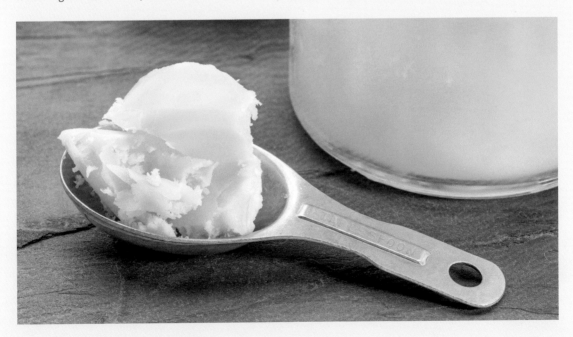

SUNFLOWER SEED BUTTER

Preparation Time: About 5 minutes

Makes enough for one 13-ounce jar

Thanks to my husband, Tom, who created this easy recipe. It can be used as a spread, but we snack on it with just a spoon.

½ cup sunflower seeds

¼ to ⅓ cup vanilla protein powder

1 teaspoon ground cardamom

¼ vanilla bean or ½ teaspoon vanilla extract

½ cup water

2 pinches KAL Stevia or 1 to 2 tablespoons maple syrup,
  to taste

COOK'S TIP: The protein powder I use in this spread is VegaLite/Vanilla from Thorne Research, which has a good reputation for product purity and is available online.

AYURVEDIC NOTE

Sunflower seeds are good for all *doshas*, in moderation. Although oily, they are lighter than nuts and are a better protein source for *kapha* than nuts. Because they are slightly cooling, they are better for *pitta* than nuts. The warmth of cardamom helps balance the spread for *vata* and *kapha*.

 Reduce cardamom to ½ teaspoon.

1. Place all ingredients in the dry blender pitcher. Blend for 30 seconds to 1 minute.

2. Transfer to a glass jar. Keeps in the cupboard up to two weeks.

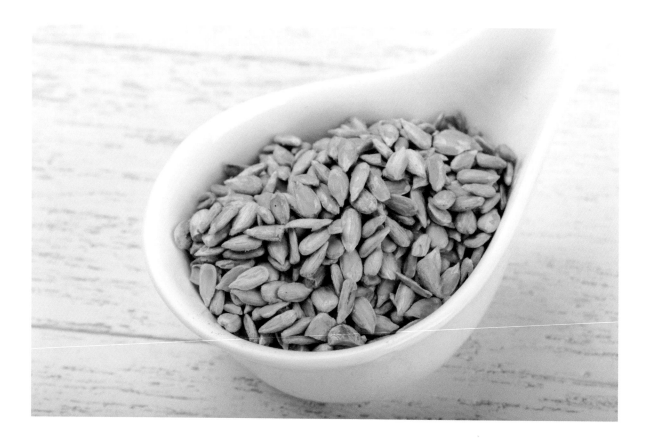

WARM QUINOA WITH FRESH ALMOND MILK

Preparation Time: About 25 minutes
Serves 4

Quinoa is a complete protein, and if you can digest it well, it's an excellent choice for breakfast.

½ cup dried quinoa

2 cups water

2 teaspoons ghee or coconut oil

¼ teaspoon Fine Ground Celtic Sea Salt

½ teaspoon ground cardamom

1 teaspoon ground cinnamon

½ teaspoon freshly grated ginger

1 teaspoon coconut sugar or 2 pinches of KAL Pure Stevia

TIME-SAVER: You can make the quinoa the night before and reheat it in the morning for two to three minutes with 1 cup almond milk.

AYURVEDIC NOTE

Quinoa is good for *pitta* and *kapha* but, because it is dry and light, can be hard to digest for *vata* types. This is why the recipe calls for more water than is customary in many recipes. The ghee and spices support *vata*, as will added ginger. If you have *vata* problems, you may want to eat quinoa no more than once a week.

V Add 1 teaspoon freshly grated ginger.

K Omit ghee. Use stevia instead of sugar. Reduce the water to 1 cup. Serve with almond milk rather than coconut milk.

1. Melt the ghee or coconut oil in a 1- or 2-quart saucepan on medium heat.

2. Rinse the quinoa in a bowl with water and strain. Add the quinoa with the rest of the ingredients to the melted ghee, and bring to a boil. Reduce the heat to medium-low, cover the pan, and cook until all the liquid is absorbed, 15 to 20 minutes.

3. Serve with Fresh Almond Milk (page 81) or unsweetened coconut milk and slivered almonds, walnuts, or pecans. Add more sweetener to taste.

VEGETABLE OMELET

Preparation Time: 10 minutes
Serves 1

I offer this recipe to illuminate the value of cumin and coriander as digestive aids, especially with eggs. This omelet is as flexible as your taste buds. I like using some chopped red bell pepper and asparagus, or a handful of fresh spinach. If you don't want to bother with perfecting an omelet, you can simply scramble your eggs with the precooked veggies.

½ to ¾ cup favorite chopped vegetables
1 tablespoon ghee or olive oil
1 large egg
2 egg whites
1 pinch Fine Ground Celtic Sea Salt
⅛ teaspoon ground cumin
⅛ teaspoon ground coriander
A few sprigs of cilantro or a small handful of basil, chopped

COOK'S TIP: You'll need only a teaspoon of fat if you use a ceramic or other nonstick pan. You can also use other favorite spices such as fresh dill or rosemary.

AYURVEDIC NOTE

Egg whites are considered beneficial for all *doshas*. Eggs with yolks can aggravate *pitta* and *kapha*. All *doshas* are supported by the cumin, coriander, and cilantro.

P Omit yolks and use a total of 3 egg whites.

1. Preheat an omelet pan or a small to medium sauté pan on medium-high heat. Add the ghee or olive oil to the pan, and sauté the chopped vegetables, covering the pan—3 to 5 minutes, depending on the thickness of the veggies. Then remove the vegetables from the pan and set aside.

2. While the vegetables are cooking, whisk the egg and egg whites together. Whisk in the salt and ground spices, and add the chopped cilantro or basil.

3. Pour the eggs into the pan. Cook undisturbed for about a minute. Reduce heat to medium. Using a spatula, push the edges of the eggs away from the side of the pan, and tip the pan so the uncooked eggs move toward the center. Cook for another 2 to 3 minutes, until the omelet is completely set and the eggs are only a little moist. Draw an imaginary line down the center of the eggs, and spread the cooked vegetables over the eggs on just one side of that line. Then use a large spatula to fold the half without vegetables over the half with. Let the omelet cook another minute and serve.

BLUEBERRY BUCKWHEAT PANCAKES

Preparation Time: About 30 minutes active, plus griddle time
Makes 16 pancakes using ¼ cup batter

¼ cup walnut oil, melted coconut oil, melted ghee, or
   melted butter
1 cup buckwheat flour
1 cup oat flour
¾ teaspoon Fine Ground Celtic Sea Salt
1 tablespoon coconut sugar
2 teaspoons baking powder
1 teaspoon ground cardamom
2 large eggs
2 teaspoons vanilla extract
1½ cups plus 2 tablespoons plain unsweetened
   almond milk
6 ounces fresh blueberries (1 generous cup)

COOK'S TIP: If you like thick pancakes, decrease the almond milk
to 1¼ cups.

AYURVEDIC NOTE
These dry and light flours balance each other with liquid and fat, making these pancakes good for *vata* and *pitta*, when eaten in moderation. *Kapha* types should save pancakes for special occasions.

K Serve with room-temperature honey instead of maple syrup.

P Omit yolks and use a total of 3 egg whites.

1. If using the ghee, butter, or coconut oil, melt it now in a small saucepan. Remove from heat to let cool.

2. Combine all the dry ingredients in a mixing bowl, and gently stir with a whisk.

3. In separate bowls, separate the eggs. Whisk the egg yolks and combine with vanilla and oil. If using cooled ghee, butter, or coconut oil, remeasure before adding. Stir in 1½ cups almond milk. Combine the liquid mixture with the dry ingredients, and mix well with a spatula.

4. Beat the egg whites with a handheld electric beater or whisk until foamy and light but not stiff or dry (1 to 2 minutes). Fold the whites into the batter, making sure it's thoroughly mixed. Let the batter rest for 15 to 30 minutes.

(RECIPE PHOTO ON PAGE 60)

5. Heat a nonstick griddle or cast-iron pan on medium heat. When the pan is hot, grease it with 1 teaspoon of ghee, and pour the batter in quarter-cup or larger rounds. Sprinkle each pancake with 1 tablespoon of blueberries. Let the pancakes cook for 5 minutes on the first side, until bubbles start to form and the pancake is well browned on the bottom; then flip and brown on the second side for 5 minutes, until the pancakes are cooked through. As the pan gets hotter, the pancakes will cook in about 3 minutes on each side. Serve immediately with pure warmed maple syrup, or keep in a warm oven until everyone can be served.

6. Before you cook each batch, stir a tablespoon of almond milk into the batter to bring it back to the right consistency.

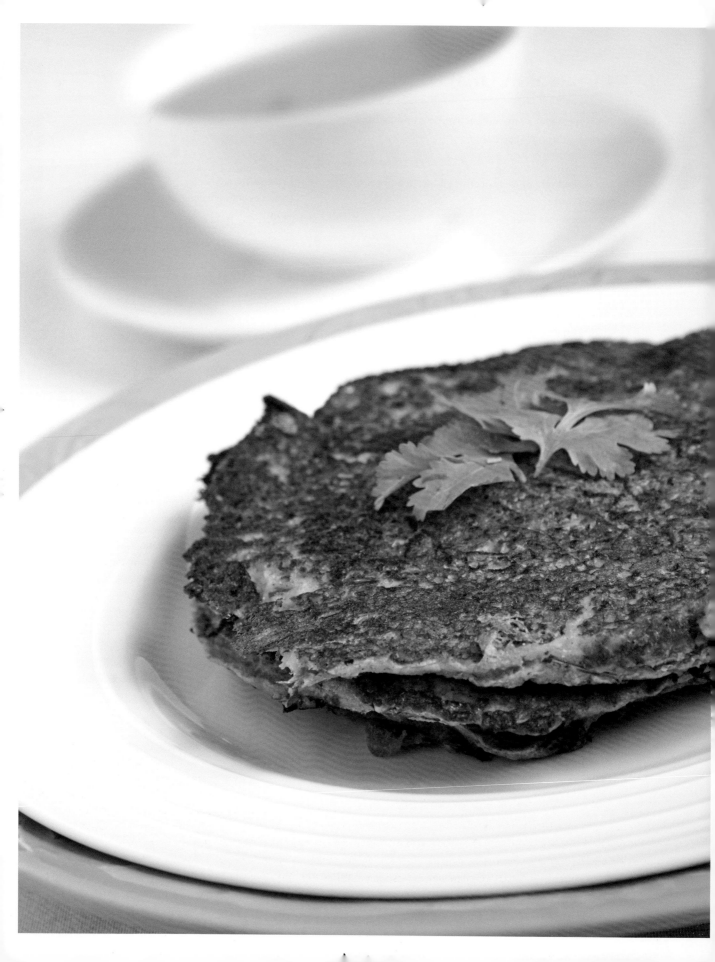

SAVORY CHICKPEA PANCAKES WITH CURRY LEAF CHUTNEY

Preparation Time: About 20 minutes, plus griddle time

Makes 8 small pancakes

When my husband and I first hosted the Ayurvedic vaidya Smita Naram in our home, she taught me to make a classic—yet simple and intensely delicious!—Ayurvedic dish: Savory Chickpea Pancakes, *which she served with Curry Leaf Chutney. Enjoy these easy-to-make pancakes as a meal or a delicious protein side dish. You'll find online videos that demonstrate the* dosa-*style pouring technique. And the chutney, I have found, can accompany a variety of dishes.*

FOR THE BATTER:

1 small zucchini

1 cup chickpea (garbanzo bean) flour

1 teaspoon ground cumin

1 teaspoon ground coriander

¼ to ½ teaspoon garam masala

¼ teaspoon ground turmeric

½ teaspoon Fine Ground Himalayan or Celtic Sea Salt

1¼ cups water

1 to 2 teaspoons freshly grated ginger

1 cup tightly packed chopped cilantro

2 teaspoons fresh lime juice

Ghee, sunflower, or coconut oil for cooking

FOR THE CHUTNEY:

8 to 10 fresh curry leaves

¼ cup raw almonds

1½- to 2-inch piece of ginger, peeled

½ to 1 cup water, according to preference

2 cups tightly packed fresh cilantro, washed

¼ teaspoon Fine Ground Celtic Sea Salt

2 teaspoons fresh lime juice, or more, to taste

AYURVEDIC NOTE

Chickpea flour is an excellent protein source for *pitta* and *kapha*, and it can be eaten in moderation by *vata* types. The spices are balancing for all *doshas*, except for the garam masala. The chutney's curry leaves and ginger are also warming, making this dish acceptable for *vata* and perfect for *kapha*, and the cilantro helps balance *pitta*.

P Omit or reduce garam masala if you're sensitive to cayenne pepper. In its place, use ¼ teaspoon each of ground cardamom and cinnamon. Use the chutney in moderation.

COOK'S TIP: This mild chutney can also be used on grilled or steamed vegetables, on a veggie burger (page 147), over Quick Tofu (page 169), or drizzled over a bean soup (page 118).

1. **Prepare the batter:** Grate the zucchini and set aside.

2. Combine the chickpea flour with the ground spices and salt in a medium-sized mixing bowl, and stir with a whisk to combine well. Add the water and whisk. Add the grated zucchini, ginger, and lime and whisk again. Wash the cilantro well before chopping, and add it to the mixture. Let the batter rest while you make the chutney. Preheat a griddle or large nonstick pan (ceramic or cast iron) on medium heat.

3. **Prepare the chutney:** Put all the ingredients in a Vitamix and process. (If you have a regular blender, you may need to grate the ginger before blending.)

4. **Make the pancakes:** Grease the pan with 1 teaspoon of ghee or sunflower oil. When the pan is hot (a drop of water will sizzle), pour 1 pancake (¼ cup or less) at a time, *dosa* style. It's best to use a round serving spoon to pour the batter; then use the flat side of the spoon to spread and smooth the batter by making small clockwise circles from the center of the pancake outward until it is thin and rounded. Cook 4 to 5 minutes on the first side; then flip and brown the other side. If the pan has become dry, you could pour a little melted ghee on it between picking up the pancake and turning it over. Cook another 4 to 5 minutes on the second side or until the batter is cooked through. As the pan gets hotter, the pancakes will cook in about 3 minutes on each side. Serve with Curry Leaf Chutney or another favorite savory sauce.

SWEET POTATO PANCAKES

Preparation Time: About 1½ hours, plus griddle time
Makes 6 large pancakes or 8 poured with a ¼ cup

This is another recipe shared with Sacred & Delicious by my kitchen mentor and longtime friend, Ellen Brock. Like me, Ellen became gluten-free late in life. She developed a pancake recipe that I adapted just a tad so I could rekindle my love affair with pancakes on a guilt-free basis! As Ellen said, "They are not for the faint of heart or dieters, but they are delicious."

1 small sweet potato, peeled, wrapped in foil and roasted (about ⅔ to ¾ cups mashed)
2 tablespoons ghee, butter, or coconut oil
⅔ cup oat flour
1 tablespoon coconut sugar or maple crystals
2½ teaspoons baking powder
¾ teaspoon Fine Ground Celtic Sea Salt
1 teaspoon cinnamon
2 eggs, separated, plus 1 egg white
1 tablespoon walnut or sunflower oil
1½ teaspoons vanilla
¼ cup plus 2 tablespoons almond or coconut milk

AYURVEDIC NOTE

Sweet potatoes are extremely grounding for *vata*, as are the eggs and oat flour. Egg yolks increase *pitta* and *kapha*. Sweet potatoes are also great for *pitta* but will increase *kapha*. The nuts and extra ghee in which they are cooked will also increase *kapha* and *pitta*, which will be served by saving these pancakes for a special occasion only!

(P) Omit yolks and use a total of 3 egg whites.

(K) Serve with room-temperature honey instead of maple syrup.

1. When the sweet potato has finished roasting (about 1 hour at 450°F), unwrap it and mash it in a bowl with the ghee, butter, or coconut oil. Stir until the fat is melted. Let it cool.

2. Whisk together the flour, sugar, baking powder, salt, and cinnamon and set aside.

3. Separate the eggs. Whisk the egg yolks and combine them with the sweet potato mixture. Add the walnut oil, vanilla, and milk to the sweet potato mixture, and whisk to combine well. Now add the potato mixture to the flour mixture, and mix well with a rubber spatula.

4. Beat the egg whites with a handheld electric mixer or with a whisk until foamy and light but not stiff or dry (1 to 2 minutes by hand). Fold the egg whites into the batter. Let the batter, which will be thick, rest for 15 to 30 minutes.

5. Heat a cast-iron skillet or a nonstick griddle on medium heat. When the pan is hot, grease the pan with 1 teaspoon of ghee, and pour the batter in ¼-cup rounds. Let the pancakes cook for 4 to 5 minutes on the first side, until bubbles start to form and the pancakes are well browned on the bottom; then flip and brown on the second side for 5 minutes. The finished pancakes will still be moist inside because of the potato. Serve immediately with pure warmed maple syrup, or keep in a warm oven until everyone can be served.

6. As you pour each batch, add 1 or 2 more tablespoons of almond milk to bring the batter to the right consistency. As the pan gets hotter, the pancakes should cook in 3 to 4 minutes per side.

FRESH ALMOND MILK

Preparation Time: About 5 minutes
Serves 4

I'll admit I was skeptical when my husband bought a Vitamix blender to add to our already well-equipped kitchen. Now, I concede it is a grand addition to the purist's home. The Vitamix is what allows me to make almond milk, and there is nothing quite like fresh almond milk. Unlike boxed milk, which has thickeners and preservatives, fresh almond milk tastes utterly pure and delicious. (With a little maple syrup, it doubles as dessert!)

1½ cups almonds
6 cups water
1 to 2 tablespoons pure maple syrup (optional)

COOK'S TIP: 1. A Vitamix allows you to use whole almonds and discard the skins when you squeeze the liquid through a nut-milk bag, which you can find in health food stores and online. **2.** If you do not own a professional-grade mixer, such as a Vitamix, soak the almonds in water over night. In the morning, pull off the skins and discard them. Or buy blanched almonds. Then follow the directions below.

AYURVEDIC NOTE
Fresh almond milk is considered *sattvic,* or pure, and it is a modest source of protein. Almonds are the easiest of all nuts to digest. Fresh almond milk without maple syrup is fine for all *doshas* on a daily basis. Maple syrup will increase *kapha.*

 Omit the maple syrup.

1. Combine all ingredients in the blender. Start on low speed and increase the variable speed quickly to 10 and then to high. Mix on high for 1 or 2 minutes.

2. Ready a pitcher by lining it with a mesh nut-milk bag. Pour liquid into the bag to strain it. Holding the top of the bag to keep it closed, squeeze the bag until you extract all the liquid.

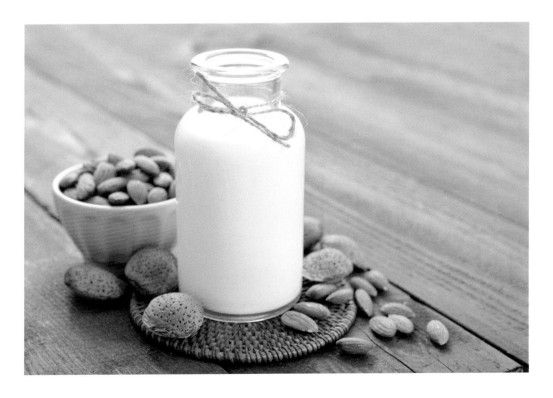

DATE ENERGY DRINK

Preparation Time: Overnight (5 minutes active)
Serves 1

This recipe was inspired by a drink I tasted in India at the Swad Shakti Café in the Ayushakti Ayurved Centre in Malad, India. Dates and figs are an excellent source of iron. Though high in natural sugar, dates are also a modest protein source for vegetarians.

2 Medjool dates, pitted and soaked
1 dried fig, soaked
1½ cups unsweetened almond milk (page 81)

COOK'S TIP: This recipe assumes that you are using dried fruit. However, if you have access to fresh fruits, they do not need to be pre-softened.

AYURVEDIC NOTE
Dried fruits increase *vata,* but once they've been soaked and softened, they are excellent for *vata* and *pitta.* This drink is energizing for *vata* and *pitta* but is best avoided or taken in moderation if you have *kapha* problems.

1. Remove the pits from the dates. Soak the dried dates and figs in a bowl of water for 4 to 8 hours—until the fruit has softened.

2. Combine all ingredients in a blender, and blend high until the mixture is creamy. Pour and serve.

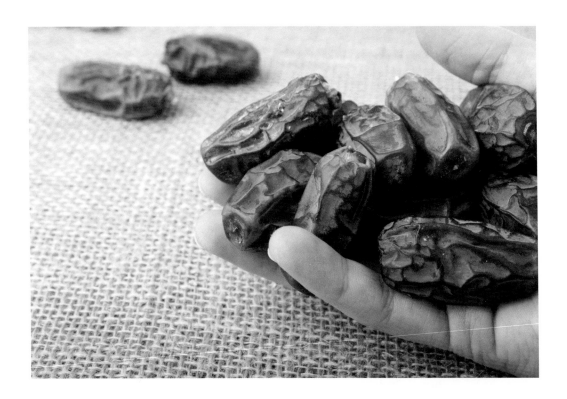

PAPAYA JUICE

Preparation Time: About 5 minutes
Serves 2

Papayas are rich in enzymes that aid digestion and help balance blood sugar. When in India at the Ayushakti Panchakarma Clinic, I drink papaya juice almost every day. Reminder: To avoid sabotaging digestion, Ayurvedic smoothies are ice-free. As I mentioned in Part One, the temperature in your belly is about 110°F so room temperature in your house is usually cool enough!

1 large ripe papaya (approximately 10 inches long)
4 cups water

COOK'S TIP: A papaya is ripe when much of it has turned from dark green to yellow, and is getting soft when you squeeze it.

AYURVEDIC NOTE
Fresh papayas are good for all *dosha*s. The juice is considered a blood thinner in Ayurvedic medicine. Papaya contains natural estrogen so Ayurvedic practitioners advise pregnant women to avoid it.

1. Cut the papaya in half lengthwise. Scrape out the seeds with a tablespoon. Scoop out the flesh and place it in a blender.

2. Add water and blend on high for 30 seconds to a minute.

(RECIPE PHOTO ON PAGE 62)

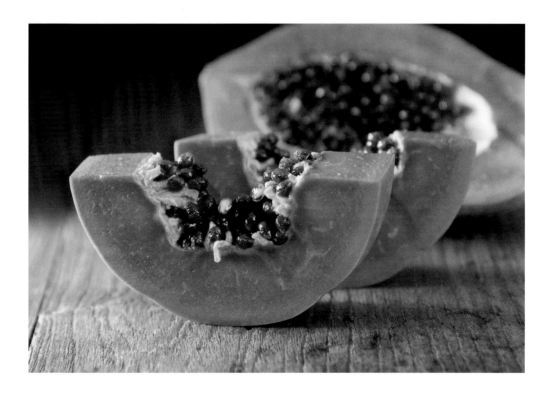

PROTEIN SMOOTHIE

Preparation Time: About 5 minutes
Serves 1

Thanks to my ever-devoted husband, Tom Mitchell, for his penchant for experimentation in the kitchen and for creating the recipe for this satisfying smoothie.

2 cups fresh almond milk or water
¼ to ⅓ cup raw sunflower seeds
1 pitted Medjool date or 1 scoop KAL Pure Stevia Extract
⅛ to ¼ teaspoon ground cardamom
1 scoop plant-based protein powder, preferably vanilla flavored

COOK'S TIP: 1. If you have freshly made almond milk in the house, as we do, I highly recommend using it as the base of this drink. It will be more delicious and substantive. Otherwise, I recommend water rather than using a boxed product with guar gum and preservatives. **2.** The protein powder I use in this drink is called VegaLite/Vanilla from Thorne Research, which has a good reputation for product purity and is available online.

1. Combine all ingredients in a blender.

2. Blend on the highest speed and serve.

AYURVEDIC NOTE
Sunflower seeds are said to be *tridoshic*, or good for all *doshas*. Cardamom is excellent for *vata* and *kapha*; less so for *pitta*, but OK in moderation. Dates increase *kapha*, so I recommend stevia for anyone with *kapha* problems—but it's fine to have a date on occasion! If you are an Ayurvedic purist, you may not wish to imbibe protein powder because it is not fresh food. This is a worthy ideal; however, many vegetarians require a protein boost once or twice a day, especially in their youth and as they age past fifty.

P Use ¼ cup sunflower seeds and reduce cardamom to ⅛ teaspoon or a pinch.

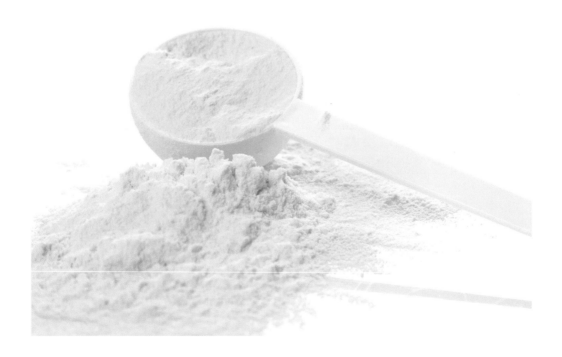

SUMMERTIME TEA

Preparation Time: 1 hour (less than 5 minutes active)
Serves 6 to 8

I owe this recipe to the tradition of Ayurveda, as passed on by Dr. Vasant Lad. At the Ayurvedic Institute in New Mexico, a tea made of cumin, coriander, and fennel is served daily as a digestive aid. I added the mint to tempt American taste buds while increasing the tea's cooling appeal during the hot months.

FOR THE CUMIN-CORIANDER-FENNEL MIXTURE (C-C-F):
½ **cup cumin seeds**
½ **cup coriander seeds**
½ **cup fennel seeds**

FOR THE SUMMERTIME TEA:
8 cups water
2 tablespoons C-C-F mixture
2 to 4 large handfuls of fresh peppermint leaves or
  2 peppermint tea bags

COOK'S TIP: 1. I keep a jar of C-C-F in my cupboard so it's always available. **2.** Boil the water in a 3-quart or larger pot, preferably one with a pour spout. Do not steep the herbs in a teakettle, as the herbs will permanently flavor the pot.

AYURVEDIC NOTE
Cumin and coriander seeds are used in most Ayurvedic dishes to balance the digestive enzymes. Cumin seeds aid digestive sluggishness and nutrient absorption. Coriander seeds kindle *agni* without increasing *pitta* or causing acid indigestion. Both are helpful for bloating. Fennel seeds also aid digestion, helping to avoid flatulence or gurgling in the stomach. Fennel is also used to treat nausea and low *agni*. Mint is used medicinally in Ayurveda for bloating, flatulence, ulcers, and nervous indigestion. If you need to burp or if you suffer from acid indigestion, drink a cup of this tea, and you may be able to avoid over-the-counter antacids. This tea is balanced for all constitutions, especially in the summertime. If you are suffering from a chest cold or asthma, this tea should be avoided until the lungs are clear.

 Omit the peppermint, which is cooling.

1. To prepare the C-C-F mixture, add the cumin, coriander, and fennel seeds to an empty 16-ounce glass jar. Shake it well.

2. To prepare the Summertime Tea, bring the 8 cups of water to boil in a pot. Once the water boils, remove the pot from the heat source.

3. Add 2 tablespoons of the C-C-F mixture and peppermint leaves or tea bags. Let this steep for at least 10 minutes. You can also wait until the tea cools to room temperature, which will make a stronger brew. Pour the tea through a strainer into a pitcher.

4. Serve hot or cool. The tea will taste fresh for only about 8 hours, even if refrigerated. If you wish, sweeten with coconut sugar or stevia. Use honey only after the tea has cooled.

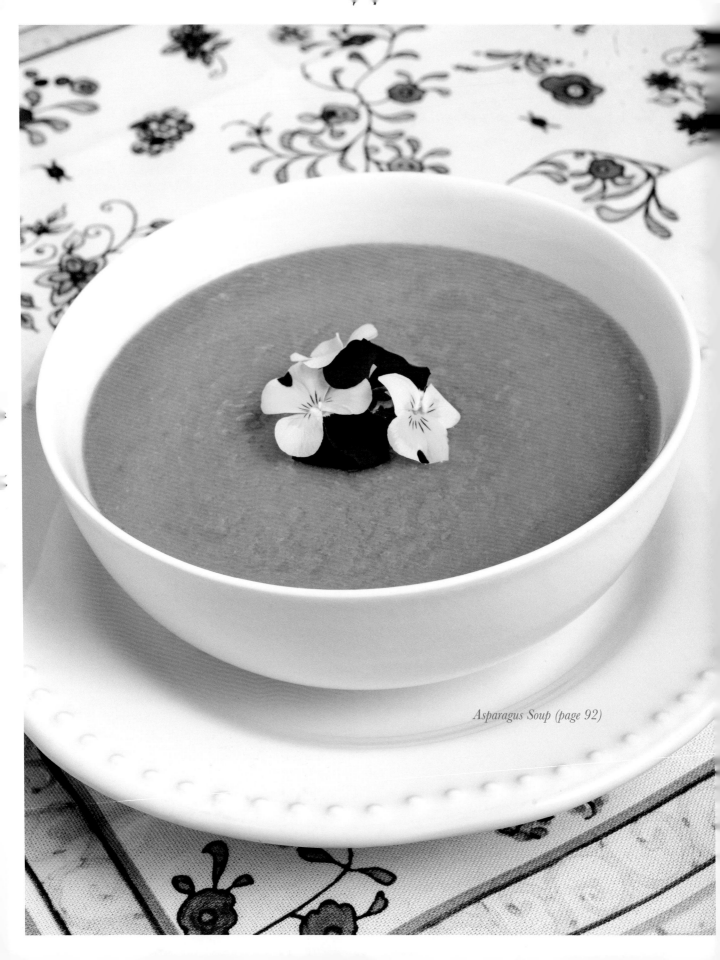

Asparagus Soup (page 92)

CHAPTER 6.

Vegetable Soups

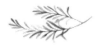

The spices are my love . . . At a whisper they yield up to me their hidden properties, their magic powers. Yes, they all hold magic, even the everyday American spices you toss unthinking into your cooking pot. You doubt? Ah. You have forgotten the old secrets your mother's mothers knew.

— Chitra Banerjee Divakaruni, *The Mistress of Spices*

Homage to Soup: The True Comfort Food

To my mind and sensibilities, true comfort is a steaming bowl of soup. As the autumn nights turn chilly and the cold of winter settles in to stay awhile, people across the globe turn to soups, stews, or chili to warm themselves from the inside out.

We know instinctively that hot soup with warming spices sustains health during the cold season. Ayurveda explains this truth by way of the fundamental principle discussed earlier (page 19): **like increases like; opposites create balance.** During autumn and winter, when it's cold outside, the *vata* and *kapha doshas* naturally increase because they are characterized by cold. To find balance, we crave warm foods and heating spices.

If you happen to suffer from *vata*-related conditions throughout the year—osteoarthritis, chronic pain, insomnia, constipation, or anxiety (to name a few)—warm soup can play a key role in your healing process and help restore your quality of life. Soup, when made correctly, is just what the doctor ordered to support the recovery from many chronic illnesses. Warm soup calms *vata*, strengthens *agni* (the digestive fire), and helps clear *ama* (toxins).

Using healing spices such as ginger, garlic, and turmeric will strengthen the immune system, which is often under attack during the cold season. If you're fighting off a cold or flu or already suffering from the unpleasant symptoms, hot soups with ginger, garlic, and turmeric can hold illness at bay or, at the very least, shorten your misery by calming *kapha* and *vata* and by helping the body detoxify.

And if your goal is to trim pounds, soups are also great for helping you lose weight. Focus on nondairy soups, such as those found in *Sacred & Delicious,* and dals, which are filling and protein-rich.

Better Water, Better Soup

You may have purchased a water filter long ago, but if not, I encourage you to do so. Your soups and soup stocks can only taste as good as the water with which they are made—a chlorine-free water means much better-tasting soup! Filtered water is also much better for your health.

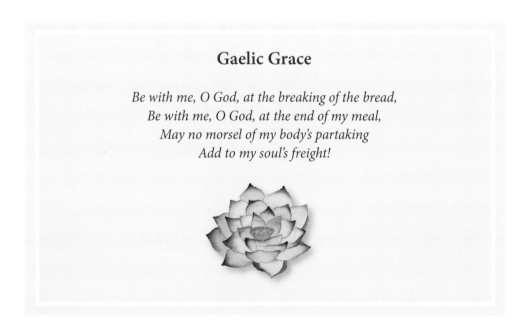

Gaelic Grace

Be with me, O God, at the breaking of the bread,
Be with me, O God, at the end of my meal,
May no morsel of my body's partaking
Add to my soul's freight!

General Notes about Soup Stock

I like to make my own stock for several important reasons. First and foremost, it's fresh. Nothing compares to the taste or healing power of a fresh soup stock created from pristine vegetables teeming with nutrients. According to Ayurveda, fresh food has much higher *prana*, or life force, so fresh soup stock made with fresh vegetables supports health and well-being better than anything that's been premade. Second, all the boxed or canned stocks and flavor cubes I've come across contain some kind of preservative and, I find, leave an undesirable aftertaste. This can undermine an otherwise delicious recipe.

Many cookbooks state that a soup stock will last in the refrigerator up to six days, but I prefer to keep a stock for no more than three or four days. It only takes about 10 minutes to throw together a simple stock, either on your stove top or in a slow cooker. Ideally, you will start the stock an hour before cooking a soup, but if you like, you can wash and chop the rest of the vegetables for your meal while the stock simmers.

If you use a store-bought stock as a base for *Sacred & Delicious* recipes, it will likely be quite salty, much saltier than what you would make yourself. For this reason, I always suggest that when using a boxed or canned stock, you need to save the addition of salt and Bragg Liquid Aminos (which is also salty) until the end of the recipe, after you've tasted the soup, and add them judiciously. Finally, if you use a packaged stock, I also suggest that you cut the amount of stock to 1 or 2 cups and add water to fulfill the liquid requirement called for in the recipe. Some prepared stocks' flavor is overpowering and will undermine the flavor intended in these soups.

EASY VEGETABLE SOUP STOCK

Preparation Time: 1 hour (10 minutes active)
Makes 6 to 10 cups

In addition to its fundamental job as a soup starter, stock serves nicely as a base for many other recipes to create a more textured flavor—including many side dishes, beans, stews, rice dishes, or gravy. I often make a large batch so that I have enough for two soup recipes.

1 large sweet yellow onion, such as Vidalia
1 fennel bulb with greens
4 to 6 large carrots
4 to 6 stalks celery with leaves
1 small sweet potato
8 to 12 cups water
Handful of shiitake mushrooms (optional)
2 handfuls of fresh basil (or 3 teaspoons dried)
3 to 4 sprigs fresh marjoram or oregano
**   (or 1 teaspoon dried)**
1 to 2 fresh bay leaves
2 teaspoons Light Grey Celtic Sea Salt
1 teaspoon ground turmeric or 1-inch piece of
**   peeled tumeric root**

COOK'S TIP: Feel free to add bits and pieces of other veggies still fresh in the fridge. Ayurveda cautions against using nightshades: tomatoes, eggplants, and peppers.

AYURVEDIC NOTE

When onions are boiled, they're somewhat heating to the metabolism, which may increase *pitta*. Fennel is cooling and will balance these flavors, making this stock fine for all *doshas*. Turmeric has an antibacterial capacity and acts as a preservative, so the stock can be kept up to four days in the refrigerator.

V Add a 2-inch piece of peeled fresh ginger or a whole clove of garlic.

P Replace onion with 2 leeks (the bulbs plus an inch of the light-green shank) or roast the onion before adding it.

K Add a 2-inch piece of peeled fresh ginger. Add ½ teaspoon sweet paprika, if you like.

S Replace onion with 2 leeks (the bulbs plus an inch of the light-green shank) or roast the onion prior to using it in the stock.

1. Peel the onion and wash all the vegetables. Cut off the fennel stalks and add them to the pot (or save them for another recipe). Halve or quarter the onion, fennel bulb, carrots, celery, and sweet potato.

2. Combine all the ingredients in an 8-quart stock pot with the water and cover the pot. Bring to a boil; then reduce the heat to medium or medium-low heat.

3. Once the stock is simmering, add the whole mushrooms to the stock pot (discarding any stems that don't look fresh). Rinse the fresh herbs and add them to the stock pot along with turmeric and salt.

4. Simmer for at least 30 minutes and up to 90 minutes. Let cool; then strain.

ROASTED VEGETABLE BROTH

Preparation Time: About 1¾ hours (20 minutes active)
Makes 14 cups

This recipe was inspired by my neighbors, Marvin and Gena Brown, who kindly cater to their vegetarian friends when hosting a Passover Seder by offering Matzo Ball Soup (page 110) without the traditional chicken stock. I prescribe a large batch of this broth, because holiday meals often include eight or more people around the table. It can be used up to three days for any freshly made soup or casserole.

2 tablespoons ghee, butter, or olive oil
2 medium leek bulbs plus an inch of the light-green shank
2 medium Vidalia or yellow onions
8 medium or 6 large carrots
6 stalks celery
3 parsnips
2 large cloves garlic
8 to 10 large shiitake mushrooms
16 cups water
2 fresh bay leaves
¼ cup basil leaves
2 to 2½ teaspoons Light Grey Celtic Sea Salt

AYURVEDIC NOTE

Onions are heating and so, to a lesser degree, are leeks. When roasted, however, onions and leeks sweeten and do not increase *pitta*. Mushrooms can aggravate arthritic conditions, but I find that shiitakes do not have this effect.

K Reduce ghee to 2 teaspoons, using it only to grease the roasting pan.

1. Preheat the oven to 425°F. Melt ghee, butter, or olive oil in a small saucepan. Cover one or more large roasting pans or stainless steel baking sheets with parchment paper. (This will make the pan easier to clean.)

2. Cut off the leeks' large green leaves; wash and dry the remaining bulbs. Peel the onions and cut them in half. Clean and dry the carrots, celery, and parsnips. Remove the ends and cut the vegetables in half. Peel the garlic cloves.

3. Brush the parchment paper with ghee, and place all the vegetables (except the mushrooms) in the pans. Use the rest of the ghee to brush the vegetables. Place the pans in the oven, uncovered. Let the vegetables roast until they are completely tender and nicely browned, about 1 hour. Shake them every 15 minutes or so to keep them turned.

4. While the veggies roast, clean the mushrooms and add them to an 8-quart stock pot with the water. Transfer the roasted vegetables to the stock pot along with any drippings from the roasting pan. Add the bay leaves, basil leaves, and 2 teaspoons salt. Bring to a boil. Reduce the heat and let the broth simmer for 45 minutes to an hour. Remove the vegetables and leaves with a long-handled flat strainer, or strain the liquid into a second large pot, retaining only broth for serving. Add salt if needed.

STOCKS

Vegetable Soups 🪷 91

ASPARAGUS SOUP

Preparation Time: About 40 minutes
Serves 4

When I initially crafted this soup, my intention was to make a creamy version, but it smelled so good before I added milk that I served it dairy-free and have ever since. This recipe is quick, and it's easy to make. It is a consistent crowd-pleaser and is especially easy to digest. It is also one of the few vegetable soups that I enjoy at room temperature on a warm day.

SOUPS

4 cups Easy Vegetable Soup Stock (page 90), heated
6 to 7 cups asparagus (about 2 pounds before trimming)
1 medium leek bulb plus an inch of the light-green shank
2 tablespoons ghee
2 tablespoons coconut flour
3 stalks of lemongrass (or ½ teaspoon lime juice)
1 tablespoon fresh tarragon leaves plus sprigs for garnish
   (or 1 teaspoon dried)
½ teaspoon Light Grey Celtic Sea Salt
1 tablespoon Bragg Liquid Aminos

COOK'S TIP: 1. Thick asparagus stalks have more flavor and, whenever available, are best for a soup. **2.** Whatever the thickness, prepare the asparagus by breaking off the woody section at the bottom of the spear, which is the lower quarter or so. **3.** Look for aging asparagus tips, which rot easily, and break them off. **4.** If you cannot find lemongrass, add a splash of fresh lime juice to each bowl just before serving.

AYURVEDIC NOTE

Asparagus are *tridoshic*, meaning they are excellent food for everyone and are very easy to digest. If you use coconut flour, it is excellent for *vata* and *pitta*, less so for *kapha*. As leeks are the least heating member of the onion family, they do not aggravate *pitta* when cooked. *Kapha* types are advised to eat only small amounts of any oil, butter, or ghee.

 Reduce ghee and flour to 1 tablespoon each.

MENU SUGGESTION

For a light spring or summer dinner, try this soup with Sweet Potato Salad (page 220, and/or Mixed Greens with Roasted Vegetables (page 207). Need some protein? Try Quick Tofu (page 169). The soup is also delicious with Spelt Bread with Figs and Walnuts (page 65) or a piece of Gluten-Free Whole Grain Bread (page 68).

1. Break and throw away the woody lower quarter or third of each asparagus spear, and break the remaining stalk into 3 to 4 pieces.

2. Thinly slice the leek. Prepare the lemongrass: remove 2 or 3 outer layers of lemongrass and cut off the ends.

3. Heat ghee or oil on medium heat in a 5- to 6-quart soup pot. Add the sliced leek and sauté for about 5 minutes until it's uniformly golden. Add flour to the leek and stir with a whisk. Once the flour has had a chance to cook for a minute but has not begun to brown, slowly add the hot vegetable stock, about ½ cup at a time, while continually whisking to avoid creating lumps.

4. Add the asparagus, lemongrass, and tarragon. Cover and bring to a low boil. Watch the pot at this stage, since the flour can cause the soup to boil over easily. Once the soup is at a simmer, reduce heat and continue simmering about 10 minutes, until the asparagus are completely tender. Remove lemongrass. Add the salt and Bragg's. (**Note:** If you are using a boxed or canned stock, don't add salt and additional Bragg's until after you purée the soup. Taste first, and add salt or Bragg's if needed.)

5. Purée the soup with an immersion blender or transfer it to a food processor. If you prefer a thinner soup, add more stock. Serve with a sprig of fresh tarragon.

(RECIPE PHOTO ON PAGE 86)

AVOCADO AND CUCUMBER SOUP

Preparation Time: About 15 minutes
Serves 4

Simple to make, this recipe can be served slightly chilled or at room temperature on hot summer days.

4 cups Easy Vegetable Soup Stock (page 90),
   room temperature, or water
2 large ripe Hass avocados
1 medium cucumber
¾ to 1 teaspoon Light Grey Celtic Sea Salt
1 cup chopped cilantro
1 to 2 tablespoons fresh lime
Pinch of pressed garlic

COOK'S TIP: 1. If you don't have time to make stock, I recommend using water rather than substituting a box or canned stock. **2.** If you're making stock the same day you're preparing this recipe, cook the stock a few hours in advance so it has time to cool to room temperature. **3.** Avocado doesn't survive well as a leftover. If you're eating this soup the next day, try some extra lime to perk it up.

AYURVEDIC NOTE

Avocado reduces *vata* and *pitta* and increases *kapha*. Cucumber is quite cooling, increasing *kapha* and *vata*, though removing the seeds makes it easier to digest. Cilantro, while also cooling to the metabolism, does not affect *vata* and *kapha doshas* adversely, and it is fine for everyone. Lime, being somewhat sour, can increase *pitta* in sensitive people. The garlic in this soup helps balance the aggravated *kapha* and *vata*. It is best to avoid this recipe when having *kapha* problems such as cold or cough.

(V) Add a whole clove of garlic, pressed.

(P) Reduce or avoid lime.

(K) Add a whole clove of garlic, pressed.

MENU SUGGESTION

Serve with black beans and Simple Summer Squash (page 193), or a Salad Bar Entrée (page 209).

1. Peel the avocados. Chop them into roughly 1-inch cubes.

2. Peel the cucumber, cut it in half lengthwise, and remove the seeds with a spoon. Chop into chunks.

3. Place all ingredients in a blender, starting with the juice from half a fresh lime. Purée. Add more lime or salt to taste.

4. Serve with a sprig of cilantro for garnish.

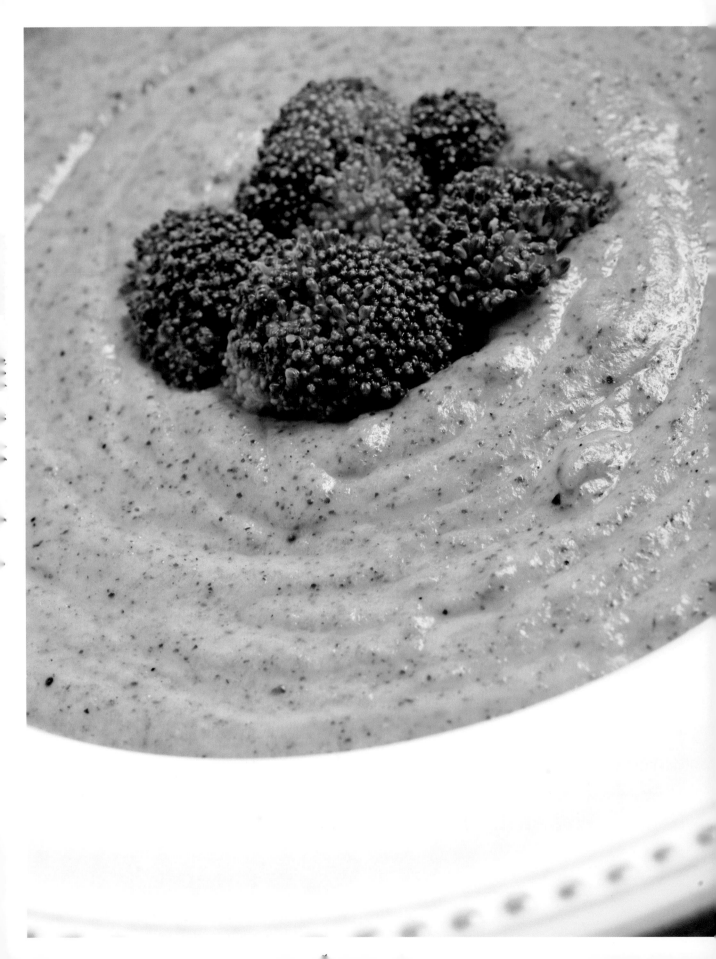

BROCCOLI AND ALMOND BUTTER SOUP

Preparation Time: 40 minutes (30 minutes active)
Serves 6 to 8

This recipe is my favorite divine inspiration! It's a showstopper for a dinner party as the soup appetizer or vegetarian entrée. It is quite rich from the almond butter, so I suggest that you save it for an occasional treat.

1 medium onion
2 tablespoons ghee or coconut oil
½ teaspoon black mustard seeds
1 teaspoon cumin seeds
1 pinch asafetida (optional)
3 large or 5 medium curry leaves
2 large parsnips
5 to 6 cups broccoli stalks plus florets (3 or 4 stalks)
4 to 5 cups Easy Vegetable Soup Stock (page 90)
1 teaspoon freshly grated ginger
2 teaspoons coconut sugar (optional)
1 cup creamy unsalted almond butter
1½ to 2 teaspoons Light Grey Celtic Sea Salt
Freshly ground pepper

COOK'S TIP: 1. Can't find organic parsnips? Substitute carrots. **2.** For the taste that matches this recipe, try Whole Foods' 365™ brand almond butter. Otherwise, you'll have the best results with a brand that uses roasted almonds and has a smooth texture.

AYURVEDIC NOTE

Broccoli is cooling and ideal for *pitta*, but it increases *vata* when eaten on its own. In this recipe the mustard seeds, asafetida, onion, ginger, and black pepper—which are all heating—balance the broccoli's cooling qualities. The spices also aid digestion. Because the almond butter is oily, it's best to eat this dish in moderation if you have any *pitta* or *kapha* problems.

(P) Reduce the almond butter to ½ cup. Omit the black pepper.

(K) Reduce the almond butter to ⅔ cup and increase the ginger to 2 teaspoons.

MENU SUGGESTION

Serve with Quick Stove-Top Maple Carrots (page 180) and Black or Wild Rice (page 162). Some people like to serve this soup over basmati rice.

1. Chop the onion and set aside.

2. Heat the ghee or coconut oil in a 6-quart soup pot on medium heat. When the oil is hot, add the mustard seeds and cover until the seeds pop like popcorn. Add the cumin seeds and cover again for about 30 seconds until these sizzle and become fragrant. Add the asafetida, curry leaves, and chopped onion. Sauté the onion on medium heat for about 5 to 10 minutes until it turns golden. Reduce the heat and sauté another 10 minutes or so until the onion caramelizes and turns light brown. Be careful not to burn.

3. While the onion is sautéing, peel and slice the parsnips. (If a parsnip is more than an inch thick, cut the thick portion in half lengthwise and remove its woody inner core, using a knife or the tip of a peeler.) Add sliced parsnips and about ¼ cup of water to the pot; cover and let the vegetables steam for about five minutes.

4. Separate the broccoli heads into florets. Peel the broccoli stems and cut them into pieces 2-inches thick. Add the broccoli to the pot with 4 cups of the stock. Bring mixture to a boil; then reduce heat to medium-low and simmer for 10 to 12 minutes, or until the broccoli is tender. Do not be concerned that the stock doesn't cover the broccoli completely, as the broccoli will cook through with the steam arising from the boiling stock.

5. Once the broccoli is tender, remove the curry leaves from the pot with tongs (if you wish). Add the ginger, sugar (if using), and almond butter, and purée the soup. If you prefer a thinner soup, you may wish to add some additional stock or water at this point. Finish the soup with salt (to taste), and mix well. (**Note:** If you are using a boxed or canned stock, taste first, and add salt only as needed.)

6. Serve with freshly ground black pepper.

The Remarkable Flavor of Curry Leaves

If you've never cooked with curry leaves, I invite you to try them. These leaves have an irreplaceable flavor—and they are not hot to the taste. English speakers call them curry leaves because they are often used in the curry dishes from South India and Sri Lanka. These leaves have no other relationship with curry. In general, the term *curry* denotes rich and sometimes complex sauces made with spice mixtures that include ground cumin, coriander, turmeric, and cardamom as well as black mustard seeds, and dried chilies. **Please do not substitute curry powder for curry leaves** in *Sacred & Delicious* recipes!

Curry leaves add a layer of complex flavor that particularly enhances vegetarian cooking. Many of my recipe testers have commented on what a difference curry leaves make in the flavor of a dish they tried, first without curry leaves and then with them. Ambitious cooks will be glad they took the time to find them locally or online.

According to Dr. Vasant Lad, the *rasa* (taste) of curry leaves is sweet, astringent, and pungent. Although these leaves are slightly heating, they have a sweet *vipak* (aftertaste). Their complexity makes them *tridoshic*, which means they are balancing for every constitution. Medicinally, curry leaves are used in Ayurveda to support digestion and lower blood sugar.

Because of their rich flavor, curry leaves can be added to many hearty American-style soups, stews, and chili dishes, as well as to bean and vegetable dishes. You can either remove the leaves before you purée or, since they have medicinal value, leave them in. According to Indian tradition, curry leaves are auspicious. One friend told me that in her family you are considered lucky when you find the curry leaf in your bowl!

Curry trees (whose biological name is *murraya koenigii*) grow wild in the foothills of the Himalayas and have been cultivated for centuries in South India and along India's western coast. More recently, curry trees have been planted in Florida to supply the Indian immigrant community. You can purchase curry leaves in Asian or international markets. Occasionally, I have found curry leaves at Harmony Farms, our neighborhood health food store, or at Whole Foods Market. You can also order them online.

You can store fresh curry leaves in a sealed bag in the refrigerator for two to three weeks—and longer if you freeze them. For best results, do not remove the leaves from their stems until you're ready to cook. Curry leaves can also be dried, but then they lose much of their flavor.

When we were visiting friends several years back, I marveled at the curry trees they had cultivated indoors to a height of about six feet. Our kind host, Pravina Baldev Thakor, graciously offered me a small cutting from one of the trees, and I named the plant Annapurna for the Indian goddess of food. I quickly learned that picking stems off the main branch encouraged growth.

Annapurna continues to thrive in a pot outside on our deck in the summer and comes inside to live with us during the cold months. She's not as happy inside, so on returning her to her outdoor abode, I always cut her way back to encourage growth. Within a month she's filling out beautifully, and within two she's become her glorious self again!

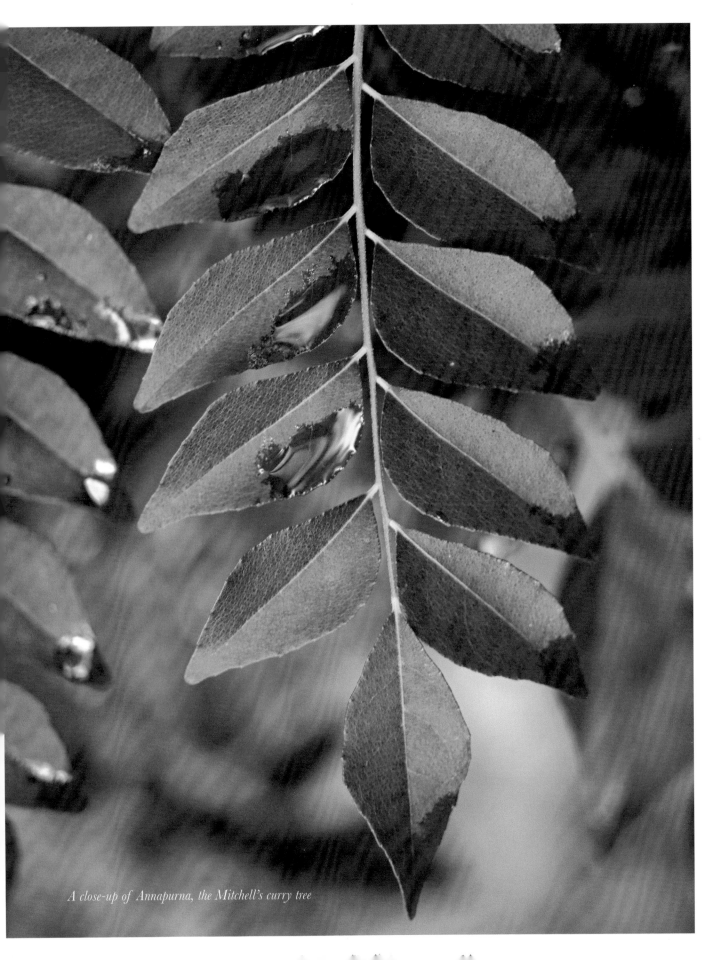

A close-up of Annapurna, the Mitchell's curry tree

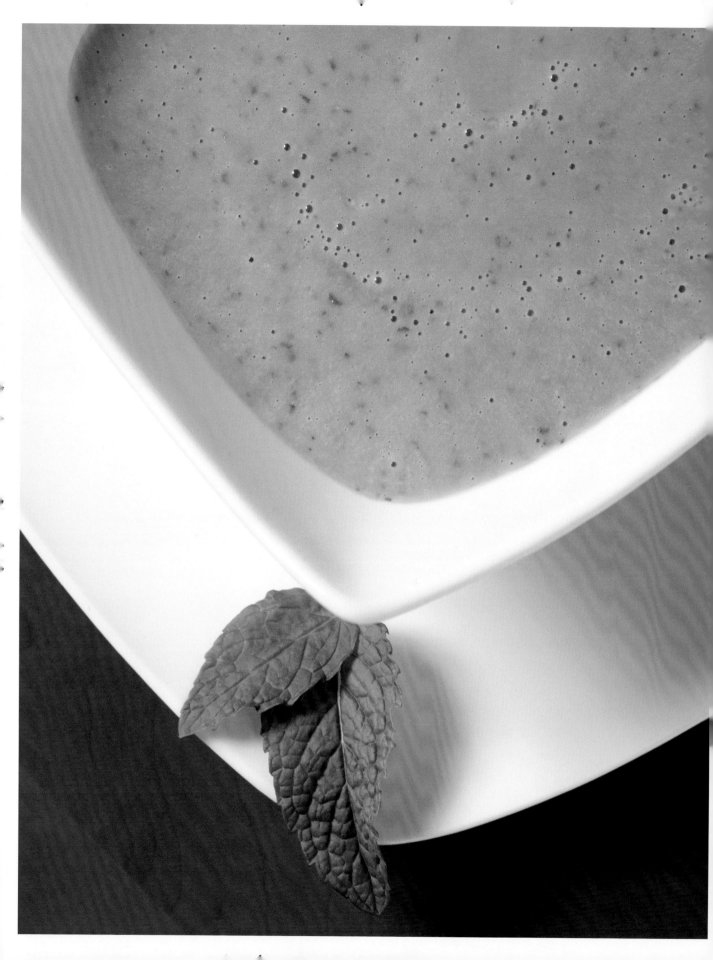

CARROT SOUP WITH COCONUT MILK

Preparation Time: About 30 minutes, plus time to cool
Serves 3 to 4

My friend Ellen Brock shared a simple yet elegant carrot soup recipe, which I have adapted. This soup is lovely when warm and works well served room temperature during the summer.

1 medium leek bulb plus an inch of the light-green shank
8 large carrots
2 tablespoons ghee or coconut oil
4 to 5 cups Easy Vegetable Soup Stock (page 90)
1 cup tightly packed chopped cilantro plus sprigs for garnish
Small handful mint leaves
1 cup coconut milk or fresh almond milk
1 teaspoon Light Grey Celtic Sea Salt

COOK'S TIP: If you have an aversion to cilantro, consider adding some fresh basil.

AYURVEDIC NOTE
Cooked carrots are excellent for all *doshas*. Mint and cilantro are excellent for cooling the metabolism during the summer months. Avoid coconut milk when you have a *kapha* condition such as a cough or cold.

(V) Add 1 to 2 teaspoons freshly grated ginger.

(K) Replace coconut milk with almond milk. Add 1 to 2 teaspoons freshly grated ginger. Use ghee or sunflower oil instead of coconut oil.

(W) Use unsweetened almond milk instead of coconut milk. Replace mint and cilantro with a handful of fresh basil and 1 to 2 teaspoons of freshly grated ginger.

MENU SUGGESTION
Serve with a Simple Green Salad (page 206) and Black-Eyed Pea Salad (Page 215), or Savory Tofu (page 170).

SOUPS

1. Wash and slice the leek. Scrub and chop each carrot into 4 or 5 chunks.

2. Heat ghee or coconut oil on medium heat in a 4-quart or larger soup pot. Add the sliced leek and sauté about 5 minutes or until it starts to turn golden. Add the carrots and 4 cups of stock, and bring to a boil on high heat. Reduce the heat to medium and simmer, covered, for 10 to 15 minutes, or until the vegetables start to become tender.

3. Add the cilantro, mint, coconut milk or almond milk, and salt. (**Note:** If you are using a boxed or canned stock, purée and taste before adding the salt; add salt as needed.) Purée the soup with an immersion blender. Add additional stock if you prefer a thinner soup.

4. Let cool to room temperature before serving with cilantro garnish.

GREEN BEAN AND SHIITAKE MUSHROOM SOUP WITH WILD RICE

Preparation Time: About 1½ hours
Serves 4 to 6

This recipe manifested as one of those delightful inventions when I threw all the veggies left in the refrigerator into the pot. Thanks to our friend Sal Corbo, a marvelous cook who helped adjust the seasonings for this hearty soup.

SOUPS

1 cup black rice or dried wild rice mixture

2½ cups water

1½ teaspoons Light Grey Celtic Sea Salt

3 cups snapped green beans

2 cups shiitake mushrooms

2 medium leek bulbs plus an inch of the light-green shank

1 large parsnip

2 large carrots

2 tablespoons ghee or olive oil

½ teaspoon ground cumin

½ teaspoon ground coriander

1 small clove garlic

½ cup red lentils

5 cups Easy Vegetable Soup Stock (page 90)

2 or 3 sprigs each of fresh thyme, tarragon, and parsley

1 fresh bay leaf

3 black peppercorns

2 tablespoons Bragg Liquid Aminos

COOK'S TIP: 1. Wild rice mixtures are available at standard grocers, and black rice is also available at organic chains and in many local health food stores. **2.** Mushroom lovers may prefer to slice and sauté the mushrooms and garlic in a separate pan and add them at the end of the recipe, after you've puréed the soup, so that you can savor the mushroom slices in every bite. If someone in your household does not appreciate the texture of mushrooms, the purée disguises them so their flavor can be enjoyed nonetheless.

AYURVEDIC NOTE

Green beans are fine for all three *doshas*. Wild and black rice will increase *vata* somewhat because it is harder and chewier than other rice, so be sure to cook it until tender. Garlic and ginger, in moderation, will pacify *vata* and *kapha* without increasing *pitta*. Mushrooms increase *vata* but are balanced by garlic and ginger.

(V) Add 1 to 2 teaspoons freshly grated ginger.

(P) Cook the garlic whole rather than pressing it into soup.

MENU SUGGESTION

Serve with Beet Salad (page 213) over red leaf lettuce, and Easy Winter Squash (page 194).

TIME-SAVER: Get a 15-minute head start by snapping beans the night before, or cook the wild rice while you're getting ready for work.

1. Rinse the wild rice mixture. Bring rice and water to a boil in a 2- or 3-quart saucepan with ½ teaspoon of the salt. Reduce heat to medium-low, and simmer covered for about 1 hour, until the rice is tender.

2. Prepare green beans by snapping off the stems and snapping the rest of the beans in halves or thirds. Rinse and drain. Peel and slice leeks. Clean and slice the parsnips and carrots.

3. Heat ghee or oil in a 6-quart soup pot on medium heat. When the ghee is hot, add the leeks and sauté them 10 to 12

minutes, stirring occasionally, until they turn golden and the edges start to brown.

4. Add the cumin and coriander, and stir. Add parsnips and carrots with 2 to 3 tablespoons of water. Cover and steam about 5 minutes. While the vegetables cook, clean the mushroom caps (discard stems) and cut into quarters. Add the mushrooms and the garlic to the pot. Cook about 2 minutes.

5. Rinse and drain the lentils. Add the lentils, the snapped green beans, and the stock to the pot. Prepare bouquet garni of thyme, tarragon, and parsley sprigs by tying their stems together, or stuff them into a spice bag and add to the pot. Add the bay leaf and peppercorns to the bag or pot. Bring soup to a low boil. Reduce heat to medium-low and simmer 15 minutes or until the green beans are completely tender. Once the vegetables are tender, remove the bouquet of spices and bay leaf.

6. Purée the vegetables and return to the pot. Then stir the cooked wild rice into the purée. Add 1 teaspoon salt and Bragg's to taste. (**Note:** If you are using a boxed or canned stock, taste first and add salt or Bragg's as needed.) If the soup is too thick for your liking, add another cup or two of water or stock, and taste again for salt before serving.

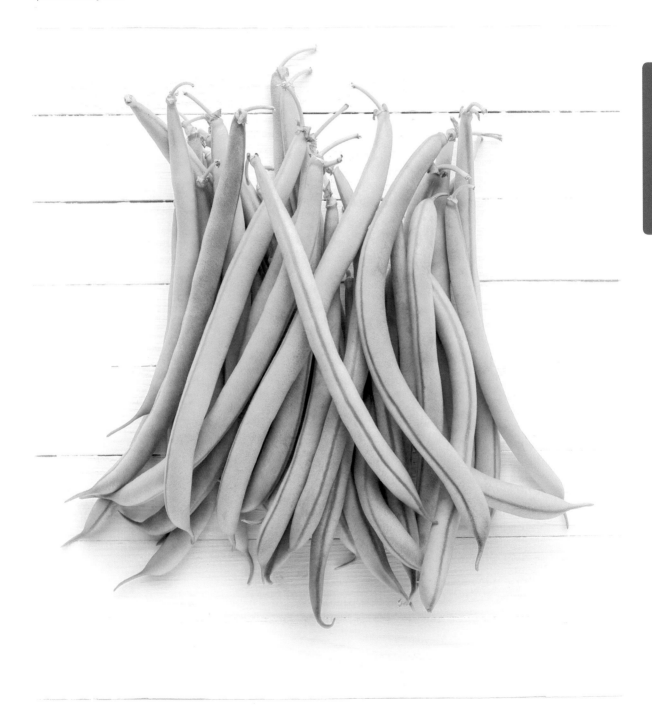

OKRA SOUP

Preparation Time: About 45 minutes (35 minutes active)
Serves 4

Although okra is as Southern as biscuits or peach pie, I never tasted okra until I was in my early twenties—and I grew up in South Carolina. There's a perfectly good explanation for this omission: my mother was a Jewish cook from New Jersey! I first experienced okra soup at a restaurant in the historic district of Charleston, South Carolina, and that's when I got hooked. This recipe is a far cry from Charleston, but my Southern friends seem to love it nonetheless!

SOUPS

½ cup uncooked quinoa
1 cup water
1½ teaspoons Light Grey Celtic Sea Salt
1 medium or large leek bulb plus an inch of the light-green shank
1 very large or 2 medium sweet potatoes
2 cups chopped okra
1 small tomato (optional) or 3 pieces of *kokum*
1 tablespoon ghee or sunflower oil
2 pinches asafetida (optional)
3 curry leaves
1 teaspoon ground cumin
½ teaspoon ground turmeric
1 teaspoon ground coriander
5 cups Easy Vegetable Soup Stock (page 90)
2 ears corn
2 tablespoons fresh basil (or 2 teaspoons dried)
2 tablespoons chopped parsley
2 teaspoons freshly grated ginger
1 large clove garlic, pressed
1 tablespoon Bragg Liquid Aminos
Freshly ground black pepper

AYURVEDIC NOTE

Okra and corn (as well as quinoa) are particularly likely to increase *vata,* so I've added asafetida, ginger, garlic, and black pepper to aid digestion. Be sure to cook the corn until it's tender to help *vata.* Corn reduces *kapha,* helping offset the sweet potatoes, which increase *kapha.* Sweet potatoes are excellent for balancing *vata* and *pitta.* Tomato is listed as an optional ingredient since tomatoes increase all *doshas.* But wait! Cumin is an antidote to the tomato's acidity, which makes cooked tomatoes acceptable if eaten on occasion. If you want the sour taste without tomatoes, add fresh lime juice or *kokum,* a sour Indian fruit that reduces *pitta.*

(V) Use less corn. Replace the quinoa with white or brown basmati rice.

(P) Omit the tomato. Use 2 to 3 pieces of dried *kokum* to the pot in step 4, and remove them before serving. Or add fresh lime juice, to taste.

(K) Replace the rice with quinoa.

MENU SUGESTION

This hearty soup needs nothing but Corn Bread (page 71) to fill out the meal and ensure its place on a Southern menu.

1. Rinse the quinoa and strain it. Bring the cup of water and ½ teaspoon salt to a boil in a 1-quart pot. Add quinoa, cover, and reduce heat to low until all the water is absorbed.

2. Slice the leek and chop the sweet potato, okra, and (if using) tomato.

3. Heat the ghee or sunflower oil in a 6-quart soup pot on medium heat. When the ghee is warm, add the asafetida and curry leaves, and cover immediately in case the leaves pop. After about 10 seconds, add the leeks and sauté about 10 minutes or until they turn uniformly golden. Add cumin, turmeric, and coriander, and stir for a few seconds. If using tomatoes, add them to the pot now, stir and cover. Reduce heat to medium-low and simmer for about 10 minutes.

4. Add the stock, the sweet potatoes, and the okra to the pot. Bring to a gentle boil; then reduce heat to medium-low and continue simmering for at least 20 minutes or until all the vegetables are tender.

5. While the soup is simmering, cut the corn off the cob with a sharp knife and pull out any grassy strands. Add the kernels to the soup and simmer for about 10 minutes or until the corn is completely tender.

6. Chop the basil and parsley, and grate the ginger. Add these to the soup pot along with pressed garlic. Add Bragg's and salt. (**Note:** If you are using a boxed or canned stock, taste first and add Bragg's and salt only as needed.) Add cooked quinoa to the pot and stir. Serve with a generous portion of freshly ground pepper.

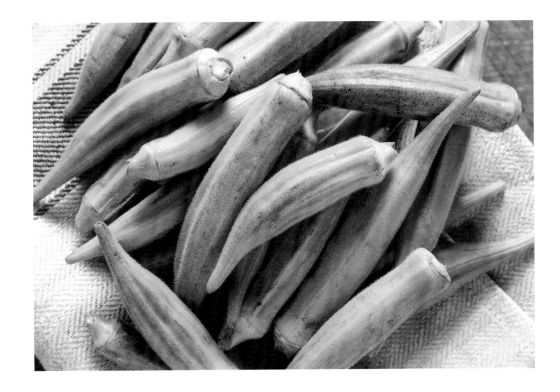

ROASTED SQUASH SOUP WITH GLAZED PECAN GARNISH

Preparation Time: About 2 hours (30 minutes active)
Serves 4

Squashes of every variety are a staple in traditional Ayurvedic cooking, primarily because they are so very easy to digest. I enjoy this dish the most when it combines the flavors of butternut and acorn squash—although you can use just one, if you prefer. Sometimes a squash will have a slightly bitter taste, in which case you may want to add just a little sugar.

SOUPS

FOR THE SOUP

- 1 large butternut squash
- 1 large acorn squash
- 2 tablespoons ghee or coconut oil
- 1 teaspoon ground cardamom
- 1 teaspoon ground cinnamon
- 1 pinch cloves
- ½ teaspoon ground cumin
- ½ teaspoon ground coriander
- 4 cups Easy Vegetable Soup Stock (page 90)
- 1 teaspoon freshly grated ginger
- 1 teaspoon Light Grey Celtic Sea Salt
- 1 to 2 teaspoons coconut sugar or maple syrup (optional)

FOR THE PECAN GARNISH (OPTIONAL)

- 2 teaspoons ghee, unsalted butter, or coconut oil
- 1 to 2 teaspoons coconut sugar
- ½ teaspoon ground cinnamon
- 1 pinch paprika
- ¼ cup chopped pecans
- 1 pinch mineral salt

COOK'S TIP: 1. Plan to finish baking the squashes at least 15 minutes before your usual cooking time so they have time to cool before you handle them. (See Time-Saver.) **2.** If you don't have a cleaver or large sharp knife, you'll wish you did when it comes time to cut any winter squash. **3.** Cutting the squash open is easier if you own a microwave. Cook each squash for 1 minute in the microwave to soften it. Or heat the squash whole in the oven for 10 minutes before slicing open. **4.** Based on the squashes' size, you may find that you need to bake them up to 90 minutes.

AYURVEDIC NOTE

Squash is one of the easiest foods to digest and is excellent for *vata* and *pitta* types. It should be eaten in moderation by people with *kapha* imbalances. The cardamom, cinnamon, and cumin, all mildly heating, are added to balance *kapha*. If you have a cold or cough, however, squash is best avoided altogether. Although nuts can increase *pitta* and *kapha*, eating such a small quantity is fine for most people.

K Double ginger and reduce ghee to 1 tablespoon. Avoid garnish.

MENU SUGGESTION

Serve with Broccoli with Caramelized Onion Masala (page 176) or Gujarati Green Beans (page 187) and Sautéed Red Cabbage (page 183).

TIME-SAVER: Prepare the squashes for baking the night before you cook. In the morning, while you're getting ready for work, bake the squashes whole on 450°F for 1 hour; then turn the oven off and let them cool while you're gone. When you return home, they will be easy to handle, so you can cut them open and scrape out the seeds and the flesh. As a second time-saver, the soup is also delicious without the pecan garnish.

1. Roast the squash: Preheat oven to 450°F. Line the bottom of a large roasting pan or baking dish with parchment paper. Cut each squash in half with a cleaver or large knife, and scoop out seeds and strings with a spoon. Place the squash with its bowl down in a baking dish. Cover with foil and roast for 1 hour, or until the squash is tender enough to scoop out. Remove from oven and let cool.

2. Make the pecan garnish: While the squash is baking, heat the ghee, butter, or coconut oil in a small saucepan or skillet on medium heat. Add the coconut sugar, ground cinnamon, and paprika to the pan. Add the chopped pecans and stir until the nuts are coated. Sprinkle with a dash of salt, and set aside to cool.

3. Prepare the soup: in a 5- or 6-quart soup pot, heat the ghee or coconut oil on medium-low heat. Add the cardamom, cinnamon, cloves, cumin, and coriander, and stir for about 10 seconds.

4. Add soup stock and stir. Scoop out the cooled squash flesh; add it to the pot and cover. Heat the soup until it is steaming. Add ginger, salt, and purée the soup. (**Note:** if you are using a boxed or canned stock, taste first, and add salt as needed.) Add additional stock or water if you prefer a thinner soup and reheat if necessary. If the squash is bitter, you may want to add some coconut sugar or maple syrup.

5. Serve each bowl with a sprinkle of pecans for garnish.

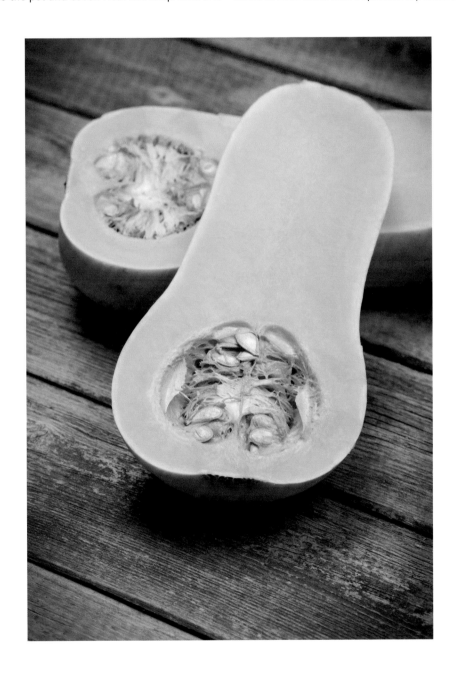

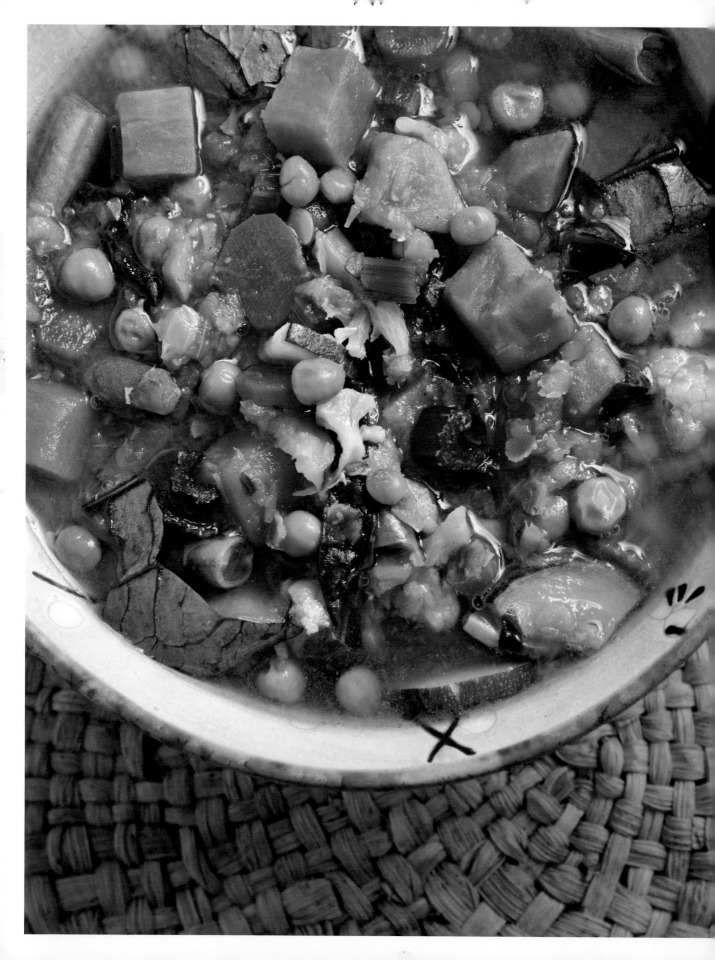

MIXED VEGETABLE SOUP

Preparation Time: About 1¼ hours
Serves 4 to 6

I once served this soup to forty people who were not familiar with Ayurvedic or vegetarian cuisine. Nonetheless, I received count-less compliments, which I attribute to the complex flavors provided by the assortment of spices. While some of these spices may be unfamiliar, I enthusiastically invite you to overcome any trepidation about cooking with spices that may seem exotic to you. That just means you haven't yet tried them. Once they're in your cupboard, you'll be glad you have them at the ready.

2 cups cauliflower florets
1 large yellow onion
2 tablespoons ghee or olive oil
½ teaspoon black mustard seeds
1 pinch asafetida (optional)
3 large curry leaves and/or 1 fresh bay leaf
2 to 3 large carrots
2 stalks celery
½ teaspoon ground turmeric
1 teaspoon ground cumin
1 teaspoon ground coriander
½ cup water
1 large sweet potato
1 cup dried red lentils
4 to 6 cups Easy Vegetable Soup Stock (page 90)
2 cups fresh snapped green beans
6 to 8 leaves of red chard
1 cup quinoa or lentil and rice pasta (optional)
1 medium zucchini
Handful or 2 of fresh basil (or 2 to 3 teaspoons dried)
¼ cup flat-leafed Italian parsley
1 teaspoon freshly grated ginger
1 teaspoon Light Grey Celtic Sea Salt
1 tablespoon Bragg Liquid Aminos
Black pepper to taste

COOK'S TIP: For a deeper flavor and improved digestion, begin by roasting the cauliflower florets and add them to the soup after they have browned a bit. Roast the cauliflower at 375°F on an oiled baking sheet for 15 to 20 minutes. If you like very thick soups, you can double the lentils.

AYURVEDIC NOTE

This soup includes a variety of tastes and spices that balance each other beautifully. The ginger, asafetida, mustard seeds, and black pepper are especially helpful in digesting the lentils, white potatoes, cauliflower, and chard—all which increase *vata* more or less and need the help of heating spices. When my *vata* feels high, I forgo the cauliflower. The red lentils make this soup a good source of iron and phosphorus, and, in combination with the rice or quinoa pasta, provide a complete protein.

V Omit or use less cauliflower. Add 1 clove of pressed garlic or more ginger.

P Reduce the black mustard seeds to ¼ teaspoon.

K Replace the sweet potatoes with white.

MENU SUGGESTION

This soup goes nicely with Corn Bread (page 71) or Gluten-Free Whole-Grain Bread (page 68).

1. Separate the cauliflower into small florets. Dice the onion.

2. In a 6-quart soup pot, melt ghee or oil on medium heat. When the ghee is hot, add the mustard seeds and cover the pot until the seeds pop like popcorn. After the seeds have finished popping, add asafetida and curry leaves, and cover immediately in case the leaves pop and the oil splatters. Add the chopped onion and sauté 5 minutes on medium heat. Reduce heat to medium-low and continue cooking another

10 minutes, until the onion turns completely golden and the edges start to brown.

3. While the onion cooks, chop the carrots and celery. When the onion begins to caramelize, add the turmeric, cumin, and coriander, and stir. Then add the carrots, celery, and water. Cover and steam for about 5 minutes.

4. While the vegetables are becoming tender, peel and dice the sweet potatoes. Add potatoes to pot and re-cover.

5. Rinse and strain lentils. Add lentils to the pot with 4 cups vegetable stock and bring it to a boil. Reduce heat to medium, add the bay leaf (if using), and cook for another 15 minutes.

6. Snap the ends off the green beans, break the beans into 1½-inch pieces, and add to the pot. Soak the chard leaves in water to clean them. Chop or hand-tear the leaves into bite-sized pieces, and add these to the pot. Chop the chard ribs, and add them to the pot also. If you're adding pasta to the soup, do so now with 1½ cups extra water. Continue to boil lightly on medium heat for 15 minutes.

7. Slice the zucchini, chop the basil and parsley, and grate the ginger. Add them to the pot and simmer until zucchini is tender, about 5 minutes. Add salt and 1 tablespoon Bragg's. (**Note:** If you are using a boxed or canned stock, taste first, and add salt and additional Bragg's to taste, as needed.) Add more water if the soup is too thick for your liking. If you wish, add freshly grated black pepper before serving.

Vegetable Soup Variations

Use whatever fresh vegetables you have in the fridge, but please avoid frozen or canned vegetables, which lack *prana* (life force). (See page 41 for more information.) I especially like to add about a cup of diced okra or some fresh corn off the cob in the summer. Or I might replace sweet potato with a small butternut squash, cubed, for a soup that is not quite so sweet. If you use a fresh tomato, please add ½ teaspoon cumin seeds or powder—because cumin is the antidote to the tomato's acidity. (Add cumin seeds at the beginning of preparation after the mustard seeds pop.)

   If you don't have lentils handy, you can make a plain vegetable soup, but the lentils really do add a much-appreciated layer of flavor. If you like a thicker soup, you can also use split mung dal in place of the red lentils. Or, if you prefer and have time to soak 2 cups of kidney beans or other legumes the night before, cook these in a slow cooker while you're at work, and they'll be ready to add to the mix. You can use a small amount for your soup, and then you'll have beans ready for another meal the following day.

SWEET POTATO AND SWISS CHARD SOUP

Preparation Time: About 1 hour (45 minutes active)
Serves 5 to 6

This soup was inspired by a cook named Ananta, whom I met at the Ayurvedic Institute in New Mexico. I mimic his adventurous use of almost every spice he had in the cabinet that day. The heaviness of the sweet potatoes and richness of the spices allows this soup to work well as an easy one-dish meal.

3 large sweet potatoes
¼ teaspoon ground cardamom
½ teaspoon ground cinnamon
1 teaspoon ground cumin
½ teaspoon ground fennel
1 pinch garam masala
1 pinch ground nutmeg
½ teaspoon ground turmeric
1 teaspoon ground coriander
2 tablespoons ghee or olive oil
5 cups Easy Vegetable Soup Stock (page 90)
8 to 10 large leaves of red chard
2 tablespoons fresh basil (or 2 teaspoons dried)
1 teaspoon fresh marjoram (or ½ teaspoon dried)
1 teaspoon freshly grated ginger
1 to 1½ teaspoons Light Grey Celtic Sea Salt
1 tablespoon Bragg Liquid Aminos
1 to 2 teaspoons fresh lime juice

COOK'S TIP: 1. This is one of the few soups that doesn't miss a base stock, so don't hesitate to make it with water on a day you have no fresh stock. **3.** You can vary both flavor and texture by serving it with chopped walnuts, cashews, pistachios, or almonds—if you think you would enjoy a little crunch. You can try 2 tablespoons of almond or cashew butter for a creamy texture.

AYURVEDIC NOTE

Chard is excellent for *kapha* and *pitta*, although its slightly astringent quality is mildly aggravating to *vata*. Sweet potatoes are excellent for *vata* and *pitta*, although they can increase *kapha*. The primarily heating spices in this soup assist both *vata* and *kapha*, so I find this soup very balanced. Because of the sweet potato emphasis, this dish is best avoided or eaten only occasionally by people with *kapha*-related problems. Nuts may increase *pitta* and *kapha* but should be fine in such a small quantity.

(P) Reduce the garam masala to a pinch or two.

(K) Add 1 clove garlic or double the ginger. Omit the nuts.

MENU SUGGESTION

Serve with Quick Tofu (page 169) or Refried Beans (page 168) for some protein. If you prefer bread, enjoy with Spelt Bread with Figs and Walnuts (page 65), Gluten-Free Whole Grain Bread (page 68), or Corn Bread (page 71).

1. Peel the potatoes and cut each of them into 4 or 5 thick chunks. Set aside.

2. Pull all the ground spices out of the cabinet and have them lined up and ready to measure. Heat the ghee or olive oil on medium-low heat in a 6-quart soup pot. When the ghee or oil is warm enough to simmer spices, add all dry spices one at a time.

3. Add soup stock or water to the pot along with the sweet potatoes. Bring the pot to a boil; then cover the pot and reduce the heat to medium-low.

4. While the potatoes cook, soak the chard in cold water to clean it. Remove the stems, chop them like celery, and add them to the pot. Hand-tear or chop the chard leaves into bite-size pieces and set aside. Chop the fresh basil and marjoram. Peel and grate the ginger.

5. When the potatoes are tender, turn off the stove, add the ginger, and purée the soup with a handheld immersion blender. After you're finished, add the chard leaves to the soup along with the basil, marjoram, and salt. (Note: if you are using a boxed or canned stock, taste first and add more as needed before serving.) Let the soup simmer on medium-low heat until the chard is tender, stirring occasionally, about 10 minutes. Add Bragg's to intensify flavor only if using fresh stock. Add lime to taste before serving.

MATZO BALL SOUP

Preparation Time: About 2 hours
Serves 5 to 8 (makes 16 small matzo balls)

For a Jewish family, no holiday meal is complete without a good matzo ball soup. When my parents moved to South Carolina in 1954 and were separated from the mishpocha *(their extended families), they began sharing holidays with new friends in our small Jewish community. This Matzo Ball Soup recipe (with the addition of asafetida and a few substitutions) comes from Doris Sopkin, affectionately known to my brother and me as Aunt Doris. Our mother's best friend of more than fifty years, Aunt Doris was like a second mom during my childhood, and she remained a close friend and confidante for the remainder of her life.*

Of course, traditionally a matzo ball soup is made with chicken broth; here I use a roasted vegetable broth as the base. I have added ghee to give this soup a little bit of the fatty flavor that makes a matzo ball soup so delicious. I've also used both spelt and gluten-free matzo meal, but this recipe works perfectly using regular matzo meal.

FOR THE MATZO BALLS:
¼ cup melted ghee
3 eggs
½ teaspoon Fine Ground Celtic Sea Salt
1 pinch asafetida (optional)
½ teaspoon baking powder
1 cup gluten-free or spelt matzo meal

FOR THE SOUP:
4 carrots, peeled and chopped into bite-sized chunks
¼ cup loosely packed flat-leaf parsley
Freshly ground black pepper
12 to 18 cups Roasted Vegetable Broth (page 91)

AYURVEDIC NOTE

Spelt matzo meal is very dry and light, which is good for *kapha* but increases *vata*. Spelt is balanced somewhat for *vata* by the ghee, asafetida, and garlic in the soup stock. Gluten-free matzo meal may increase *kapha* and requires gluten-free asafetida. If eaten on occasion, however, this comforting soup is fine for everyone.

MENU SUGGESTION
Serve with Elegant Green Beans (page 186) and Roasted Veggies (page 199) and Quick Tofu (page 169) with Nut-Butter Sauce (page 171).

TIME-SAVER: Prepare the Roasted Vegetable Broth the day before.

1. Prepare the Matzo Balls: Melt the ghee. Set aside to cool.

2. Combine matzo meal, salt, asafetida, and baking powder in a small mixing bowl. Beat the eggs in a separate bowl and add them to the dry ingredients. Add the ghee and mix well. Cover the mixture, and refrigerate for at least 30 minutes.

3. Prepare to cook the matzo balls by bringing a pot of water to boil in a 6-quart soup pot. Once the water is boiling, reduce heat to medium.

4. Pour a cup of chilled water for wetting your hands. Dip your hand in the cold water, grab about a tablespoon of the matzo meal dough, and use your hands to shape it into a small ball, about 1 inch in diameter. As you form the balls, gently drop them into the boiling water; they will expand as soon as they are immersed in the hot liquid. Reduce heat to medium-low, and cook them for about an hour.

5. Prepare the Soup: If using broth that has already been refrigerated, bring it to a boil in a separate 8-quart soup pot, and add the carrots and parsley. Reduce heat to medium-low and simmer. Taste and add salt, if needed.

6. When the matzo balls are cooked and you are ready to serve, transfer two or three balls to each soup bowl and ladle the broth and carrots into the bowl. Serve with freshly ground black pepper.

ZUCCHINI SOUP WITH PASTA AND GREENS

Preparation Time: About 45 minutes

Serves 4 to 5

This hearty soup is an easy one-dish meal that is satisfying, easy to digest, and rich in iron. Add more lentils if you prefer a very thick soup.

1 medium onion

2 tablespoons olive or sunflower oil

2 large carrots

1 to 1½ cups red lentils

5 to 6 cups Easy Vegetable Soup Stock (page 90)

1 fresh bay leaf

1 whole clove garlic, peeled (optional)

1 cup dry pasta (optional)

2 large or 3 medium zucchinis

2 cups tightly packed baby spinach leaves, arugula, or dandelion greens

2 tablespoons or more tightly packed fresh basil (or 2 teaspoons dried)

1 tablespoon fresh oregano (or 1 teaspoon dried)

1 teaspoon freshly ground ginger

1 tablespoon Bragg Liquid Aminos

1 teaspoon Light Grey Celtic Sea Salt

AYURVEDIC NOTE

Red lentils are excellent for *pitta* and *kapha*, while they may increase *vata* somewhat. To address this, I add garlic and ginger, which are both very pacifying for *vata*. Cooked carrots are excellent for all *doshas*. Zucchini is excellent for *vata* and *pitta*. Because of its liquid quality, zucchini will increase *kapha*, but the spices in this dish support *kapha*. Cooked spinach is excellent for *kapha* and *pitta* and fine in moderation for *vata*.

V Serve with black pepper.

K Add a second garlic clove. Use black pepper generously or a pinch of cayenne. Use quinoa pasta.

MENU SUGGESTION

Serve with Gluten-Free Whole Grain Bread (page 68) or Quick Tofu for extra protein (page 169).

1. Dice the onion. Heat the oil in a 6-quart soup pot on medium heat. When the oil is warm, add onions and sauté about 15 minutes until they are uniformly golden and starting to brown, stirring occasionally. While the onions are cooking, wash and slice the carrot into thin rounds. Add them to the pot and sauté for about 5 minutes.

2. Rinse the lentils in cold water a few times, and pick out stones and other debris. Add the strained lentils to the soup pot and stir to coat the lentils. Add the soup stock and bring to a boil. Add the bay leaf and garlic clove (if using). Reduce heat to medium and cover for 10 minutes, letting the lentils simmer.

3. If using pasta, add it now, re-cover, and simmer for another 10 minutes. While the pasta cooks, slice the zucchini into thin half or quarter rounds, and wash the spinach.

4. Once the pasta is cooked, reduce the heat to medium-low. Add the zucchini and spinach, and re-cover. Chop the basil and oregano, and add to the pot. Peel and grate the ginger, and add it to the pot along with Bragg's and salt. **(Note:** If you are using a boxed or canned stock, taste first, and add salt only as needed.) Simmer until the vegetables are just tender, about another 5 minutes. Taste and add more fresh basil, ginger, or Bragg's until your taste meter says "delicious."

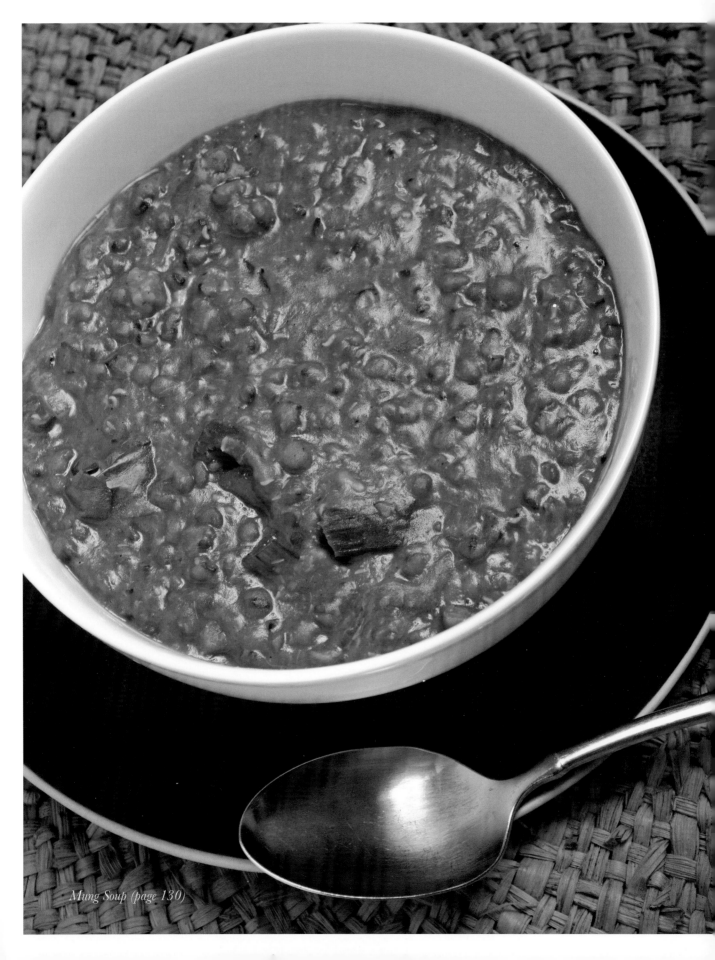

Mung Soup (page 130)

CHAPTER 7.

Legume-Based Soups and Dals

When you are aware of your hunger, that pure awareness is God.

When you are hungry, the Divine is hungry in you.

When you eat food, then there is satisfaction.

You are eating not just to fill your stomach.

You are eating to satisfy God.

That is why eating the right kind of food is a sacrifice to inner awareness.

⁓ Dr. Vasant Lad

Cooking Legumes and the Dal Tradition

Legumes

Dals

Food Notes

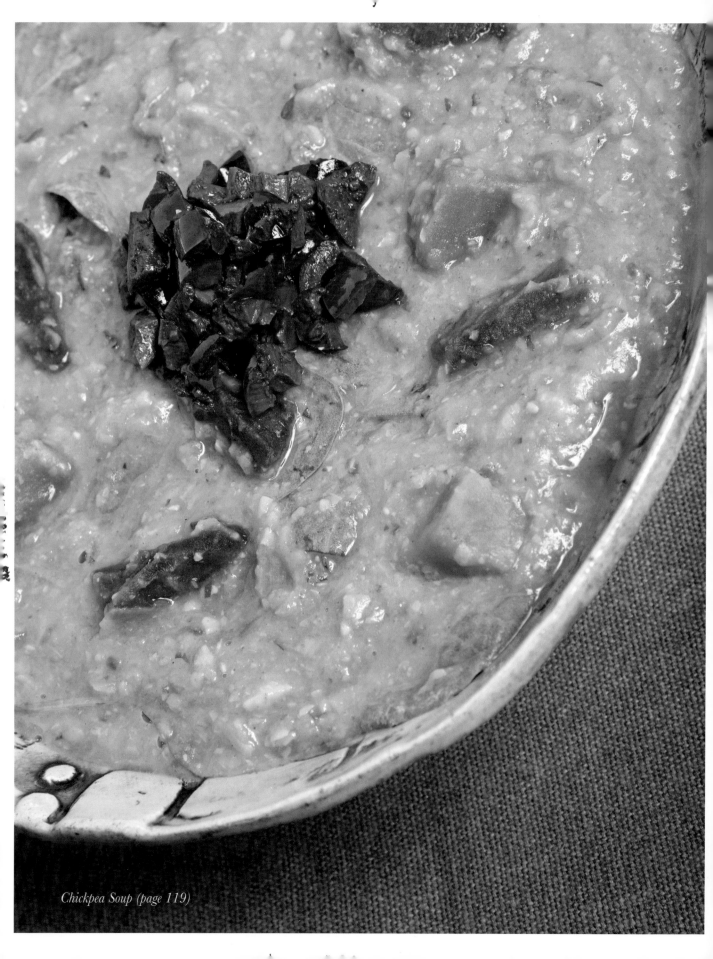

Chickpea Soup (page 119)

Cooking Legumes and the Dal Tradition

The soups built around legumes are grouped together in *Sacred & Delicious* because these require similar treatment for ease of digestion. Legumes are naturally filling and nutritious, so they serve well as a centerpiece for vegetarian meals. The legume family includes all manner of beans, such as black, kidney, navy, pinto, and lima beans, as well as lentils, peas, peanuts, and soybeans. Lesser known in the West are legumes classified as "grams," which include green gram (mung beans), their split yellow cousin (split mung), and black gram (urad dal). The grams, which are part of India's *dal* tradition, are smaller and generally easier to digest than the beans typically consumed in the United States.

Dal is the Sanskrit word for all varieties of dried legumes that are cooked with water and spice blends and served as soup. *Dal* is a distinct part of the cuisines of India, Pakistan, Nepal, Sri Lanka, and Bangladesh. *Dal* (sometimes spelled *dhal* or *dahl*) is typically served as a stand-alone soup, over basmati rice, or scooped up with flatbreads. Because dals are relatively inexpensive as well as nourishing and tasty, they are the heart of meals and are served once, twice, or three times a day in vegetarian homes throughout much of South Asia.

Mung and split mung (sometimes spelled *moong*), are considered the most essential foods in Ayurvedic cooking because they are easily digested proteins that are *tridoshic*, meaning they are good for almost everybody all the time. People who are not able to digest most beans (even when spiced properly) will typically find they can eat mung (especially the split variety) with perfect ease. From the Ayurvedic perspective, **this ease of digestion and relatively high protein value make mung the most important staple in a healthy vegetarian diet**.

Split mung dal, when seasoned correctly, is perhaps the easiest of all foods to digest, and for this reason, it is given to pregnant and nursing women as well as to patients recovering from illness or surgery. Split mung is also used as a staple food during *panchakarma*, the classic Ayurvedic therapy for eliminating toxins—which, according to Ayurveda, are a primary source of disease. Whole mung soup is also part of the Ayurvedic regimen because it, too, is a naturally detoxifying agent and is also easy to digest for most people.

All *dals* and legumes are more easily digested with the aid of asafetida, black or brown mustard seeds, cumin, coriander, and turmeric as well as with the help of lots of fresh ginger and moderate amounts of garlic, if garlic is part of your diet. All of these spices pacify *vata*, the airy culprit that is poked by legumes.

Different regions of India favor other dals in their indigenous cooking, my favorite being *toor* (sometimes called *tuver*) from the region of Gujarat. While I have learned the art of cooking dal from some of my Indian "sisters," I have not adopted their liberal use of hot chilies. As mentioned earlier, traditional Ayurvedic cooking does not recommend the use of chilies, although they are now beloved throughout much of the world.

Soaking: Yes or No?

Most legumes are more easily digested if they're soaked for eight hours prior to cooking. The soaking reduces complex hard-to-digest sugars. It also renders the legumes better able to absorb the cooking liquid, which makes them softer, which in turn makes them more digestible. This is true regardless of the pot you use.

Soaking hard beans, especially black beans and garbanzos, can also shorten the cooking time by as much as half.

Here are a few exceptions I've found to the presoaking rule:

- If you buy fresh, organic split mung, it only requires soaking for one or two hours. It will cook within 20 to 25 minutes, depending on the quantity. It's available online at Banyan Botanicals.
- Avoid soaking red and green lentils before cooking, as they can become mushy.

Sorting, Soaking, Rinsing

As a first step, sort through the dried beans and pull out any pebbles you find. These are often harvested right along with the edible seeds. You can sort them on a countertop or sift through them a handful at a time as you pour each measured cup of beans into the soaking bowl.

After sorting the beans, cover them with cold water in a large bowl, one that will hold at least three times the volume of the beans. Pour the soaking water off and rinse the beans before cooking. This process not only reduces complex sugars that can cause flatulence, but also removes any silt that may have settled in the water.

You can rinse the legumes efficiently by pouring off the murky liquid through a strainer. Refill the bowl with water and pour again through the strainer—two or three times for hard beans. With certain dals, such as *toor* and split mung, you'll need to repeat this soaking step several times, continuing until the liquid becomes clear. As you're pouring off the liquid, give another careful look for pebbles or debris you may have missed.

Technical Cooking Tips

Here is a simple list of pointers for cooking various types of legumes.

- ◉ For greatest efficiency, cook hard legumes (such as garbanzo beans or *toor* dal) in a pressure cooker. They will be completely tender in half the time it would take in a soup pot.
- ◉ Hard beans and dals can be simmered for 1 to 2 hours in a good stainless steel pot on medium-low heat after bringing the liquid to a boil.
- ◉ Softer beans, such as kidney and mung beans can be successfully cooked in a slow cooker. However, all beans must be brought to a full boil and cooked at a boiling temperature for at least 10 minutes to avoid food poisoning. According to the FDA's *Bad Bug Book*, many beans have a toxic agent known as phytohaemagglutinin or PHA. This is most highly concentrated in red kidney beans. Outbreaks of the associated sickness most often occur with undercooked beans prepared in a slow cooker or oven-baked casserole. For this reason, only prepare beans in a slow cooker if it eventually brings food to a boil on high heat .
- ◉ It is best to cook the softer legumes, such as split mung beans and all lentils, in a regular stainless steel pot or slow cooker on medium-low heat. These legumes turn to mush in a pressure cooker.
- ◉ When the legume pot is on high heat, it can boil over easily because of the foamy froth created as the starch molecules expand. I like to remove the lid and skim the carb-rich foam off two or three times. Once the boiling settles down to a low simmer, it's safe to let the beans cook undisturbed.
- ◉ To cook beans more quickly, you can add salt to the soaking water, but the texture of the beans will be more mealy than creamy, according to food writer Harold McGee. For creamier beans, add salt when you're finishing the dish.

Cooking Directions by Type of Pot

In *Sacred & Delicious* recipes, you can follow these cooking directions with all hard beans, unless the recipe directs you otherwise.

IN A PRESSURE COOKER: Place the beans in the pot with cold water or, if the recipe calls for it, with soup stock. Seal the pressure cooker and place it on high heat until it reaches maximum pressure according to the manufacturer's directions. Turn off the heat on a gas stove; on an electric stove, gently move the pot to a cool spot on the stove and allow the pressure to release as the pot cools, about 15 minutes. Finally, open the cooker when safe according to the manufacturer's directions. (If you're in a hurry, some cookers can be safely placed under cold running water until the pressure releases, but check your manufacturer's directions before doing this.) When the cooker is opened, the beans should be tender, but if they are still tough, continue to cook the beans on medium heat covered, but without the seal.

IN A STAINLESS STEEL SOUP POT: Bring the beans to a boil in cold water or (if the recipe calls for it) in soup stock. Reduce the heat to medium or medium-low, and simmer the beans, covered, 1 to 2 hours (depending on your altitude and humidity and on how long the beans have been stored). As the beans cook, stir them occasionally. Cook until they are fully tender.

IN A SLOW COOKER: Place the beans into the slow cooker with cold water or, if the recipe calls for it, with the soup stock. Use 4 cups of liquid for every 1 cup of legumes in a slow cooker. If the recipe calls for a bay leaf, curry leaves, or a whole garlic clove, add these to the pot now. Cover the pot, and turn the slow cooker to a high heat for at least 1 hour and up to 5 hours. Then reduce the heat to low for the rest of the day or until the beans are completely tender. If at the end of the cooking time the beans seem to have too much liquid, take out the excess with a ladle before adding spices.

Be sure to sauté a recipe's onions and spices in a separate pan before adding them to the slow cooker or a standard pot—but do this only about a half hour before serving. When combining all the ingredients in cold water at the beginning of the cooking, the soup will taste flat. Also, the spices may burn if you add them too early in the cooking process.

Finishing Dal with Spice Mixtures

To finish your dal, you will be making what is called the *tarka* (also spelled *tadka* or called the *chaunk* or *thalimpu,* depending on which of the Indian languages is being spoken). The *tarka* is herbs and spices that have been sizzled in hot oil to release their full fragrance before being added to the pot of cooked legumes as a finishing touch. You can certainly use more spice than I call for in the recipes; I find, however, that most Americans are not accustomed to heating spices and are better served by the mild doses I suggest.

The *tarka* spices all aid digestion. These spices typically include asafetida (to help avoid flatulence), black mustard seeds, cumin, coriander, and turmeric. Turmeric also has antimicrobial powers that keep cooked foods fresher longer. Please note that gluten-free asafetida is not sold in American supermarkets or Indian grocers but can be found online.

Here are some tips about finishing your dal successfully:

- Look for a 1-quart stainless steel covered saucepan with a pour spout.
- Heat the ghee or oil on medium heat until it is hot.
- Add the black or dark-brown mustard seeds and cover immediately because they will pop. (Do not replace black or dark-brown mustard seeds with yellow.)
- Though many cookbooks suggest adding mustard seeds and cumin seeds at the same time, I've found it better to add the cumin seeds just after the mustard seeds stop popping because cumin burns easily. Remove the pot from the heat and while the oil is still hot, add the cumin seeds, and let them sizzle and become fragrant.
- Add any additional ground spices one at a time and let them simmer collectively for only 10 to 15 seconds before pouring them into your pot of hot legumes.

After you've poured the spice mixture into the larger pot, ladle some of the hot dal and its liquid back into the spice pot; then swirl the spice pot and pour this mixture with the spice residue into the larger pot of legumes. This will allow you to retrieve the full measure of spice.

BLACK BEAN SOUP WITH WINTER SQUASH

Preparation Time: 8 hours soaking, plus 1½ to 2 hours cooking (40 minutes active)
Serves 6 to 8

When you soak the beans and use the right spices, black bean soup is very satisfying and easier to digest than it might be otherwise. If you don't have soup stock, this soup will still sparkle with flavor.

3 cups dried black (turtle) beans

7 cups water

1 medium sweet or red onion

2½ tablespoons olive oil

⅛ teaspoon asafetida (optional)

5 large curry leaves (or substitute 1 fresh bay leaf but not curry powder!)

1 small butternut squash

1½ teaspoons ground cumin

1 teaspoon ground coriander

2 teaspoons freshly grated ginger

2 small cloves garlic, pressed

3 teaspoons Light Grey Celtic Sea Salt

Dash red pepper flakes or 1 small slice poblano pepper

MENU SUGGESTION

Serve with Quick Sautéed Asparagus (page 173), a dollop of Guacamole (page 219), or over basmati rice.

AYURVEDIC NOTE

Black beans are good for *pitta* and *kapha*. Along with garbanzo beans, black beans are among the most *vata*-increasing legumes—in other words, they are likely to cause flatulence. The longer you soak them prior to cooking, the easier they are to digest. The asafetida and other heating spices, such as the garlic, ginger, and red pepper flakes, help mitigate the beans' airy effect. Also, the winter squash is added to help balance the soup for *vata*.

(V) Double the garlic or ginger. Go easy on red pepper.

(P) Eliminate the red pepper flakes and, if you wish, serve with freshly ground black pepper instead. If you're sensitive to garlic, cook the whole clove in the pot for 10 to 15 minutes, then remove the garlic before puréeing

(S) Eliminate the red pepper flakes. Add a cup of chopped cilantro at the end of the recipe.

1. Soak the beans in cold water for 8 to 12 hours. After soaking, rinse the beans well and strain.

2. Cook the beans with water in a stainless steel pot or pressure cooker according to directions on pages 116 and 117. If using a pressure cooker, the beans will need to be cooked an additional 30 minutes or more on medium heat after the pressure releases.

3. While the beans are cooking, dice the onion. Heat 2 tablespoons of oil in a sauté pan on medium heat. Add the onion, asafetida, and curry leaves to the pan and sauté for 10 to 15 minutes, stirring occasionally, until most of the onion is uniformly golden and starting to brown. Reduce heat to medium-low and continue cooking another 10 to 15 minutes until the onion caramelizes more completely. When they are ready, remove from heat.

4. Peel and cut the squash into bite-sized cubes, 1½ to 2 cups. (If you end up with extra squash, save for a stir-fry or roast for a salad.)

5. When you can open the pressure cooker (or when the beans have cooked for an hour in a standard pot), check the beans for tenderness. If they are still hard, cook for another 30 minutes on medium heat; then add the squash to the pot. (If using poblano pepper, add the slice now.) Cover, and continue to cook until the beans and squash are completely tender.

6. Returning to the onions, return the pan to the burner on medium heat. When the pan is warm, add ½ tablespoon of oil along with the cumin and coriander, and stir for about a minute. Transfer the onions and spice mixture to the soup pot only when the beans and squash are completely tender. Ladle hot liquid from the soup into the spice pan and swirl to maximize the amount of spices you're able to collect from the pan.

7. Add the ginger, garlic, salt, and pepper flakes. If using poblano pepper, remove it now. Use a handheld immersion blender to purée about one-third of the beans, leaving the soup a little chunky.

LEGUMES

CHICKPEA SOUP

Preparation Time: 8 hours soaking, plus 1½ to 2 hours cooking
Serves 5 to 6

I first created this recipe for my blog; it was such a hit that I added it to these pages just before going to press. This is satisfying as a soup or stew—and either way it serves well as a one-course meal. Also, it's one soup that doesn't require stock, though if you have some homemade stock in the fridge, feel free to use it.

2 cups dried chickpeas

3 cups Easy Vegetable Soup Stock (page 90)

2 to 3 cups water

2½ to 3 cups cubed sweet potatoes (1 large potato)

1 cup diced shallots (2 large)

2 tablespoons olive oil or ghee

1 or 2 pinches asafetida (optional)

1 teaspoon ground cumin

1 teaspoon ground coriander

10 reconstituted sun-dried tomatoes, or 2 teaspoons of fresh lime

20 pitted kalamata olives, chopped finely

5 to 6 ounces baby spinach

Handful of chopped parsley

1 large clove garlic, minced or pressed

2 teaspoons freshly ground ginger

2 handfuls of chopped fresh basil

2 to 3 teaspoons Light Grey Celtic Sea Salt

Black pepper, to taste (optional)

AYURVEDIC NOTE

Chickpeas can be difficult to digest, so they must be cooked until quite tender. The asafetida, garlic, and ginger are all needed to aid digestion. If you react to nightshades, it's best to avoid the tomatoes, though the small amount in this recipe is balanced by the cumin.

V Omit or decrease tomatoes. Add 1 to 2 tablespoons of fresh lime juice.

P Omit or decrease tomatoes. Add 1 tablespoon of fresh lime juice.

K Add a dash of cayenne powder or red pepper flakes.

MENU SUGGESTION

Serve with Gluten-Free Whole Grain Bread (page 68).

1. Soak the chickpeas in cold water for 8 to 12 hours. After soaking, rinse the beans well and strain. Cook the peas with stock and water (or just water) according to the directions for a stainless steel pot or pressure cooker on pages 116 and 117. Use 5 cups of liquid for stew and 6 cups for soup.

2. Chop the sweet potatoes. The timing of adding these chopped potatoes to the chickpeas depends on your pot. For a pressure cooker, add them once you can open the cooker, and then cook on medium heat (unsealed) until the potatoes are tender. For a standard pot, add the potatoes after the chickpeas have cooked 1 hour and let them finish the last 15 minutes of cooking time together. For a slow cooker, steam the potatoes in a separate pot, and add them at the end.

3. Dice the shallots and sauté them in the olive oil or ghee on medium heat until they are uniformly golden and starting to brown. Add the asafetida, cumin, and coriander, and stir for about 30 seconds. Set aside until step 5.

4. Slice the tomatoes (use more or less, to your liking), and set them aside. Chop the olives and set aside.

5. Once the potatoes are tender, transfer the shallot mixture to the soup pot. Use an immersion blender to purée about half of the soup or stew. Then add the rest of the ingredients, except for the olives, and stir. (If you omit tomatoes, add lime now, starting with 1 teaspoon and adding more to taste.) Add another cup of water if you prefer a thinner soup. Adjust the salt to taste. Top each serving with a spoon or two of chopped olives.

(RECIPE PHOTO ON PAGE 114)

STEWED LENTILS

Preparation Time: 4 hours (40 minutes active)
Serves 4 to 6

This recipe comes from our friend Raffaella DiGiorgio and her mother, Serafina. They graciously shared the family recipe for this traditional slow-cooked dish from Puglia, the southern region of Italy. These simple ingredients allowed to simmer for 3 to 4 hours will make your finished meal molto buono—very good!

1 medium or large onion
2 cloves garlic
3 tablespoons olive oil
⅛ teaspoon asafetida (optional)
1 stalk celery
2 large carrots
2 cups uncooked green or brown lentils
3½ cups water
2 cups Easy Vegetable Soup Stock (page 90)
1 fresh bay leaf
1 large Yukon Gold potato
2 to 3 cups of fresh kale or chard
2 teaspoons Light Grey Celtic Sea Salt
Dash of red pepper flakes or freshly ground black pepper

COOK'S TIP: If you don't have any homemade stock available, start the recipe with 5½ cups of water.

AYURVEDIC NOTE

Brown lentils, white potatoes, and garlic are excellent for *kapha*, which is why it is such a natural dish for chilly autumn and early spring nights, the *kapha* times of year. They will increase *vata* as lentils and potatoes are dry, and potatoes and celery are naturally cooling. However, the onion, asafetida, garlic, and pepper are all heating, balancing this dish for all *doshas* when eaten on occasion.

V Use black pepper instead of the red pepper flakes. Omit the potato.

P Reduce the garlic to 1 clove. Use black pepper instead of the red pepper flakes.

K Replace the olive oil with sunflower oil. Omit the potato.

MENU SUGGESTION

This dish works well as a one-pot meal, but if you're serving company, I suggest adding either the Simple Green Salad (page 206) or the Quick Sautéed Asparagus (page 173) and Gluten-Free Whole Grain Bread, warmed (page 68).

1. Dice the onion and mince the garlic.

2. Heat the olive oil in a 6-quart soup pot on medium heat. Add the onion and asafetida to the pot, and sauté for 10 to 15 minutes, stirring occasionally, until the onions are almost uniformly golden.

3. While the onion sautés, dice the celery and carrots. Add these, along with the garlic to the onion. Cover and cook for about 10 more minutes, stirring once or twice, until the celery and carrots are tender and the onion is starting to brown. The onion should caramelize without burning.

4. Rinse the lentils in cold water a few times and strain, picking out stones and other debris. Add strained lentils to the soup pot with water, stock, and bay leaf. Cover and bring to a boil; then reduce heat to medium-low or low so that the lentils are just simmering. Simmer covered for 3 to 4 hours. While you should check the pot occasionally, do not stir. If you do, the lentils will get mushy.

5. After 2 hours, peel and dice the potato and add to the pot. Also clean the greens, hand-tear into bite-size pieces, and add to the soup. Stir the pot once. Continue to simmer for another hour or longer. You will know the lentils are ready when they become thick and are darkening, like gravy. Close to serving time, add salt to taste. Serve with a dash of red pepper flakes or a generous portion of freshly ground black pepper.

LEGUMES

FRESH PEA SOUP

Preparation Time: About 1 hour (45 minutes active)
Serves 4

One sure sign that winter is turning to spring is the arrival of fresh peas in the grocery store. I can never pass them up, even though they require some labor. I find that shelling them is well worth the effort, although this seems to be part of a lost culture. I hope you'll try it sometime, as the taste of frozen peas just can't compare. I shell the peas the night before, and then cooking is a cinch the next day.

3 cups freshly shelled English peas
1 leek bulb plus an inch of the light-green shank
2 stalks lemongrass
2 tablespoons ghee or coconut oil
1 pinch asafetida (optional)
½ teaspoon ground cumin
½ teaspoon ground coriander
2 tablespoons coconut flour
3 cups Easy Vegetable Soup Stock (page 90), heated
1 tablespoon Bragg Liquid Aminos
1 teaspoon Light Grey Celtic Sea Salt
1 large fresh bay leaf
5 whole cloves
3 large mint leaves
1 teaspoon freshly grated ginger
Freshly ground black pepper

COOK'S TIP: 1. If you can't find lemongrass, add a small splash of lime to each bowl when serving. **2.** It takes about 1 pound of peas in their pods to net 1 cup of shelled peas. I like to shell peas after dinner the night before, watching a romantic comedy. *Please* avoid tragedies and violence while preparing food!

AYURVEDIC NOTE
Fresh peas are excellent for *pitta* and *kapha*. They increase *vata* somewhat, but they are pacified by the asafetida and ginger.

 Add 1 clove pressed garlic.

MENU SUGGESTION
Serve with Oven Oven-Baked Sweet Potato Chips (page 198) and Simple Summer Squash (page 193).

1. Shell the peas; rinse and drain them. Dice the leek. Peel and discard a few of the outer layers of the lemongrass.

2. Heat 1 tablespoon of the ghee or oil in a 5- to 6-quart soup pot, on medium heat. Once the ghee is hot, add the asafetida. Reduce the heat to medium-low. Add leek to the pot and sauté for 10 to 15 minutes, stirring occasionally, until it is uniformly golden. Add cumin and coriander and stir.

3. Add the flour and stir with a whisk. Slowly add the hot stock to the pot a little at a time, whisking to keep lumps from forming. Once all the stock has been added to the pot, add the shelled peas, lemongrass stalks, Bragg's, and salt. (**Note:** If you are using a boxed or canned stock, taste the soup once it's finished, and add salt only as needed.) Bring to a gentle boil; then reduce the heat to medium-low, cover the pot, and simmer for 12 to 15 minutes until the peas are completely tender.

4. While the soup is coming to a boil, make a bouquet garni of bay leaf, cloves, and mint leaves by placing them in a cheesecloth bag. Add the bouquet to the pot. After the peas are tender, remove the bouquet and the lemongrass.

5. Peel and grate the ginger, and add it to the pot once the peas are tender. Purée the soup with a handheld immersion blender. Or transfer the vegetables and about a cup of the liquid to a food processor or blender, purée, and return the puréed mixture to the pot, mixing well with the remaining liquid. Serve with a little freshly ground pepper.

HEARTY SPLIT PEA AND ZUCCHINI SOUP

Preparation Time: 8 hours soaking, plus 1½ to 2 hours cooking (1½ hours active)

Serves 6

2 cups dried split peas

4 cups Easy Vegetable Soup Stock (page 90)

1 cup water

3 large carrots

2 medium or 1 large leek bulb plus an inch of the light-green shank

1 thin slice of poblano pepper (optional)

1 large clove garlic

10 to 12 Swiss chard or kale leaves

3 tablespoons ghee or coconut oil

2 medium zucchini

2 teaspoons freshly grated ginger

¼ cup tightly packed chopped Italian parsley

1 to 2 tablespoons Bragg Liquid Aminos

½ teaspoon black mustard seeds

⅛ teaspoon fenugreek seeds

⅛ teaspoon asafetida (optional)

5 large curry leaves (or substitute 1 fresh bay leaf—but not curry powder!)

¼ teaspoon garam masala

½ teaspoon ground turmeric

1 teaspoon ground cumin

1 teaspoon ground coriander

2 teaspoons Light Grey Celtic Sea Salt

Freshly ground black pepper

COOK'S TIP: If you don't have a pressure cooker, plan this soup for a weekend when you have the afternoon to let the split peas cook on the stove on medium heat for 1½ hours or more before you assemble the soup. If you do not have fresh stock available, this recipe works fine using only water.

AYURVEDIC NOTE

Split peas and white potatoes are excellent for *kapha* and *pitta*. These same foods increase *vata*, but all the spices in this recipe aid digestion, and their warmth is beneficial for *kapha* as well as *vata*. If you have blood sugar issues, omit white potatoes.

V Double the garlic. Omit white potato and replace with chopped Swiss chard.

P If you're sensitive to garlic, cook the clove whole and remove it before serving or puréeing. Also, omit the poblano pepper, or cook the slice whole with the vegetables and remove it before serving.

K Double the garlic.

MENU SUGGESTION

Serve with Gluten-Free Whole Grain Bread (page 68) or Our Daily Bread (page 67).

1. Soak split peas in cold water for 8 hours. After soaking, rinse them well a few times until the water is clear, and then strain them. Cook the split peas with stock and water according to directions on pages 116 and 117, about 20 minutes in a pressure cooker and 1½ hours in a regular pot.

2. While the split peas are simmering, wash and slice the carrots and slice the leeks. Mince the slice of poblano pepper and the garlic clove. Rinse the Swiss chard and slice the stems like celery; then stack the leaves and chop them into 2- or 3-inch pieces.

3. In a small sauté pan, heat 1½ tablespoons of ghee or oil on medium heat. Add the leeks to the pan and cook for about 10 minutes, stirring occasionally, until they turn uniformly golden. In the last few minutes before the leeks are golden, add the minced garlic. Once the leeks are done, remove the pan from the heat.

4. When you can open the pressure cooker or the split peas are close to tender in a regular pot, add the leeks, carrots, and chard or kale. Continue cooking on medium heat, without the pressure cooker seal, about 15 minutes or until the vegetables are tender.

5. Slice the zucchini, peel and grate the ginger, and chop the parsley. Once the carrots are almost tender, add the zucchini, ginger, and parsley to the pot with 1 tablespoon Bragg's. Cook about 7 more minutes until the zucchini is also tender.

6. While the zucchini is cooking, heat 1½ tablespoons ghee or oil in a small saucepan on medium heat. When the ghee is hot, add the mustard seeds and cover until the seeds pop like popcorn. When the seeds finish popping, add the fenugreek seeds, asafetida, and curry leaves (or bay leaf); cover in case the oil splatters; and reduce heat to low (or remove the pan from an electric burner). Uncover and add garam masala, turmeric, cumin, coriander, and poblano pepper. Swirl the pan for a few seconds; then pour the spice mixture into the soup pot. Ladle some hot liquid from the soup into the sauce-pan and swirl again to maximize the amount of spices you're able to retrieve from the pan.

7. Add salt and more Bragg's to taste. (**Note:** If you are using a boxed or canned stock, add salt only as needed.) Add more water or stock if you prefer a thinner soup. Serve with a generous portion of black pepper in each bowl. For a more refined dish, you may wish to purée the soup with a handheld immersion blender before serving.

Hindu Blessing

Om brahmarpanam brahma havir
Brahmagnau brahmana hutam
Brahmaiva tena ghantavyam
Brahmakarma samadhinaâ

The act of offering is Brahman.
The offering itself is Brahman.
The offering is done by Brahman
in the sacred fire which is Brahman.
He alone attains Brahman who, in all actions,
is fully absorbed in Brahman.

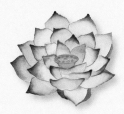

SMOKY WHITE BEAN SOUP

Preparation Time: 8 hours soaking, plus 1½ to 2 hours cooking (1½ hours active)
Serves 4

Campbell's Bean with Bacon Soup was a standard in our house for a quick winter Saturday lunch when I was growing up, and I tried to capture the essence of this hearty fare with a vegetarian recipe. Admittedly, Smoky White Bean Soup is not a quick version and may best be saved for a weekend cooking project. If you have the luxury of time, start the soup early enough in the day that you can let it sit on low heat for another hour after it has been assembled. The longer the flavors mingle, the better.

2 cups dried northern white or navy beans
5 cups water
1 to 2 teaspoons smoked salt
1 medium onion
1 stalk celery
2 carrots
1 clove garlic, minced
2 tablespoons ghee or coconut oil
1 teaspoon black mustard seeds
⅛ teaspoon asafetida (optional)
5 large curry leaves (optional—that's *leaves*, not powder!)
1 teaspoon ground cumin
1 teaspoon ground coriander
½ teaspoon ground turmeric
1 medium tomato
1 teaspoon freshly grated ginger
1 tablespoon fresh thyme (or 1 teaspoon dried)
1 tablespoon fresh dill (or 1 teaspoon dried)
1 teaspoon mild paprika
1 to 2 cups Easy Vegetable Soup Stock (page 90)
1 large fresh bay leaf
2 tablespoons Bragg Liquid Aminos
Freshly ground black pepper

COOK'S TIP: Try Artisan Salt Company's Salish Smoked Salt.

AYURVEDIC NOTE

On the plus side, white beans will reduce *pitta* and *kapha*. However, beans and tomatoes will increase *vata*. Asafetida, garlic, ginger, and onions, aid digestion to help balance *vata*. Cumin is the antidote for the tomato's acidity, which increases *pitta*, and coriander also balances *pitta*.

P If you're sensitive to garlic, cook the clove whole and remove it in step 7. Reduce mustard seeds by half.

MENU SUGGESTION

Serve with Wilted Baby Spinach (page 195) and Corn Bread (page 71).

1. Soak the beans in cold water 8 to 12 hours. After soaking, rinse the beans well, and strain them.

2. Cook the beans with water and salt according to directions (pages 116–117), about 20 minutes in a pressure cooker, and 1½ hours in a regular soup pot or until the beans are tender.

3. While the beans are cooking, dice the onion, celery, and carrots. Mince the garlic.

4. In a separate 3-quart or larger soup pot, heat the ghee or coconut oil on medium heat. When the ghee is hot, add the mustard seeds and cover until the seeds pop like popcorn. Add the asafetida and curry leaves and, again, quickly cover in case the oil splatters. Uncover and add the diced onion to the pan and sauté for 10 to 15 minutes, until it is almost uniformly golden and starting to brown.

5. Add the carrots and celery to the onion. Cover the pot to cook the vegetables for about 10 minutes—or until they are tender and the onions are caramelizing. Then add the garlic, cumin, coriander, and turmeric. Stir for about a minute and remove from heat.

6. While the vegetables sauté, chop the tomato. (If you wish, remove the seeds before chopping.) Peel and grate the ginger. Add the tomato, ginger, thyme, dill, paprika, and ¼ cup soup stock to the vegetable pot. (If you are using a whole clove of garlic vs. minced—see ⓟ in Ayurvedic Note—add it now.) Cover and simmer until the tomatoes are cooked. Remove from heat.

7. When the beans are tender, drain and rinse twice in cold water, and then drain them again. Return all but 2 cups of the beans to the bean pot or pressure cooker, and add the 2 cups beans to the sautéed vegetable pot. Purée the vegetables and beans (but not a whole garlic clove—see ⓟ in Ayurvedic Note) with a handheld immersion blender. If you do not own this device, let the mixture cool and purée it in a food processor.

8. Transfer the purée to the bean pot. Add 1 cup vegetable stock, bay leaf, and Bragg Liquid Aminos. (**Note:** If you are using a boxed or canned stock, taste first, and add Bragg's only as needed.) If you'd like a thinner soup, add more stock. Cover and reheat. Serve with freshly ground black pepper.

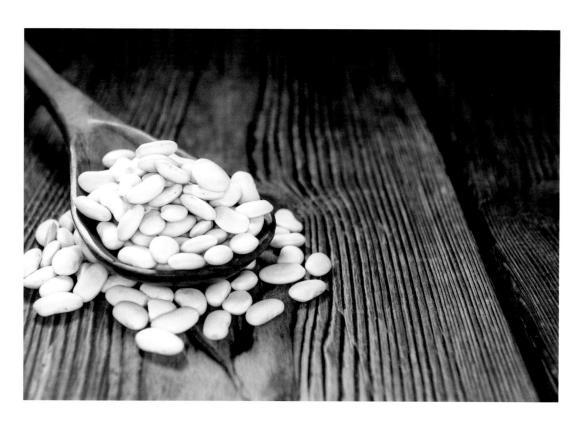

CLASSIC SPLIT MUNG DAL

Preparation Time: 1 to 8 hours soaking, plus ½ hour to 1 hour cooking
Serves 2 to 4

Split mung dal is the easiest of the dals to make because it cooks quickly and does not require a pressure cooker. Traditionally, dal is served as soup or over basmati rice. This particular recipe is inspired by my friend Alka Singh, an altogether remarkable cook, who adds some browned onions to her dal for a flavor that hails from North India.

1 cup split-mung dal
3 cups water
1 small onion (optional)
2½ tablespoons ghee or coconut oil
¼ teaspoon black mustard seeds
½ teaspoon cumin seeds
1 pinch asafetida (optional)
3 curry leaves (or substitute 1 fresh bay leaf—
**   but not curry powder)**
¼ teaspoon ground turmeric
½ teaspoon ground coriander
½ to 1 teaspoon freshly grated ginger
1 teaspoon Light Grey Celtic Sea Salt
A handful or 2 of fresh cilantro, chopped
1 tablespoon unsweetened shredded coconut (optional)

COOK'S TIP: See the sidebar "Split Mung: The Occasional Bad Batch" (page 127) for recommendations about purchasing and soaking split mung dal.

AYURVEDIC NOTE

This dish is *tridoshic*, meaning it is good for *vata*, *pitta*, and *kapha*. The spices aid digestion and balance each other. Split mung dal spiced mildly, as it is in this recipe, is one of the best healing dishes on the planet, according to Ayurvedic literature and masters.

V Increase ginger.

K Increase ginger and avoid coconut.

MENU SUGGESTION

Serve with Simple Toasted Millet (page 160), or Indian Rice with Cashews (page 163), and Savory Cauliflower and Carrots (page 185).

1. Rinse the dal until the water comes clear; then strain the dal and place it in a soup pot with 3 cups of water. Cover and bring to a gentle boil; then reduce heat to medium-low and simmer, covered, for 20 to 40 minutes (depending on the quality of the dal). Cook it until the dal is completely tender. As the starch creates foam during the first 15 minutes, skim this from the top of the pot with a large spoon two or three times to avoid the pot's boiling over. Stir often until the cooking is finished, as this dal has a tendency to stick to the bottom of the pot.

2. While the dal is simmering, dice the onion. Heat 1½ tablespoons of ghee or oil in a sauté pan on medium heat. Add the onion to the pan and sauté for 10 to 15 minutes, stirring occasionally, until the onion is almost uniformly golden and starting to brown. Reduce the heat to medium-low and continue cooking the onion another 10 to 15 minutes until it caramelizes more completely.

3. When the dal is close to tender, prepare the *tarka*: In a small saucepan, heat 1 tablespoon of ghee or oil on medium heat. When the ghee is hot, add the mustard seeds and cover until the seeds pop like popcorn. When the seeds finish popping, add the cumin seeds, cover, and remove from heat to prevent the seeds from burning. After the cumin seeds sizzle and become fragrant, add asafetida and curry leaves (if using), and quickly cover, in case the oil splatters. Add the turmeric and coriander. Swirl the spices in the pan for a few seconds to mix them, and then add the *tarka* to the soup pot. Ladle some hot liquid from the soup into the *tarka* pan and swirl again to maximize the amount of spices you're able to retrieve from the pan.

4. Add the sautéed onion, grated ginger, and salt. Add some cilantro to each serving. The shredded coconut may be added for a sweet taste. Serve as a soup or over brown or white basmati rice.

Dal Variations

You can make many interesting variations of the Classic Split Mung Dal and *Kitchari*. For instance, I like to add diced sweet potato or winter squash to the dal as it comes to a boil to sweeten the mixture. I also add sliced zucchini and/or 1 to 2 cups of baby spinach, shredded Swiss chard, or kale in the last 10 minutes of cooking time. You can add any vegetables you like. Use leftover soup stock to deepen the flavors, and mix it up a bit with familiar American herbs such as fresh basil.

Clarification of Indian Spice Terms

Many Indian dishes, especially dals, are cooked with layered spices called the *tarka* (or the *tadka*, *chaunk,* and other terms from the many languages of India). These all mean "tempering," the common Indian practice of briefly sautéing whole spices and other ingredients (which can include chopped onion, ginger, sugar, etc.) in hot ghee to release their essential oils and enhance their fragrance and flavor. The sautéed ingredients, with their cooking oil, are then added to a dish as the final step in its preparation.

Two other common spice terms from India—*masala* and *curry*—have been explained in varied and sometimes conflicting ways. Both names are given to dried spice mixtures in which whole spices have been roasted and then ground to a powder. These can be stored in a cupboard for two or three months before losing their freshness and potency.

The masala (mixture) or garam masala (heating mixture) is a combination of several warming spices—often dried chilies, coriander seeds, cumin seeds, cardamom seeds, cinnamon stick, whole cloves, and fennel—roasted, ground together, and then added, usually at the end of the cooking process.

The Anglicized term *curry*—which comes from the Tamil word *kari*, meaning "sauce"—properly means the gravy-like sauce that includes a complex mélange of as many as twenty ground spices: most of the masala spices as well as turmeric, tamarind, saffron, peppercorns, curry leaves, and/or a number of others. The spices are mixed with water in the dish to make a sauce—hence the name.

Traditional masala and curry spice mixtures are made from scratch by roasting and grinding fresh spices, and every Indian family seems to have their own special blend with its own unique flavor. When you buy a commercial jar of masala or curry powder, you are getting a particular blend of spices. Though I prefer to hand-select spices for the dishes I prepare, I keep a small jar of both curry and garam masala powders in my pantry for those times when I need to cook quickly or a little extra "fire power" is called for at the last minute.

Split Mung: The Occasional Bad Batch

High-quality split mung dal found in Indian stores can be soaked for several hours and still maintain a perfect consistency when cooked, so you can put it on to soak when you leave the house for the day, and it will be primed for cooking when you return. Split mung also remains easily digestible if soaked only 1 hour before cooking, so you can use it without as much planning as you may need for other dals.

The exception is when the split mung is inferior in quality, which sometimes occurs for mung that was farmed in drought conditions. This can happen with other legumes as well, but it is more common with split mung. These legumes simply do not cook.

I have purchased bags of split mung that will not cook through, even if simmered two hours, despite soaking for several hours. For this reason, and to ensure high quality, I've begun purchasing an organic split dal online that is always edible when cooked, and does not need to be soaked. See banyanbotanicals.com.

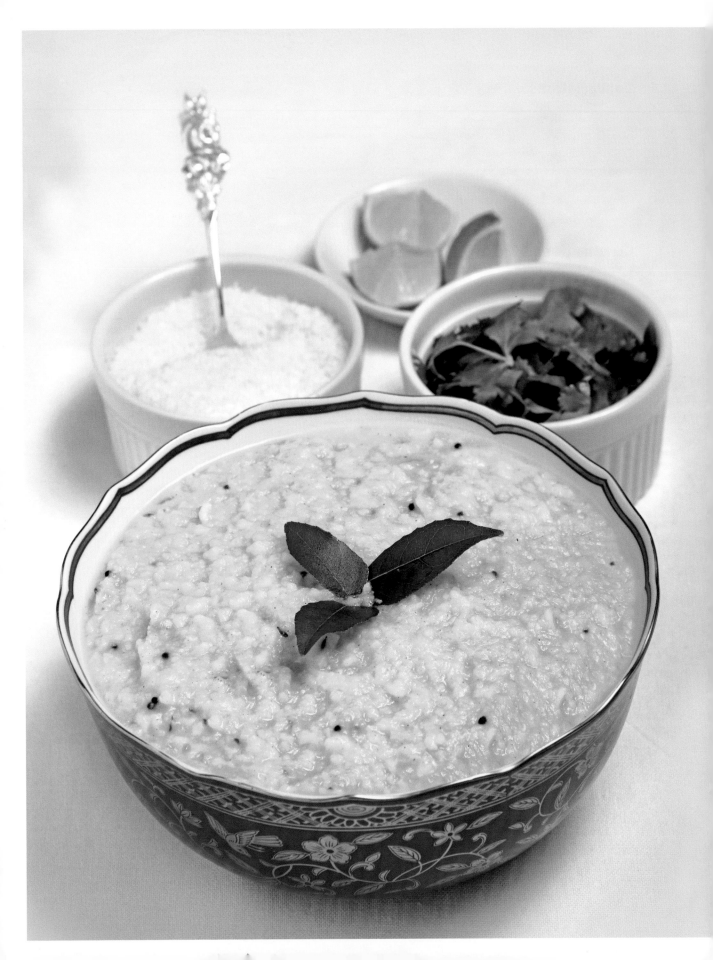

KITCHARI

Preparation Time: 30 minutes
Serves 5 to 6

No cookbook based on Ayurveda would be complete without a recipe for kitchari, *which is sometimes called kitchadi. A combination of split mung dal and rice,* kitchari *is completely satisfying and, at the same time, it allows the body to heal and detoxify. This combination of qualities makes* kitchari *Ayurveda's quintessential comfort food in the best sense of the term. Whenever my digestion is off or I feel unwell for other reasons, I often turn to* kitchari *to help settle my stomach and my mind. Traditional* kitchari *recipes have a 1:1 ratio of dal and rice. Because I've had blood sugar problems, I have developed this recipe with a 2:1 ratio to lower the carbohydrate count.*

2 cups yellow split mung dal

9 cups water

2 teaspoons Light Grey Celtic Sea Salt

1 fresh bay leaf or 3 curry leaves

1 cup uncooked California organic white basmati rice

2 tablespoons ghee or sunflower oil

½ teaspoon black mustard seeds

1 teaspoon cumin seeds

¾ teaspoon ground turmeric

½ teaspoon ground cinnamon

1 teaspoon ground coriander

7 whole cardamom pods (or ½ teaspoon ground cardamom)

2 tablespoons shredded unsweetened coconut (optional)

1 teaspoon freshly grated ginger

Cilantro for garnish

COOK'S TIP: Use 2 cups split mung, 1 cup brown basmati rice, and 9 cups water if you have diabetes or insulin resistance. Also, *kitchari* develops a skin as it cools. This can, however, be stirred back into the rice with additional water to bring it to the desired thickness once again.

AYURVEDIC NOTE

Kitchari is considered *tridoshic*, meaning it is good for most people any time. It is easy to digest, gives strength and vitality, and is considered a complete food that is high in protein.

(P) Reduce the mustard seeds to ¼ teaspoon or omit altogether.

(K) Eliminate the coconut and reduce the ghee to 1 tablespoon. Double the ginger.

(W) Eliminate the coconut.

MENU SUGGESTION
Serve with Roasted Veggies (page 199) or Easy Winter Squash (page 194).

DALS

1. Soak the split mung dal in water for 2 to 8 hours. Prior to cooking, rinse the dal until the water is clear. Strain the dal and place it in a soup pot with the water, salt, and bay leaf or curry leaves on high heat. Once it comes to a boil, reduce heat to medium-low. Rinse and add the rice, and continue to simmer, covered, for 20 to 30 minutes altogether (depending on the freshness of the dal).

2. In the first 15 minutes, the starch in the dal will create foam; skim this from the top of the pot with a large spoon two or three times to avoid the pot boiling over. Stir the soup often until it's finished cooking, as this dal tends to stick to the bottom of the pot.

3. If using vegetables (see Dal Variations on page 127), prepare them and add them to the pot after the first 15 minutes. If using spinach, you can add this in the last 5 minutes, just before making the *tarka*.

4. After the vegetables are tender and the dal and rice are soft, prepare the *tarka*: In a small saucepan, heat the ghee or oil on medium heat. When the ghee is hot, add the mustard seeds, and cover until the seeds pop like popcorn. When the seeds finish popping, add the cumin seeds, cover, and turn off the gas (or remove the pan from an electric burner) to prevent the seeds from burning. Let the cumin seeds sizzle and become fragrant, and add the turmeric, cinnamon, coriander, and cardamom pods. Swirl the spices in the pan for a few seconds and add the *tarka* to the soup pot. Ladle some hot liquid from the soup into the *tarka* pan and swirl again to maximize the amount of spices you're able to retrieve from the pan.

5. The finished dish will be like a thick porridge. If you prefer, you can add some water to make it thinner. Add ginger. Add salt to taste. Garnish with coconut and cilantro.

MUNG SOUP

Preparation Time: 8 hours soaking, plus ½ hour to 8 hours cooking (20 minutes active)
Serves 6 to 8

I tasted this divinely spiced bean soup on my first trip to India in 2004. While there, I spent five weeks in the Ayushakti pancha-karma clinic established by Drs. Pankaj and Smita Naram on the outskirts of Mumbai. Housed in the clinic is a lovely restaurant that serves a bountiful menu of delicious and healing recipes, including this one, which was developed by Dr. Smita Naram.

Dr. Naram is an accomplished Ayurvedic physician, known in India as a vaidya. A pulse master, pharmaceutical herbalist, and educator, she excels equally in the art of Ayurvedic cuisine. I've been especially impressed with the way she seasons food without overwhelming the senses. In fact, the traditional Ayurvedic cooking that she practices does not favor the hot chilies that are used so liberally by most modern Indian cooks.

2 cups whole green mung beans

7 to 9 cups water

1 large fresh bay leaf or 3 curry leaves (not curry powder!)

2 tablespoons ghee or sunflower oil

½ teaspoon black mustard seeds

1 pinch asafetida (optional)

1 teaspoon ground cumin

1 teaspoon ground turmeric

1 teaspoon ground coriander

⅛ teaspoon garam masala

2 teaspoons freshly grated ginger

1 large garlic clove, pressed (optional)

2 to 2½ teaspoons Light Grey Celtic Sea Salt

½ cup freshly chopped cilantro

Lime wedges (1 for each serving)

COOK'S TIP: If mung beans are soaked in advance for several hours, they can be cooked successfully in about 20 minutes with a pressure cooker or 1 hour in a regular soup pot. The beans have a distinct and lovely flavor, however, when cooked 7 to 8 hours in a slow cooker.

AYURVEDIC NOTE

Whole mung beans are one of Ayurveda's preferred foods for detoxification. If you need to lose weight, mung soup is a safe food for dieting when combined with vegetables. Whole mung is classified as *tridoshic*, meaning it's good for all *doshas*. I find, however, that whole mung increases *kapha* if I have a cold or cough. All of the spices support digestion.

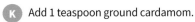 **(P)** Increase the ginger and omit the garlic. Replace garam masala with ⅛ teaspoon cinnamon.

(K) Add 1 teaspoon ground cardamom.

MENU SUGGESTION
Serve with Sweet and Savory Quinoa with Carrots (page 161), Smoky Swiss Chard (page 201), or Elegant Green Beans (page 186)

1. If you're using a slow cooker, rinse the beans, strain them, and place them in the cooker with the water. If the beans were soaked for 8 hours, start with 7 cups of water; otherwise, use 8 cups. Turn the cooker on the high setting for 5 to 6 hours. If you are at home, you can reduce the heat to low once you see the beans start to split. If you're going to be away from the cooker for 7 hours or longer, start with 8 cups of water and keep the cooker on high until you return.

If you're cooking mung beans in a pressure cooker or standard pot on the stove, soak them for 8 hours before cooking. Rinse the beans well before cooking, and start with 6 cups of water. Add more water at the end, if you like a thinner soup.

2. About 30 minutes before serving the soup, add the bay leaf (if using) and coconut sugar.

3. At this point prepare the *tarka*. In a small saucepan, heat the ghee or oil on medium heat. When the oil is hot, add the mustard seeds and cover until the seeds pop like popcorn. Turn off the gas (or remove the pan from an electric burner) to prevent the seeds from burning. If using curry leaves, add them to the hot oil. Add the asafetida, cumin, turmeric, coriander, and garam masala. Swirl the spices in the pan for a few seconds to mix, and then pour the mixture into the soup pot. Ladle some hot liquid from the soup into the *tarka* pan and swirl again to maximize the amount of spices you're able to retrieve from the *tarka* pan.

4. Add fresh ginger and garlic. Add salt to taste and stir well. Add more water if you prefer a thinner consistency. Serve each bowl with a small handful of cilantro and a wedge of lime.

(RECIPE PHOTO ON PAGE 112)

DALS

FAVORITE *TOOR* DAL

Preparation Time: 8 hours soaking, plus 45 minutes cooking (20 minutes active)
Serves 2 to 4

This is my favorite dal recipe, and I learned to cook it from my friend Alpa Bhatt, an Ayurvedic physician from Gujarat state in India. I met Alpa in the years she lived in North Carolina, when she generously offered to be my first Ayurvedic cooking mentor. Her native Gujarati cuisine subtly combines sweet and sour tastes along with pungent Indian spices to create distinctive and enticing dishes.

Although toor *dal is often served over basmati rice, my favorite way to eat it is as a simple soup with vegetable side dishes. As a note on the amounts, if you're serving this as a soup, the 1 cup dried dal will fill only 2 or 3 bowls. If you ladle the cooked dal over rice, however, this same 1 cup of dried dal will feed up to 4.*

1 cup *toor* dal (also known as split pigeon peas)
3 cups water
1 tablespoon ghee or sunflower oil
½ teaspoon black mustard seeds
½ teaspoon cumin seeds
2 pinches asafetida (optional)
1 pinch fenugreek seeds
3 to 5 fresh curry leaves (not curry powder!)
½ teaspoon finely chopped poblano pepper (optional)
¼ teaspoon ground turmeric
½ teaspoon ground coriander
1 to 2 teaspoons coconut sugar or lump of jaggery
1½ teaspoons Light Grey Celtic Sea Salt
1 teaspoon freshly grated ginger
½ cup freshly chopped cilantro
1 to 2 tablespoons fresh lime juice

COOK'S TIP: *Toor* dal will not become tender in a slow cooker, even if you cook it on high for 8 hours. If you don't have a pressure cooker, prepare this soup in a standard soup pot.

AYURVEDIC NOTE

Although *toor* dal is excellent for *vata* and *kapha* types, it should not be eaten more than once a week by people with *pitta* constitutions or *pitta* problems.

P Eliminate the poblano pepper or cook a slice in the spices and remove the slice from the pot before serving. Also reduce the black mustard seeds to ¼ teaspoon. Avoid jaggery, which is heating.

S Eliminate the poblano pepper, or eat this soup only once or twice a month.

MENU SUGGESTION

Serve with Gujarati Green Beans (page 187) and Simple Toasted Millet (page 160), or serve over basmati rice.

1. Soak the dal in cold water for 8 to 12 hours. Prior to cooking, rinse the dal several times until the water becomes clear; then strain it.

2. Cook the dal with the water and salt according to directions (pages 116–117), about 20 minutes in a pressure cooker and 45 minutes in a regular pot.

3. Prepare the *tarka*: In a small saucepan, heat the ghee or oil on medium heat. When the ghee is hot, add the mustard seeds and cover until the seeds pop like popcorn. When the seeds finish popping, add the cumin seeds, and turn off the gas (or remove the pan from an electric burner) to prevent the seeds from burning. After the cumin seeds sizzle and become fragrant, add asafetida and fenugreek seeds. Add the curry leaves and quickly cover, in case the oil splatters. Return the pan to low heat, add the poblano pepper, and sauté about two minutes. Add the turmeric and coriander. Swirl the spices in the pan for a few seconds to mix, and then pour mixture into the soup pot. Ladle some hot liquid from the soup into the *tarka* pan and swirl again to maximize the amount of spices you're able to retrieve from the pan.

4. Add the coconut sugar to the soup pot along with the ginger and salt to taste. Stir well. If the soup is too thick for your taste, add more water. Finish the soup by adding cilantro and lime to the pot or to the individual servings.

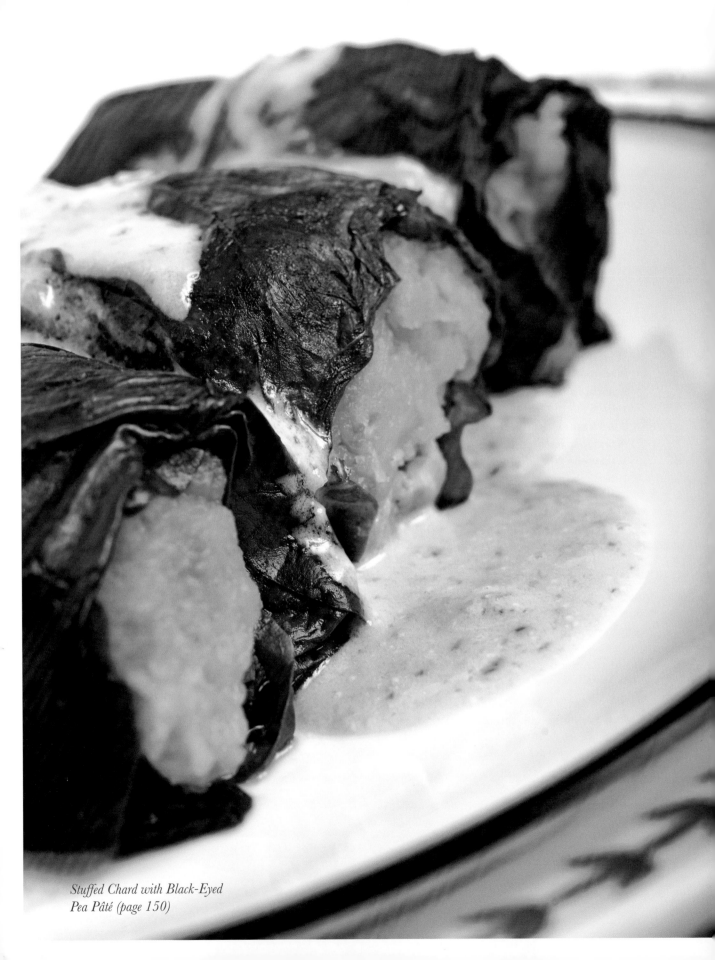

Stuffed Chard with Black-Eyed Pea Pâté (page 150)

CHAPTER 8.

Entrées

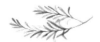

Love your loved ones—the people, the vegetables—as much as you can.
You never know if this is the last of them for you. Eat all the asparagus.

⌒ Bethany Jean Clement

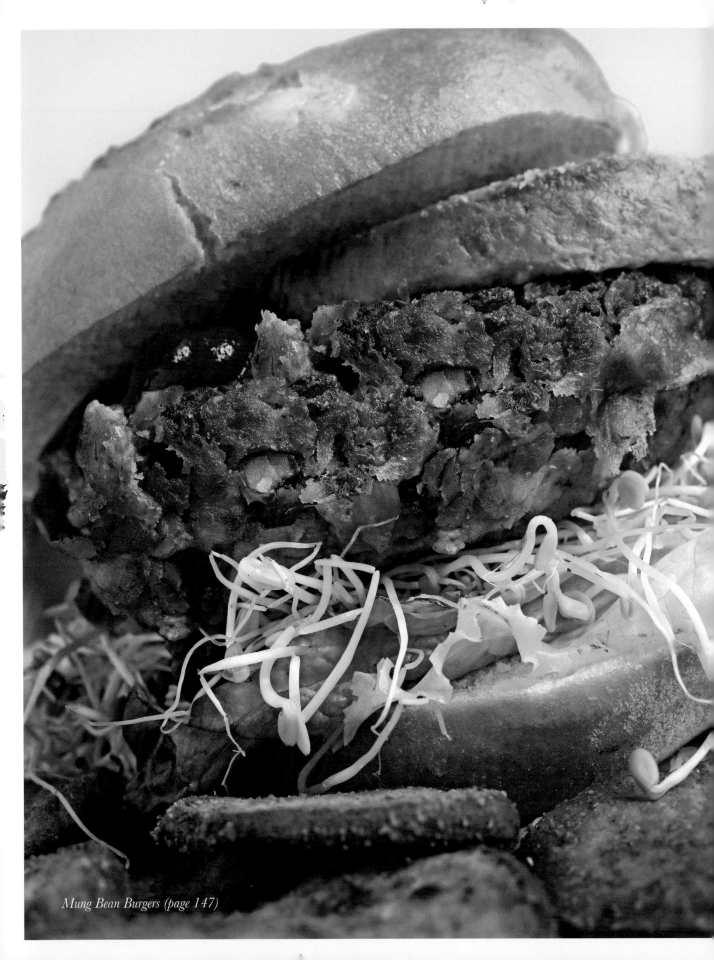

Mung Bean Burgers (page 147)

A Vegetarian Approach to Entrées

The term *entrée* has come to mean many different things depending on culture, climate, and individual food preferences. Typically, North Americans think of an entrée as a large hunk of meat or fish on a plate surrounded by a couple of side dishes—perhaps rice or potatoes and a green vegetable. In French cuisine the entrée either precedes the main course or is served between two other courses of a meal. For instance, a mushroom-cheese tart might be served as an entrée after a small piece of fish and before the roast!

Traditional Ayurvedic cooking has no entrée. Rather, there are several small servings of various foods at both the noon and evening meal. Each of the foods is served in a small dish or bowl, about a half-cup in size. In an Indian restaurant this kind of meal is called a *thali*, the Hindi word for "plate." You're served a large, often metal, plate holding bowls of, usually, a *dal* (like a lentil soup), a vegetable soup, one or two vegetable dishes (such as roasted squash and cauliflower), and a sweet (like *khir,* rice pudding) as well as a serving of basmati rice and some sort of flatbread. Naturally, a meal like this requires many hands and many hours to prepare.

Modern vegetarian households often serve one-dish meals—particularly legume-based soups or stews that bring together protein and vegetables—because they are so efficient to make. Many days a simple legume-based soup with vegetables will serve as the centerpiece of our meal, accompanied by a salad or grain dish. On occasion, though, you may want to feature a main dish, something like eggplant Parmesan or a veggie stir-fry, and this is what I'm calling an "entrée."

In *Sacred & Delicious* entrées include a legume-based "burger," a potpie, pasta loaded with vegetables, a risotto, stuffed chard leaves, and a spaghetti squash boat filled with black-eyed peas and vegetables that have been smothered in a rich tahini sauce—yum! Such entrées can serve as the centerpiece of a meal and need only a side salad to make dinner an impressive occasion.

Of course, some of these dishes require more time and labor than you might want to invest during the workweek, so I've divided the entrées into two groups, based on how much time will be needed. **Weekday Entrées** can be whipped up in 30 minutes to an hour; **Weekend and Special Occasions** recipes may take up to 2 hours. A recipe for veggie burgers that takes about 90 minutes is ideal for a Sunday afternoon, when you're cooking ahead with a couple of lunches in mind. And remember, pull out your pressure cooker if you're cooking hard beans. It will cut your cooking time in half!

RED BEANS AND RICE

Preparation Time: 8 hours soaking, plus 45 minutes to 8 hours cooking (30 minutes active)
Serves 6 to 8

Beans and rice make an excellent vegetarian entrée because, when served together, they provide protein, iron, and all the essential amino acids. You may wish to serve the kidney beans and spice mixture as a separate side dish without the rice.

3 cups dried kidney beans or red chana dal
4 to 12 cups water (See Cook's Tip)
3 to 4 cups Easy Vegetable Soup Stock (page 90, optional)
1 fresh bay leaf
5 fresh curry leaves (optional)
1 medium or large onion, chopped
2 thin slices poblano pepper, diced or whole (optional)
2 tablespoons olive or coconut oil
⅛ teaspoon asafetida (optional)
1½ teaspoons ground cumin
¾ teaspoon ground turmeric
1½ teaspoons ground coriander
3 tablespoons freshly chopped basil (or 1 tablespoon dried)
1 tablespoon fresh oregano leaves (or 1 teaspoon dried)
2 teaspoons freshly ground ginger
2 cloves garlic
1 tablespoon Celtic Sea Salt
1½ cups cooked basmati rice, white or brown (¾ cup dry)
Lime wedges

COOK'S TIP: 1. Cook the kidney beans in a slow cooker with 12 cups of liquid for several hours, but make sure they come to a boil for 10 minutes. **2.** If cooking the beans in a pressure cooker or a regular pot on a stove, use a total of 8 cups of liquid—either 8 cups of water or a mixture of water and stock. **3.** If fresh soup stock is not available, this dish will still taste delicious cooked with only water.

AYURVEDIC NOTE

Kidney beans pacify *pitta* and, when soaked and correctly spiced, may be tolerated by *vata*. They will increase *kapha* and should be avoided if you have a cold or cough.

P Omit poblano pepper or cook whole strips of poblano in the pan with the onions to flavor the oil and then remove them before serving. Also, if you're sensitive to garlic, cook the clove whole with the beans, and remove it before serving.

K Add a dash of cayenne pepper.

MENU SUGGESTION

Serve with Sautéed Okra (page 189) or Smoky Swiss Chard (page 201).

1. Soak the beans in cold water for 8 hours, then rinse them well and strain before cooking.

2. When ready to cook the beans, place them in a slow cooker with 4 cups stock (if available), plus 8 cups water, bay leaf, and curry leaves. If you have an herb bag, you can place the bay leaf and curry leaves in the bag so they are easier to remove before serving; otherwise, place them directly in the water. Turn the cooker to high. The beans can cook on high for several hours in a slow cooker, or if you are home, reduce the heat to low once the beans are tender.

If using a regular pot, bring the beans and liquid to a boil; then reduce heat to medium, add the bay leaf and curry leaves, and simmer covered until the beans are fully tender. If using a pressure cooker, add the herbs after the cooker has cooled, and let them simmer in the beans at least 10 minutes.

3. Cook rice with 3 cups of water. Bring to a boil; cover the pot and simmer on low heat until all the liquid evaporates.

4. Prepare the onion and spice mixture: Chop onions and poblano pepper and set aside. Heat the oil in a large sauté pan on medium heat. Add asafetida, poblano pepper, and onions.

Sauté the onion mixture about 10 minutes until the onions start to turn uniformly golden. Reduce heat to medium-low and continue to cook the onions another 10 minutes or more until they begin to brown and caramelize. When the onions look ready, add ground cumin, turmeric, and coriander to the pan and stir for about 30 seconds. Pour onion-spice mixture into the pot of beans, being sure to capture all the spices.

5. Chop basil and pull oregano leaves off their stems. Add these herbs to the pot of beans during the last 15 minutes the beans are cooking. Add freshly ground ginger and garlic that has been pressed. Add salt and stir. Serve over brown or white basmati rice with a dash of lime.

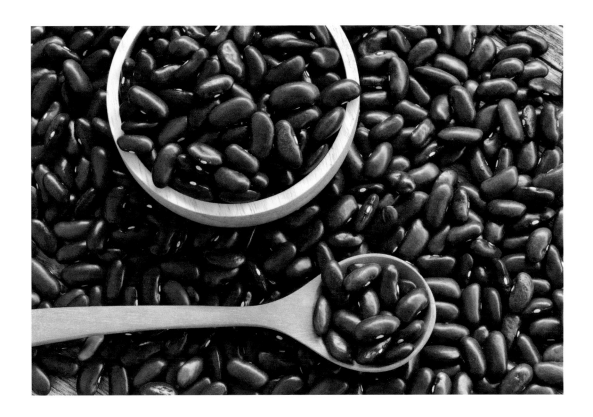

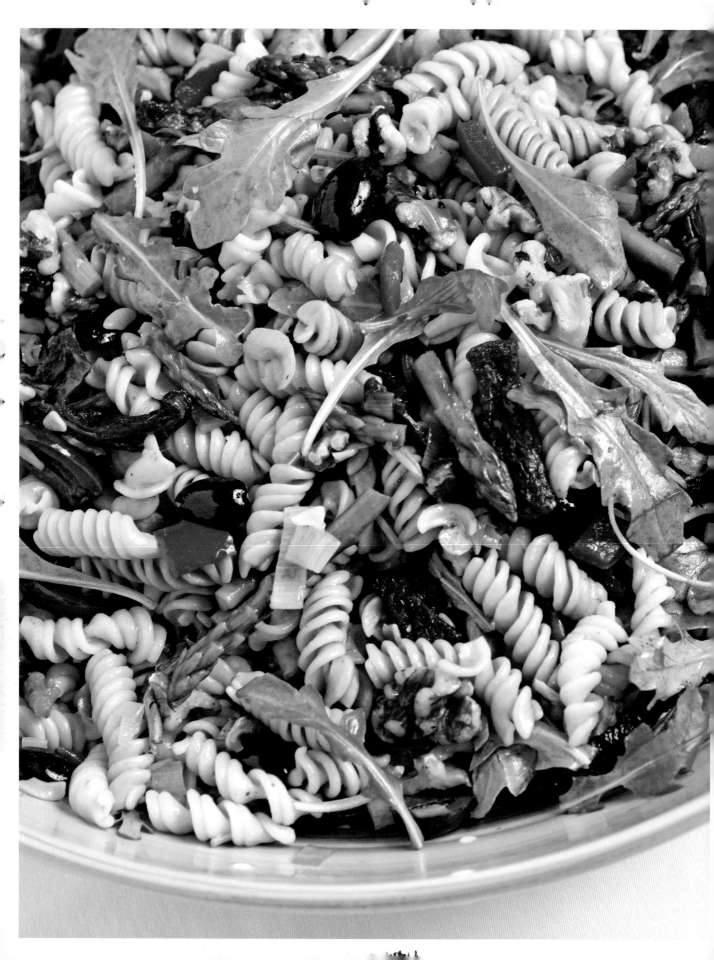

ASPARAGUS AND RED PEPPER PASTA WITH SUN-DRIED TOMATOES

Preparation Time: About 45 minutes

Serves 4 to 6

Avoid or reduce tomatoes if you suffer from arthritis

This pasta feeds four as an entrée and six or more if it is a side dish. It is delicious hot, but it can also be served at room temperature, making it ideal party fare.

1 leek bulb plus an inch of the light-green shank

1 red bell pepper

1 cup reconstituted sun-dried tomatoes

1 pound asparagus

2 teaspoons Light Grey Celtic Sea Salt

2 tablespoons olive oil, plus more to drizzle

8 ounces spelt or gluten-free pasta

24 pitted kalamata olives

2 to 3 tablespoons Bragg Liquid Aminos

¼ cup tightly packed fresh basil (or 2 tablespoons dried)

½ cup chopped walnuts

½ cup crumbled goat feta cheese (optional)

6 to 8 ounces arugula, washed

1 large or 2 small cloves garlic

COOK'S TIP: 1. Look for reconstituted sun-dried tomatoes soaked in olive oil in your grocery store to save some cooking time. **2.** To reconstitute the tomatoes yourself, pour 2 cups of boiling water over the dried tomatoes, which have been placed in a pot or stainless steel bowl. Soak 30 minutes until tender. **3.** Serve over a red lentil or quinoa pasta, so you have more protein with the meal.

AYURVEDIC NOTE

This recipe can satisfy your desire to eat Italian-style pasta while not relying too heavily on tomatoes, garlic, or hard cheeses, all of which increase *pitta* problems. Cheesy pasta dishes also increase *kapha* and can contribute to *ama* (toxins).

(V) Cook the pasta until quite tender rather than al dente. Avoid or reduce tomatoes if you suffer from arthritis.

(P) Avoid or reduce tomatoes if you suffer from arthritis. Reduce garlic. Rinse the olives in water to wash off the brine and vinegar in which olives are often soaked. Also, see menu suggestion below.

(K) Eliminate or reduce cheese, and add more garlic.

MENU SUGGESTION

Serve with Summertime Tea (page 85), which pacifies *pitta*.

1. Clean and dice the leek and bell pepper. Slice the sun-dried tomatoes into bite-sized pieces. Rinse and break asparagus spears into pieces about 1-inch long. (Use only the tender top two-thirds of the asparagus; offer the rest to Mother Nature.) Chop olives in half (optional).

2. Bring 2 quarts of water to a boil in a large soup pot in which you will later cook the pasta.

3. Heat olive oil on medium-low heat in a large sauté pan. Add leeks and sauté them for 5 to 7 minutes or until they start to turn golden. Add red peppers and sauté 5 minutes.

4. When the pasta water comes to a boil, add pasta and 1 teaspoon salt. Follow cooking directions for al dente pasta (about 8 minutes). Test to make sure the pasta is cooked but not mushy.

5. While the pasta is cooking, add the tomatoes, asparagus, and olives to the sauté pan. Add 1 teaspoon salt and 2 tablespoons Bragg's, and cook on medium heat for 5 to 10 minutes (depending on the thickness of the asparagus), until the asparagus stalks are just tender.

6. Chop basil and walnuts. Crumble the feta, if necessary.

7. When the pasta is ready, drain it and wash with cold water to halt the cooking. Drain again and transfer to a large mixing bowl. Drizzle with a little olive oil, and stir gently. Add the sautéed vegetables to the pasta. Add arugula, garlic, basil, and walnuts. Toss and taste, adding more Bragg's or salt to taste. Finish with a sprinkling of feta cheese.

BUTTERNUT SQUASH RISOTTO

Preparation Time: About 1 hour (30 minutes active)
Serves 4 as an entrée, 6 as side dish

This risotto recipe is an adaptation of a dish created by my friend Dr. Ellen Brock, whom I credit not only with teaching me vegetarian cooking but also with inspiring me to enjoy cooking as a form of play. When Ellen cooks, her eyes fill with delight, and when she serves a new dish, she grins with pleasure as everyone oohs and aahs.

1 small butternut squash (about 3 cups cubed)
1½ cups dried Arborio rice
4 cups hot Roasted Vegetable Broth (page 91)
1 large leek bulb plus an inch of the light-green shank
1 tablespoon minced fresh sage
1 tablespoon minced fresh rosemary
2 to 3 cloves garlic
⅔ cup good white wine
2 tablespoons olive oil
¾ teaspoon Light Grey Celtic Sea Salt
Small block of Parmesan or goat cheese (optional)

COOK'S TIP: 1. If you have more than 3 cups roasted butternut squash, save some of it to top a salad. Just add a little salt to the squash before serving. **2.** During the spring and summer, I substitute asparagus for squash and use basil and mint instead of sage and rosemary. **3.** Ellen makes this risotto using a French lentil stock that she found in *The Greens Cookbook*.

AYURVEDIC NOTE

This dish is fine for all types, on occasion, although less so for *kaphas*—particularly those with diabetes. Risotto rice, olive oil, and cheese all increase *kapha*, so *kapha* types may want to save this dish for a rare treat.

(P) Reduce garlic to 1 clove and reduce alcohol to ½ cup.

(K) Add an additional clove of garlic.

MENU SUGGESTION

Serve with Elegant Green Beans (page 186). During spring and summer months, also serve with Summertime Tea (page 85) or simple peppermint tea, which will balance the heat of the garlic.

1. Preheat oven to 375°F. Peel squash and cut in half. Scoop out seeds. Cut squash into strips and then into bite-sized cubes.

2. Place squash cubes on a baking sheet covered with parchment paper. Bake for 30 minutes or until the squash cubes are just tender. Remove from the oven and set aside.

3. Rinse rice with water a few times and pour into a strainer to let the rice air-dry.

4. If the soup stock you will be using is not already hot, heat the stock in a covered saucepan until it is steaming. Keep stock on low heat until the recipe is finished.

5. Slice the leek. Mince the sage, rosemary, and garlic. Uncork the wine.

6. Heat olive oil in a 3- to 4-quart pot on medium heat. Add sage and rosemary and sauté about a minute.

7. Reduce heat to medium-low. Add garlic and diced leeks and continue to sauté until the leeks are turning golden.

8. Add rice and stir well for about a minute to coat the grains in oil. Add wine and stir well until the wine evaporates.

9. Add ½ cup of hot stock and stir constantly, if possible (or every few minutes if you're dashing around the kitchen making other dishes). As stock evaporates, continue to add ½ more cup of stock at a time, continuing to stir. With the last cup of stock, add salt and butternut squash. Continue to stir until all the stock is evaporated and the squash is tender. Serve immediately with cheese, if you wish.

OLD-FASHIONED SPAGHETTI

Preparation Time: About 30 minutes
Serves 4

When I was a child, one of my family's favorite Saturday night dinners was Chef Boyardee spaghetti from a box. My mother jazzed it up with a fried onion and baked it casserole-style. To this day I think of spaghetti as a star in the category I call "fun food," although I've returned to an old-fashioned freshly made sauce.

FOR THE SAUCE:
½ cup chopped onion
1 clove garlic, chopped or pressed
1 cup chopped fresh basil leaves
1 tablespoon fresh oregano (or 1 teaspoon dried)
3 tablespoons olive oil
10 medium or 8 large heirloom tomatoes
1½ to 2 teaspoons ground cumin
1 fresh bay leaf
1 tablespoon coconut sugar
1 teaspoon Light Grey Celtic Sea Salt
Freshly ground Parmesan or goat cheese crumbles (optional)
Freshly ground black pepper

FOR THE PASTA:
1 teaspoon Light Grey Celtic Sea Salt
16 ounces gluten-free or spelt pasta

AYURVEDIC NOTE
Because tomatoes disturb all *doshas* (see notes on page 142), I save this dish for a treat at the peak of tomato season. I use heirloom tomatoes because they are often the least acidic varieties and are, therefore, better for most people.

(P) Try cooking with orange and yellow tomatoes, which typically have a lower acid content.

(K) Reduce olive oil to 2 tablespoons; avoid cheese. Substitute spaghetti squash for wheat or rice pasta.

MENU SUGGESTION
Serve with Simple Green Salad (page 206) and Lime Vinaigrette (page 210) or Mediterranean Root Vegetables and Greens (page 208). Also serve with Summertime Tea (page 85) to counteract the tomatoes' acidity.

1. Bring a large pot of water to boil for the pasta with 1 teaspoon salt.

2. Chop onion, garlic, basil, and oregano.

3. Heat olive oil in a small soup pot or large skillet on medium heat. Add onions to the pan and sauté about 10 minutes or until the onions just start to turn golden. Add the garlic and stir for about 30 seconds; then turn off the heat or move the pan off the burner.

4. While the onions are sautéing, cut the tomatoes in half. Squeeze each half through a strainer over a bowl to retain the tomato juice. Shake the pulp to discard the seeds; then chop the remaining pulp. Add tomatoes to the pot, along with the cumin and bay leaf. Sauté tomatoes uncovered for about 10 minutes.

5. Meanwhile, when the water comes to a boil, add the pasta to the water and cook it according to the directions on the box, until tender but still firm. Drain the pasta and rinse with cold water.

6. Returning to the sauce: If you want a more refined dish, you can pinch the tomato skins away from the flesh as they start to separate, or you can pull them out with a fork when they float to the surface. Or you can simply leave the skins in the sauce. Add most of the basil (leave some for garnish) and all of the oregano, coconut sugar, and 1 teaspoon salt to the sauce. Simmer another 10 minutes, then taste and add more salt, if needed.

7. Toss the pasta with the sauce and serve with basil as a garnish. Add freshly ground Parmesan (optional) and fresh pepper to taste.

8. If you like, you can bake the dressed pasta in the oven à la Bonnie Cagan (my mother) on 375°F for 30 minutes, in which case you'll want to boil your pasta only until it is barely tender.

Balancing Tomato Love

If you're like me, few pleasures rival that of picking a tomato ripe off the garden vine and eating it on the spot—plain or with a shaker of salt in hand. I've eaten more than my share of raw and cooked tomatoes, especially in Italian and Tex-Mex food. During my fifteen years living in Dallas, I must have consumed several vats of homemade tomato salsa! At Zuzu's, my favorite casual spot in Dallas, the salsa was prepared in plain view, and I used to love watching the cooks stir a cauldron of that delectable brew of fresh tomatoes, onions, and cilantro.

So are tomatoes good for us? On the plus side, tomatoes are full of antioxidants. Tomatoes also have some healing qualities, which are acknowledged in Ayurveda. In *Ayurvedic Cooking for Self-Healing*, coauthor and Ayurvedic physician Vasant Lad lists several home remedies using tomatoes. However, he also explains that tomatoes increase all *doshas*, particularly *pitta*. People with strong constitutions may be able to tolerate a lifetime of tomatoes without distress. Only you can judge whether or not eating tomatoes works for you. In my experience, eating tomatoes is fine when I do it only once in a while, and it's easiest on my body when the tomatoes are cooked with the right spices, especially cumin. Dr. Lad claims that cumin is the antidote for tomatoes. But too many tomatoes always result in joint pain for me.

Ayurveda suggests that anyone with arthritis, sciatica, kidney stones, or gallstones avoid tomatoes and all other nightshades. People suffering from osteoarthritis and rheumatoid arthritis may find that their symptoms are aggravated when they indulge in tomatoes. Modern medicine has recognized that tomatoes and other nightshades contain a chemical called alpha-solanine, which triggers inflammation and joint pain in many. Be advised that acid indigestion and acid reflux disease are also greatly aggravated by tomatoes, whether raw or cooked.

Finally, Ayurveda suggests that we avoid combining tomatoes with dairy, because the combination is especially difficult to digest and can lead to toxic buildup in the body, particularly if you have weak digestion.

Oy! For all these reasons, I rarely eat tomatoes now, but life without *any* tomatoes would be too ascetic for me! My advice, once again: don't worry about the occasional spaghetti sauce—just enjoy! It's what you eat day-in and day-out that has a long-term impact on your health.

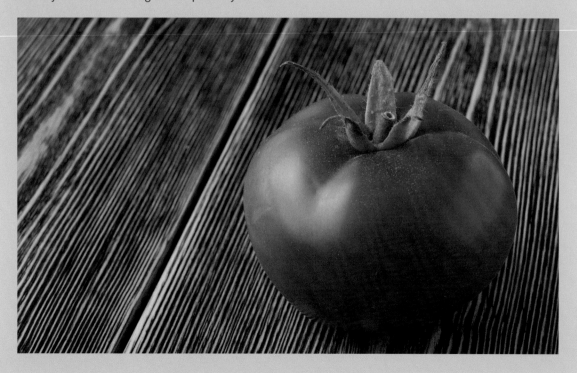

SWEET POTATO STIR-FRY

Preparation Time: About 30 minutes
Serves 2 to 3

My husband, Tom, created this easy stir-fry that I embellished with almond butter for a quick tasty meal.

1 large sweet potato
1 medium red bell pepper
1 tablespoon sunflower oil
1 teaspoon ground cumin
1 teaspoon ground coriander
2 cups broccoli florets
1 large zucchini squash
2 tablespoons Bragg Liquid Aminos
½ cup almond butter
1 teaspoon freshly ground ginger
1 cup water

AYURVEDIC NOTE
Sweet potatoes and zucchini are very calming for *vata* and *pitta*, but are best eaten in moderation by people with *kapha* problems. Broccoli and bell pepper are good for *kapha* and *pitta* but increase *vata*, which is mitigated by the ginger. While almond butter increases *kapha*, the small amount used in this recipe is fine on occasion.

V Substitute 1 or 2 carrots for the red pepper. Increase ginger and/or add fresh garlic.

K Use ¼ cup almond butter. Add a clove of garlic.

MENU SUGGESTION
Serve over Indian Rice with Cashews (page 163).

1. Peel sweet potato and cut into small cubes. Slice bell pepper.

2. Heat oil on medium heat in a large sauté pan or wok. When the oil starts to get hot, reduce heat to medium-low and add cumin and coriander to the pan. Add the sweet potato cubes and cover for 10 minutes. Add bell pepper and cover another 5 minutes.

3. While the potatoes and bell peppers get tender, separate broccoli florets and slice zucchini into rounds. Add broccoli, zucchini, and Bragg's to the pan. Cover about 5 minutes, or until the zucchini and broccoli are just tender. While the vegetables sauté, whisk the almond butter, ginger, and water in a small bowl or 1-cup measuring cup with a spout. Pour sauce over the vegetables and serve immediately over quinoa, pasta, or rice.

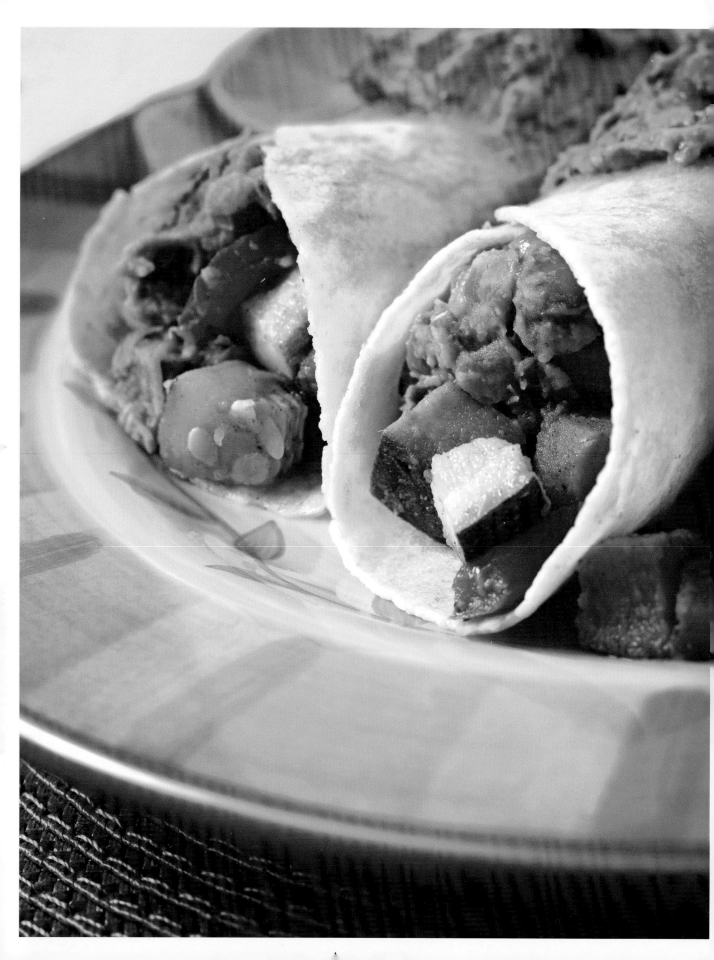

SWEET POTATO BURRITOS

Preparation Time: About 35 minutes
Serves 4

This is one of my favorite quick meals. I make it at least two or three times a month in the summer as a way to sop up guacamole. You may have begun to notice that I use a lot of sweet potatoes in recipes, and I do, for three great reasons. First and foremost, I find them delicious! They also serve as a wonderfully grounding food for vata, *because they are heavy, among vegetables. Finally, sweet potatoes are considered a good carb for anyone who is managing diabetes or insulin resistance.*

1 extra-large sweet potato or 2 medium sweet potatoes
1 medium red bell pepper
2 tablespoons olive oil
1 teaspoon ground cumin
1 teaspoon ground coriander
1 large zucchini
½ teaspoon Fine Ground Celtic Sea Salt
8 packaged gluten-free almond-flour or corn tortillas

AYURVEDIC NOTE
Because of the sweet potatoes and zucchini, these particular burritos are very easy to digest as well as filling. They are pacifying to *vata* and *pitta*. *Kapha* types should eat them in moderation.

K Add 1 clove garlic to vegetable mixture. Avoid Guacamole; try a little salsa instead.

MENU SUGGESTION
Serve with Refried Beans (page 168) or add the beans inside the tortillas. Definitely serve with Guacamole (page 219) and blue corn or bean chips. Also Summertime Tea (page 85).

1. Peel the sweet potato and chop it into bite-sized cubes or strips. Slice the red pepper into ½ -inch strips.

2. Heat the oil on medium heat in a large frying pan. When the oil is hot, add the cumin and coriander; then add potato strips or cubes, and cover. After about 5 minutes, stir and turn the heat down to medium-low for another 5 minutes, stirring occasionally to ensure that the potatoes do not stick or burn.

3. Add red bell pepper to potatoes and re-cover. While the bell peppers cook, chop the zucchini into bite-sized cubes, or strips. Add the zucchini to the vegetable mixture with salt and stir. Cover for another 5 minutes or until the zucchini is just tender.

4. Preheat the oven to 400°F and minimally oil a baking dish. Assemble tortillas by spooning vegetables onto the first third of a tortilla. Roll the tortilla up around the filling and place in the baking dish. Bake for 5 to 8 minutes or until the tortillas just start to brown.

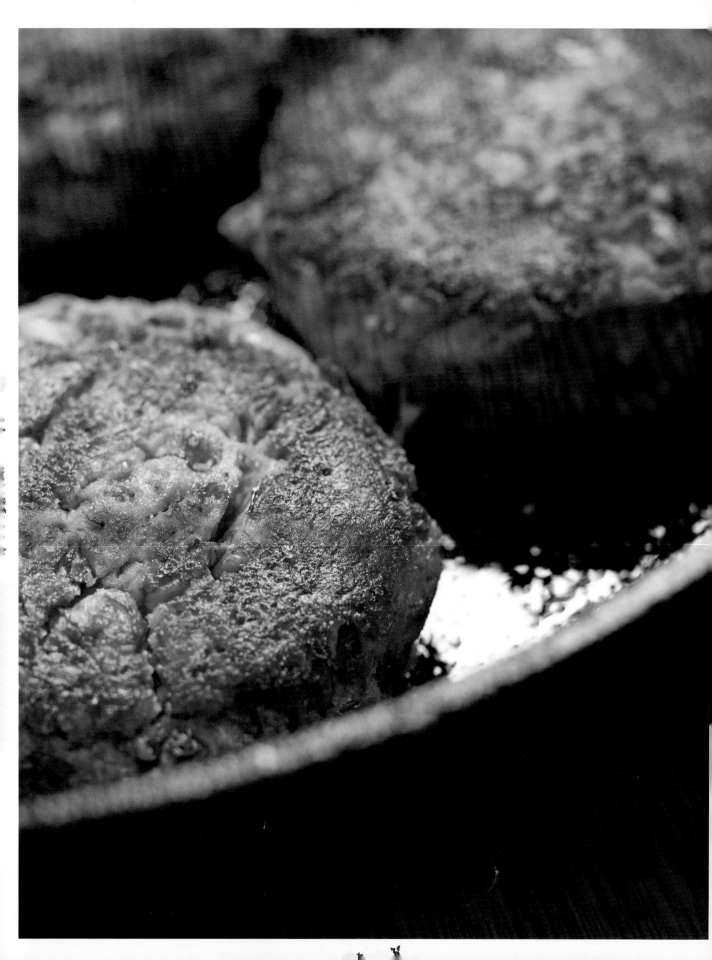

MUNG BEAN BURGERS

Preparation Time: 8 hours soaking, plus 1½ to 2 hours cooking (45 minutes active)
Makes 12 patties

I developed this burger as a fun food that's easy to digest. The onion and garlic definitely add flavor but are not absolutely required. The burger is still quite tasty without them—which is good, because some forms of meditation require practitioners to forgo such rajasic *flavoring.*

FOR THE BEANS:
2 cups dried mung beans
4 cups water

FOR THE CAKES:
1 medium or large Vidalia or red onion (optional)
2 tablespoons olive or sunflower oil for onion mixture, plus more if you brown and reheat patties in a fry pan
1 teaspoon black mustard seeds
5 curry leaves (optional)
1 teaspoon ground cumin
1 teaspoon ground coriander
1 teaspoon ground turmeric
2 pinches asafetida (optional)
1 to 1½ teaspoons Fine Ground Celtic Sea Salt
1 clove garlic, pressed (optional)
2 teaspoons freshly grated ginger

COOK'S TIP: 1. If you digest quinoa well, you can add cooked quinoa to the burgers for additional nutrients. Start with ½ cup uncooked quinoa and 1½ cups water. **2.** Store extra patties before they are browned to avoid drying out.

AYURVEDIC NOTE
Mung beans are among the easiest foods to digest and are especially agreeable for *vata* and *pitta*. They increase *kapha* somewhat, which is helped by the heating quality of garlic and ginger. If you add quinoa it increases the protein but is difficult to digest for *vata* types.

(V) Increase ginger and garlic.

(P) Reduce mustard seeds. Reduce garlic or replace it with more ginger.

(K) Increase ginger and garlic. Cook with quinoa.

SERVING SUGGESTION
Serve with or without a bun with Curry Leaf Chutney (page 79) or Guacamole (page 219). Or go all-American with mustard, ketchup, and pickles! Good with Oven-Baked Sweet Potato Chips (page 198), any of the salads (beginning page 203), or Quick Sautéed Asparagus (page 173).

(ADDITIONAL RECIPE PHOTO ON PAGE 134)

1. Soak beans 6 to 8 hours. Rinse the beans well and strain them. (See pages 116–117 for cooking directions in a pressure cooker or regular soup pot.)

2. Chop the onion. Heat the oil in a large sauté pan on medium heat. When the oil is hot, add the mustard seeds and cover until the seeds pop like popcorn. When the seeds finish popping, add curry leaves and cover immediately, as the leaves may pop. Add asafetida and onions and then sauté on medium about 10 minutes or until the onions turn golden. Reduce heat to medium-low and continue to sauté until the onions turn brown and caramelize—as much as an additional 20 minutes. When the onions are done, add the cumin, coriander, and turmeric. Stir for several seconds to combine spices with the onions and oil. Set aside.

3. Returning to the beans: When the beans are tender, strain them with a basket strainer over a mixing bowl for at least 10 minutes. Once they are well strained, return them to the pot and mash them with a potato masher. Freeze the mash for 15 minutes to chill it and allow the beans to congeal.

4. Once the beans are chilled, add the sautéed onion mixture to the chilled, mashed beans along with the salt, garlic, and ginger. Remove the curry leaves if you wish. Stir well. Taste and add more salt, if needed. Form into patties with your hands, using ½ cup mixture per patty, and set these on a plate.

5. Sauté the patties in a pan with hot oil, 3 to 5 minutes per side. Or grill for 3 to 5 minutes per side, cooking until the burgers are reheated and start to brown without drying out. Or bake in a preheated oven at 450°F for 5 minutes; then broil for another 3 to 5 minutes.

Blackfeet Indian Prayer

*The following prayer is excerpted from a rare and precious
document that was given to Jack Gladstone, an award-winning
singer, songwriter, lecturer, and storyteller who is a member of the
Blackfeet Nation. Jack's great-great-grandfather was Red Crow
(1830–1900), a legendary chief of the Blood Tribe, which is part of
the Blackfeet Nation in Northwest Montana.*

*Jack said that this sacred medicine prayer was given to his
great-grandfather by Bird Rattler (1860–1909), one of the tribal
elders. The prayer is included in an unpublished memoir that was
transmitted orally by Jack's great-grandfather, Jack Wagner (1876–
1917), and was later committed to writing and translated into English.*

*In explaining the prayer, Jack said, "In Blackfeet culture the sun
is regarded as the primary spiritual symbol of the Great Mystery."
By generously sharing this prayer, Jack offers the gift of his rich
tradition to all who honor the sacred mystery of life.*

Oki, Tshak-u-may-tah-pi! I greet you, oh Mother Earth!
It is you who have given us our food.
You have fed and protected the green grass,
The sweet roots, the berry bushes, the trees.
With rich grass you have fed the buffalo,
The deer, the antelope, the elk, and all creatures.
All these things you have given us
That we may make pemmican to eat;
That we may have clothes to warm us;
That we may build ourselves lodges
Where our friends may visit us
And warm their hearts.
It is you who feed and protect us.
And when the Great Spirit shall call us
To follow after the buffalo,
You will take into your arms our tired bodies,
Like the ashes of this sweetgrass,
And give them rest . . .

Oki, Na-tosi! I salute you, oh Sun Spirit!
Great gift of the Great Above All Person!
It is you who first planted the seed
In the heart of Mother Earth.
It is you with your great power
Who called the seed into life,
And with light and warmth caused it to grow . . .

Enter this lodge, oh Sun, that we may share your strength.
Our friends are before us.
They have proposed great things.
They have undertaken difficult tasks.
Make plain their trails before them.
Bring them health and strength and good fortune.
Keep their minds and hearts toward all people
As straight as this pipe stem;
Their deeds and thoughts are fragrant
As the incense of this sweetgrass.
Give their eyes the vision of the eagle
To see the needs of all people;
Their ears the alertness of the deer
To hear the cries for help and understanding;
Put into their minds the will to serve
And into their hearts the courage of the bear,
To speed to the relief of distress
Swift as the flight of an arrow;
Make them strong like the bull buffalo
That swerves not from its course
But overcomes all obstacles
That stand in its path.

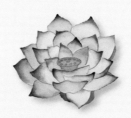

STUFFED CHARD WITH BLACK-EYED PEA PÂTÉ

Preparation Time: *1 hour soaking, plus about 3 hours cooking (2 or more active)*
Serves 6 to 10

Black-eyed peas and greens share a long tradition in the South as the New Year's culinary messengers of abundance. Being a Southern Jewish foodie, I'm proud to offer this uniquely gourmet approach to an old classic: the meat-stuffed cabbage for which Jewish cooks are renowned! This dish is an elegant entrée for vegetarians or omnivores alike.

FOR THE CHARD AND STUFFING:

- 3 cups dried black-eyed peas
- 1 large or 2 small butternut squashes
- 1 large or 2 small acorn squashes
- 1 large sweet onion
- 3 tablespoons olive oil
- 16 to 20 large red chard leaves, plus stalks
- 1½ teaspoons ground cumin
- 1½ teaspoons ground coriander
- 1 tablespoon Bragg Liquid Aminos
- ¼ cup white wine
- 1 clove garlic
- 2 teaspoons freshly grated ginger
- 2 teaspoons Himalayan salt

FOR THE SAUCE:

- ¼ pound shiitake mushrooms
- 2 tablespoons ghee or coconut oil
- 1 leek bulb, sliced thinly, plus 1 inch of green stalk
- ½ cup white wine
- 1 cup black-eyed pea cooking water
- 2 cups plain almond milk (freshly made, if possible)
- 1 fresh bay leaf
- 2 teaspoons fresh thyme
- 1 teaspoon fresh rosemary
- ½ to 1 teaspoon Fine Ground Celtic Sea Salt
- 1½ tablespoons arrowroot powder

AYURVEDIC NOTE

Like all legumes, black-eyed peas will increase *vata*, but this is mitigated somewhat by soaking and cooking the peas until they're quite tender and adding garlic and ginger. Cooking with ghee and combining beans with winter squash make this dish more easily digestible.

V Add ⅛ teaspoon asafetida powder.

P Reduce or omit garlic and reduce wine.

K Reduce or omit squash.

(RECIPE PHOTO ON PAGE 132)

1. Make the stuffing: Soak black-eyed peas in water for 1 to 4 hours. When ready to cook the peas, rinse them, and bring them to a boil with 8 to 9 cups of water. Reduce heat, cover, and cook on medium heat for 30 minutes or until the peas are completely tender.

2. While the peas are cooking, preheat the oven to 450°F. Cover a baking sheet or large baking dish with parchment paper. Prepare the squash by cutting each squash in half and raking out the seeds and moist strands around them. Cut each half again and arrange the quarters on the baking sheet with the flesh down. Bake for 1 to 1½ hours, until the squashes are completely tender.

3. Dice the onion and sauté in olive oil in a large pan on medium heat until golden. Lower heat and continue to cook the onion slowly for another 20 minutes or so until it starts to brown and caramelize.

4. While the onion cooks, soak the chard leaves in water to remove any dirt. Shake off the water and let the chard dry on paper towels. Remove the stems from all of the leaves. Slice 6 of these stems in half lengthwise, then dice finely, like celery. When the onions have caramelized, add the sliced chard stems with the cumin, coriander, Bragg's, wine, garlic, ginger, and 1½ teaspoons salt. Stir and simmer uncovered on medium-low heat. Let this mixture cook 10 to 15 minutes until the stems are just tender and the liquid evaporates.

5. When the peas are tender, strain them, saving 1½ cups of the cooking water. Mash the peas and, if they seem dry, add some of the saved cooking liquid while saving 1 full cup for the mushroom sauce. Add the onion mixture to the peas and mix well with a large spoon. Let the pea mixture rest for at least 30 minutes or chill if you want to finish the dish at a later time. This will allow the peas to congeal before stuffing the leaves. (If you're making a shepherd's pie version of the recipe, you can omit the step of chilling the peas.)

6. Once the squash is tender, let it cool for 15 minutes so you can handle it easily. Retrieve the flesh and throw away the skins. Mash the squash, and strain any liquid. Then mix with ½ teaspoon salt and set aside.

7. **Make the sauce:** Wash the mushrooms and pat dry. Remove the stems. Chop the mushroom caps or process in a food processor so the mushrooms are very finely chopped. Wash and slice the leeks. Heat a medium saucepan (preferably with a spout) on medium heat. Sauté the leeks in ghee or coconut oil until they turn golden, then add wine and mushrooms. Simmer on medium-low for about 10 minutes until the wine cooks off. Add black-eyed pea cooking water, 1½ cups of almond milk, bay leaf, thyme, rosemary, and salt. Raise heat to medium high, stirring occasionally until the sauce is steaming. Reduce heat to medium-low.

8. Place arrowroot in a small cup or dish with ½ cup cold almond milk, and combine with a fine whisk to stir out the lumps. Return the arrowroot mixture to the sauce, and stir well for 5 minutes or so until the sauce thickens. Let the sauce stay on low heat to remain warm if serving soon. (Otherwise, set aside and reheat later.)

9. **Prepare to assemble the chard rolls:** Bring 8 cups of water to a boil in a soup pot. Prepare a large mixing bowl with several cups of water and ice. Oil a casserole dish with olive or coconut oil. If you plan to serve the chard rolls shortly after assembling them, preheat the oven to 350°F.

10. Slice the bottom ¼ inch off each chard leaf to remove the remaining part of the hard red stem so that it will be easier to roll. Then, one at a time, dip each chard leaf into the boiling water for 10 to 15 seconds. Remove and plunge the leaf into ice water for 5 seconds. Shake it off, and drain the leaf on a paper towel. Repeat this process with all of the leaves. Once the leaves are ready, set up an assembly line with the leaves, black-eyed pea mixture, and mashed squash. Taking one leaf at a time, place it on a plate or board. Place two heaping tablespoons of the pea mixture at the large base of the leaf's triangle and mold the mixture into a small log. (Use less of the mixture if you have smaller leaves.) Place about 2 tablespoons of squash over the peas. Then roll upward from the base, tucking the sides. Place the rolls in the casserole dish. Cover the dish, and heat the rolls in the oven for 30 minutes. Serve the rolls with a generous portion of mushroom sauce.

Variation: If you want to save time and make a shepherd's pie version of this dish, you will not need to blanch the chard leaves. Follow all the cooking directions above. Prior to assembly, chop all of the chard leaves into strips, and steam them until tender, about 10 minutes. Layer the casserole starting with sauce on the bottom, followed by black-eyed peas, more sauce, steamed chard, more sauce, and finish with a layer of squash. If you wish, finely chop ½ cup almonds and sprinkle across the top of the squash. Bake for 30 minutes or until the casserole is heated all the way through. Serve immediately.

The Lowdown on Mushrooms

Ayurveda classifies mushrooms as *tamasic*, which means they have a dulling effect. According to Dr. Smita Naram, mushrooms deplete *ojas*, "the residual pure energy generated at the end of the metabolic cycle."

Mushrooms are also known to increase *vata*. Some Ayurvedic experts say that soaking mushrooms overnight in milk prior to cooking them transforms the mushrooms so that they have no ill effect.

Western nutritionists and practitioners of Chinese medicine take a more positive view of mushrooms. There is much research citing the medicinal benefits of mushrooms, which are rich in antioxidants. Shiitakes in particular are lauded in some literature for their support of the immune system. Nonetheless, Western health-care practitioners also recommend staying off mushrooms if you are trying to heal from a fungal condition.

Who to believe? If you love mushrooms, you might want to observe how you feel after eating them. They may work for you, and you can be the judge. I find that my occasional arthritis symptoms are increased by certain mushrooms; I always feel pain in my hands the day after eating them. However, I do not experience these symptoms when I eat shiitakes, which is why I use them in my soup stock and a few other recipes.

SPAGHETTI SQUASH BOATS

Preparation Time: 8 hours soaking, plus 1¾ hours cooking (1 hour active)
Serves 4

This is a pasta-like dish without the high carbs but with plenty of flavor. It can make an impressive one-dish meal for company. I like to use black-eyed peas because they cook quickly, but you can use other beans or use tofu for protein instead.

FOR THE SQUASH BOATS:

1½ cups dried black beans

2 teaspoons Fine Ground Celtic Sea Salt

2 medium spaghetti squashes

1 leek bulb plus an inch of the light-green shank

1 whole red pepper, diced (optional)

2 tablespoons olive oil

1 teaspoon ground cumin

1 teaspoon ground coriander

1 pound fresh baby spinach (1 large box)

FOR THE SAUCE:

1½ cups organic tahini (or nut butter)

¾ cup water

3 tablespoons Bragg Liquid Aminos

2 teaspoons freshly grated ginger

1 large clove garlic, pressed

1½ teaspoons coconut sugar (optional)

1 tablespoon freshly squeezed lemon or lime juice

1 bunch cilantro (1½ to 2 cups)

TIME-SAVER: A quicker option can be made by serving peas and veggies with sauce over gluten-free pasta, which cooks in less than 10 minutes.

AYURVEDIC NOTE

Spaghetti squash is an excellent food for *kapha*, but can increase *vata*. Black-eyed peas are good for *pitta* and *kapha* but increase *vata*, as do bell peppers. The warming spices, tahini, oil, and spinach are all good for *vata*, bringing balance to the dish. Tahini is heating and oily, which increase *pitta*, which is why I add the cooling cilantro.

(V) Substitute rice noodles for squash.

(P) Replace half or more of the tahini with vegetable stock.

(K) Replace half or more of the tahini with vegetable stock. Add a clove of fresh garlic.

MENU SUGGESTION

Serve with Quick Sautéed Asparagus (page 173) or simply with Summertime Tea (page 85).

1. Soak the black beans for 8 hours before cooking. When ready to cook, strain the beans and rinse them a few times. Place them in a soup pot in 5 cups of water and bring to a boil. Reduce to medium-low heat and simmer the beans for about an hour until they are tender but not mushy. (You can also cook the beans in a slow cooker for several hours with 6 cups water.) When the beans are done, strain them. Add 1 teaspoon salt, stir, and set aside

2. While the beans are cooking, preheat the oven to 450°F. Cut each squash in half. Remove and discard seeds and the darker colored strands around them. Place the halves flesh down in a baking dish lined with parchment paper. Cover with foil and bake for about 90 minutes. Once the squashes are very tender, remove them from the oven and let them cool for 10 minutes

3. About a half hour before you take the squash out of the oven, sauté the other vegetables: chop the leeks and red pepper (if using). Heat the tablespoon of oil on medium heat in a large (5½ quart) sauté pan or soup pot. Sauté leeks about 5 to 7 minutes, or until they turn golden. Reduce the heat to medium-low. Add the red pepper (if using) and cover for 5 minutes. Add the cumin and coriander, and stir. Add the spinach to the vegetable mixture with 2 or 3 tablespoons of water. Cover for about 3 minutes until the spinach is wilted. Add 1 teaspoon salt and stir. Set aside until ready to assemble.

4. Make the sauce: Wash the cilantro well. Combine all ingredients for the sauce in a food processor or blender. Pulse a few times until the sauce is well mixed and the cilantro is chopped. Set aside.

5. Combine the spaghetti with sauce: Rake the cooked spaghetti squash with a fork to delicately pull the strands away from the sides of the shell. Move the strands of squash into a large mixing bowl (or a pot, if the squash is no longer warm enough for serving). Pour half of the tahini sauce over the spaghetti squash and mix well. Rewarm the mixture if necessary. If you wish, warm the remaining half of the sauce in a separate sauce pan

6. Assemble the entrée: Spoon a serving of squash back into each squash boat or, if you prefer, onto 4 plates. Place a large serving of vegetables on top of the squash. Next, place a serving of black beans over the vegetables. Pour remainder of the sauce in divided portions over each serving. Garnish each serving with a slice of lime and serve.

Tahini Alert

Tahini is a delicious paste made from ground hulled sesame seeds. Unfortunately, sesame is one of the most common allergens in the United States.

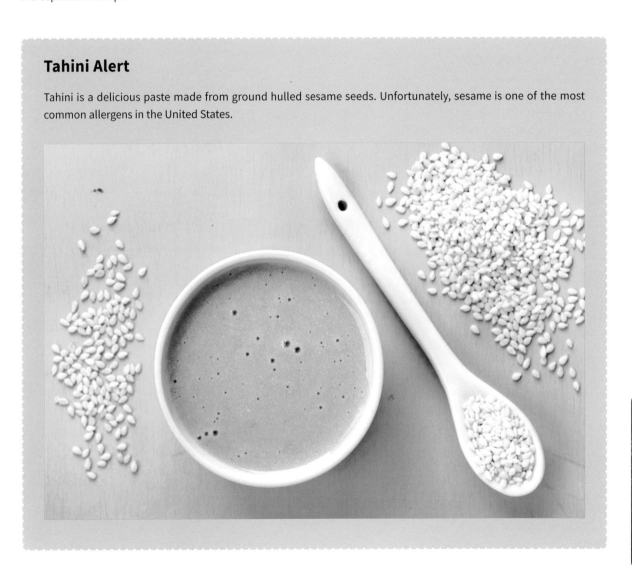

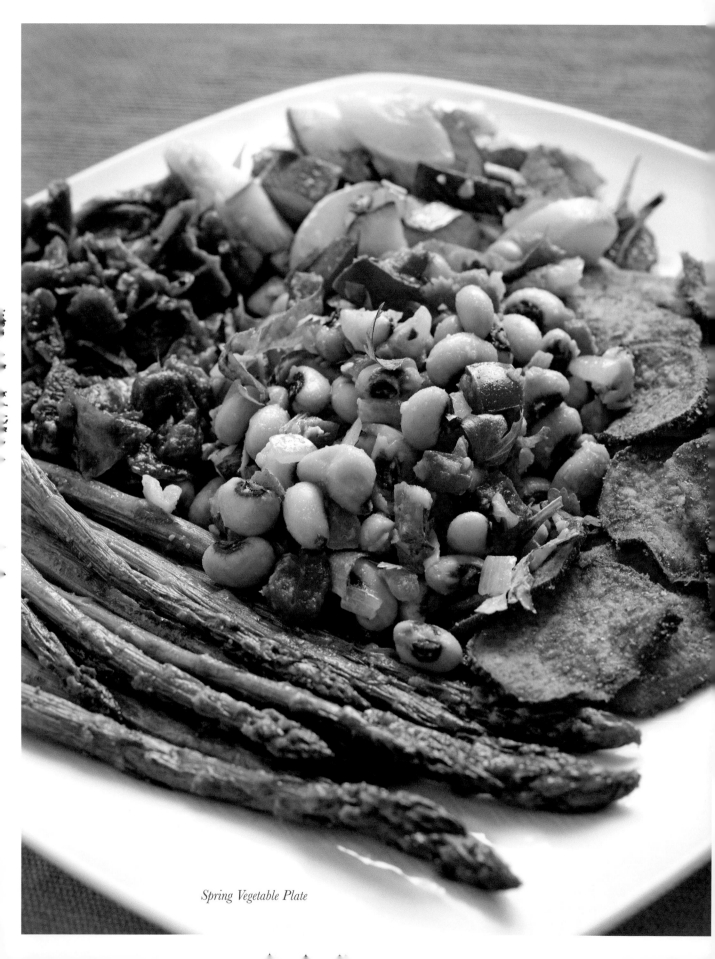

Spring Vegetable Plate

CHAPTER 9.

Side Dishes

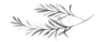

Today
The vegetables would like to be cut
By someone who is singing God's Name.

— Hafiz

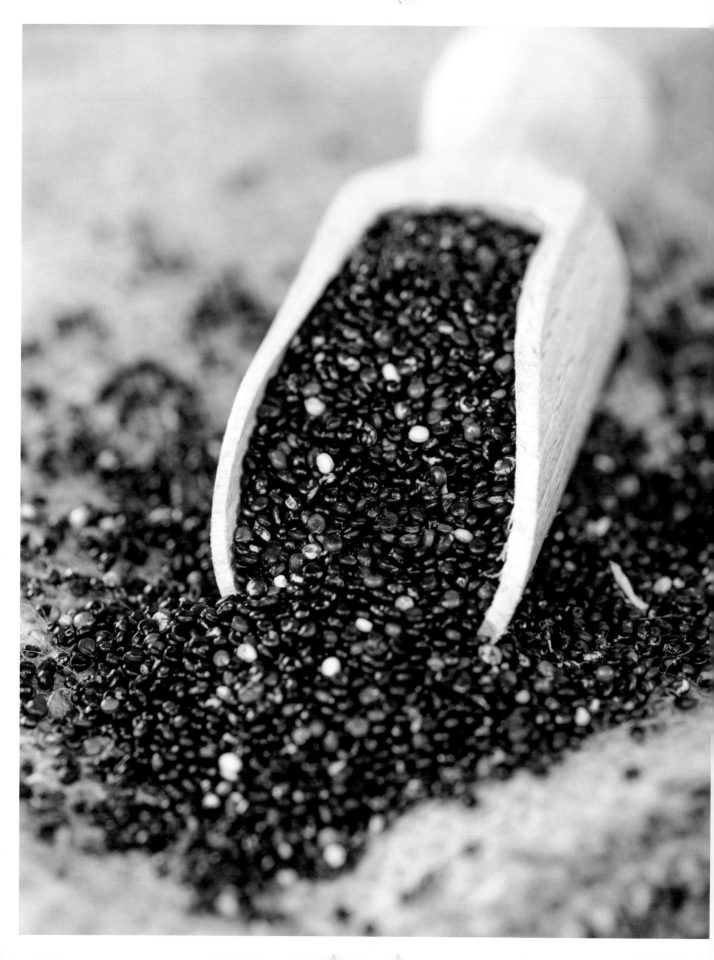

Resurgence of Ancient Grains

Anyone fortunate enough to shop in today's upscale food markets has seen packages of grains that most of us never heard of in our childhoods. These are not new foods but very old ones, with names like millet, quinoa, black rice, red rice, sorghum, spelt, and teff. These diverse and ancient grains can perk up an otherwise ordinary menu. Typically, they have excellent nutritional benefits, and they are widely available today in American grocery stores and online. The options do narrow some if you follow a gluten-free diet—note that spelt, kamut, barley, rye, triticale, and bulgur all contain at least some gluten. Nonetheless, the presence of such a variety of grains on the global market is especially welcome now with recent revelations about health risks associated with white and brown rice, which I discuss below.

Many of the rediscovered grains are ground into flour and used in baking or pancakes. Some, like millet and quinoa, offer a better protein-to-carbohydrate ratio than other grains used as side dishes, making them attractive to those who feel best when eating a low-carb diet.

Quinoa, an edible seed, is now widely treated as a grain and is considered a "superfood" by most food writers, nutritionists, and marketers. Quinoa is especially appealing to vegetarian health enthusiasts because it is a complete protein—that is, it contains all the essential amino acids and significantly greater amounts of the amino acids lysine and isoleucine than other grains. Eating quinoa can help balance blood sugar and energy levels throughout the day. Unfortunately, many people find quinoa difficult to digest. Looking at quinoa through the lens of Ayurveda, this problem can be explained by its light and dry qualities and astringent taste, which cause quinoa to increase *vata*. These problems can be mitigated somewhat when you cook quinoa in a way that balances these qualities, especially using ghee or oil and a ratio of 3:1 water to dry quinoa. Even so, I can't eat it more than once a week. So, as I frequently say, trust your gut! Eat what works for you.

Millet is a small-seeded grass that is served far less frequently than quinoa in American homes, restaurants, and deli cases. I find millet much easier to digest than quinoa, and it too is a good protein source. Millet also may increase *vata* (because it is light and dry) as well as *pitta* (because it is slightly heating). For these reasons, it's best to eat millet in the cooler months.

Despite these caveats, it is helpful—even essential—for vegetarians to have alternatives to the most traditional grain, rice, because of the unsettling information that has surfaced in recent years about the cultivation of this Ayurvedic mainstay.

The Troubling Story of Modern Rice

Rice has become a complex topic in the twenty-first century for everyone who is enthusiastically choosing healthy food. But what *is* healthy food? Basmati rice has been a staple of Ayurvedic food for millennia because rice has long been considered nourishing, grounding, and delicious. What legumes lack in the essential amino acids that make up protein are balanced by the essential amino acids in rice, helping vegetarians maintain adequate protein in their diets. For these reasons as well as others I enumerate later in this chapter, ancient and modern Ayurvedic practitioners have recommended eating at least some rice as essential to health—that is, until very recently.

Toxicologists have been analyzing levels of arsenic in rice cultivated throughout the world for more than a decade. Yes, I did say *arsenic*, a known carcinogen. In 2012 *Consumer Reports* magazine released data about high concentrations of arsenic in rice and rice products (such as baby food, cereals, and cookies), warning the public—particularly pregnant women and parents of young children—to reduce rice consumption. The 2012 report suggested that eating rice once a day can increase the body's arsenic levels by 44 percent. For millions of people throughout the world who eat rice two or even three times a day, this information is deeply troubling.

Some organic arsenic occurs naturally in the environment, but the more toxic, inorganic arsenic—which is used in pesticides—now contaminates soil and water worldwide. Such pesticides have been used heavily in cotton farming, compromising the soil in the American South, where much of the US rice crop is grown.

According to the US Food and Drug Administration (FDA), "Long-term exposure to high levels of arsenic is associated with higher rates of skin, bladder, and lung cancers, as well as heart disease." As this book goes to press, the FDA encourages the public to eat a diversified diet of healthy grains and not to have concern about the levels of arsenic found in the food it sampled, which they deem too low to cause "short-term" health problems. It is, of course, the long-term effects that are worrisome.

Of all food crops, rice is particularly vulnerable to this kind of contamination because it is grown in water. Highly processed instant rice has the lowest levels of arsenic but also has the lowest nutrition level of the various forms of rice. Brown rice, lauded in recent decades by nutritionists as the healthiest rice because its fibrous outer hull has not been removed, actually has the highest arsenic counts of all the sampled rice—and precisely because of its hull, which gets the most exposure to the contaminated water in which it is grown. Rice pastas also rank high in arsenic levels, which is bad news for the gluten-free crowd. Most disappointing of all, organic rice does not test better than nonorganic.

Such findings turn upside down a lot of what was thought to be true about healthy eating—and reminds us, as health-conscious consumers, that we must always know where our food comes from. In this day of industrialized farming, when government protects industry more readily than it does consumers, each of us has the responsibility to take care of ourselves and our families as well as we can. In such times, options for the poor are shamefully limited.

What sort of steps can you take? As you've read, Ayurveda recognizes toxic buildup as one of the primary causes of disease and chronic pain. Given this fact, I'm wary of eating much rice, even though it has always been a part of a traditional Ayurvedic diet. Until there is much stricter regulation of rice farming, I suggest the following:

- Diversify your diet with more of the ancient gluten-free grains like millet and quinoa, and, if you tolerate gluten well, also barley and couscous.
- When you choose to eat rice, eat only small amounts. Instead of eating a half cup or more, eat two or three tablespoons to augment the protein in legumes.
- Buy rice grown in California, which has been shown to have much lower levels of arsenic than rice grown in the American South and India.
- Before cooking white rice, soak it for 20 to 30 minutes. Then pour off the soaking water, and rinse the rice in water a few times before cooking.
- Boil brown rice in a lot of water and then pour off the excess. According to the Environmental Working Group, evidence shows this method can lower arsenic levels.
- Consider eliminating rice from your diet altogether—particularly if you have any kind of chronic health problem, including chronic pain.

There are other good reasons to avoid or greatly limit rice. People who have trouble managing their weight and/or have blood sugar problems often feel better and are able to lose weight more easily by dropping rice and other carbohydrates from the diet. For these reasons, I eat rice rarely. When I do, it's white or brown basmati grown in California, and I eat only a couple of tablespoons. That is enough, I feel, to supplement the legumes in my diet.

Since rice has historically been—and remains—so much a part of classic Ayurveda, I've kept one classic rice recipe in this section.

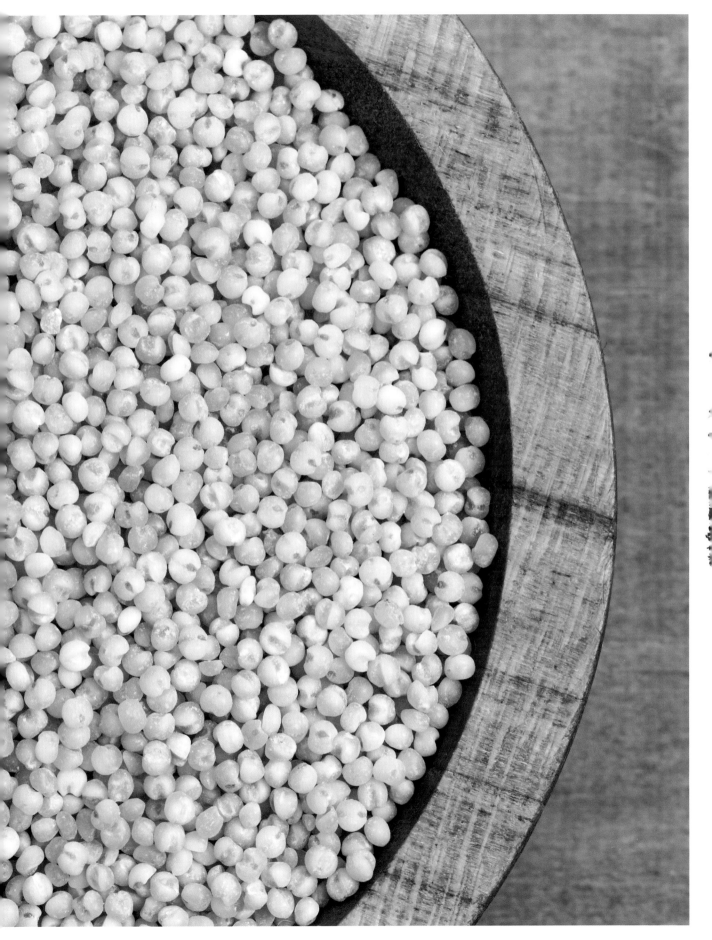

SIMPLE TOASTED MILLET

Preparation Time: About 35 minutes (10 minutes active)
Serves 4 to 6

The texture of this millet is similar to grits, if you use three cups of liquid. It's more like polenta if you add an extra cup of liquid. Like rice and quinoa, millet alone doesn't have much taste. Given enough ghee or butter, it reminds me of grits, and like all of the above, it benefits from any of your favorite herbs.

1 cup millet
3 to 4 cups Easy Vegetable Soup Stock (page 90) or water
1 teaspoon chopped rosemary
1 teaspoon chopped thyme
¾ teaspoon Grey Celtic Sea Salt
2 teaspoons ghee
½ cup chopped walnuts, pecans, or pistachios (optional)

AYURVEDIC NOTE
Millet is dry and light, which will increase *vata*, but this grain is relatively good for *kapha* for the same reasons. The herbs and ghee help balance *vata*. Millet is mildly heating but is fine for *pitta* in moderation.

V Cook with 4 cups of liquid.

P Reduce or omit nuts.

K Reduce or omit ghee. Add black pepper.

1. Rinse and strain the millet. Place the millet in a 2- or 3-quart pot on medium heat, and toast the kernels for a few minutes, stirring occasionally, until the millet starts to become more golden and fragrant. Add liquid and bring to a boil. Cover and reduce the heat to medium-low. Cook until all the liquid is absorbed, about 30 minutes.

2. While the millet is cooking, chop the herbs and add them to the pot, along with salt and ghee. If you like, add nuts when the millet is ready. Stir and serve.

SWEET AND SAVORY QUINOA WITH CARROTS

Preparation Time: About 35 minutes (15 minutes active)
Serves 4 to 6

This recipe is modeled after a traditional Indian dish made with rice, and you can certainly make it with basmati. I've adapted the recipe using quinoa, and I toned down the heat for the Western palate by dramatically reducing—and sometimes eliminating—the chili. That second shift transforms a savory curry to a savory-sweet side dish. You may want to try this recipe both with and without the poblano pepper to discover how you like it best. Special thanks to Latha Sabesan for sharing a rice recipe that inspired this dish.

1 cup dry quinoa

2 cups water

½ teaspoon Light Grey Celtic Sea Salt

1 large carrot

1 tablespoon ghee or coconut oil

½ teaspoon brown mustard seeds

½ teaspoon ground cumin

½ teaspoon ground coriander

½ teaspoon ground turmeric

1 teaspoon minced poblano pepper or
   pinch cayenne pepper (optional)

Handful of cilantro

AYURVEDIC NOTE

This dish is fine in moderation for all *doshas*.

V Cook quinoa with 3 cups of liquid for easier digestion.

P Omit cayenne or poblano pepper, or instead of mincing the pepper, sauté a whole slice, and then remove it before serving.

1. Rinse and strain the quinoa. Place quinoa, water, and salt in a 2- to 3-quart pot. Bring the pot to a boil, cover, and reduce heat to low.

2. Slice the carrot down the middle; then slice each half in half again. Slice each quarter into thin pieces, and add the carrots to the quinoa as it finishes cooking.

3. Heat the ghee or oil in a small saucepan on medium heat. When the ghee or oil is hot, add the mustard seeds and cover the pan until the seeds pop like popcorn. When the seeds stop popping, reduce heat to medium-low. Add cumin, coriander, and turmeric, and stir. If using poblano pepper, add it now and sauté for 1 minute. Add spices to the pot of cooked quinoa. Stir and serve with cilantro garnish.

BLACK OR WILD RICE

Preparation Time: About 1¼ hours (15 minutes active)
Serves 3 to 4

Black rice, found in many markets now, is often purplish in color, is chewy, and has a slightly nutty flavor. Wild rice, which is indigenous to North America, is actually classified as a grass rather than a grain. This dish can serve as a side or as a stuffing for peppers or squashes.

- 1 cup black rice or wild rice mix
- ½ cup sliced shallots or 1 sliced leek bulb plus an inch of the light-green shank
- 1½ tablespoons olive or coconut oil
- 2 cups Easy Vegetable Soup Stock (page 90)
- 1 cup water
- 1 fresh bay leaf
- ½ teaspoon Light Grey Celtic Sea Salt
- 1 tablespoon Bragg Liquid Aminos
- ¼ cup chopped parsley
- 1 to 2 tablespoons of basil, tarragon, thyme, or rosemary
- 2 tablespoons chopped blanched almonds or pistachio nuts

COOK'S TIP: 1. Soak black rice for 30 minutes before cooking, and it will cook in about half the time. **2.** Stuff rice inside a baked squash or a roasted red pepper, or eat plain as a side dish. **3.** Also see Wild Rice Salad with Winter Squash (page 221).

AYURVEDIC NOTE

Although not part of any traditional Ayurvedic cuisine, wild rice offers an interesting change of pace as a complement to vegetables. Since wild rice tends to be chewy, it can increase *vata*. This dish is fine in moderation for all *doshas*.

V Soak rice prior to cooking. Add 1 teaspoon grated ginger, or 1 clove pressed garlic, or half of each.

1. Soak the rice overnight to help remove potential arsenic residue. Strain and rinse the rice prior to cooking.

2. Slice the shallots or leeks. Heat the oil in a 2- to 3-quart saucepan on medium heat. Sauté onions until they start to turn golden, about 10 minutes.

3. When the onions are golden, add the rice to the pot, and stir for 20 seconds or so. Add the stock, water, bay leaf, salt, and Bragg's. (**Note:** If you are using a boxed or canned stock that is salted, do not add salt and Liquid Aminos until the end of the recipe. Taste first, and add salt and Bragg's as needed.) Bring to a boil; then reduce heat to medium-low, and simmer covered, 1 to 1¼ hours, until the rice is tender.

4. While the rice is cooking, chop the parsley, additional herbs, and nuts. When the rice is tender, remove the bay leaf. Add parsley and nuts. Fluff with a fork and serve.

INDIAN RICE WITH CASHEWS

Preparation Time: 30 minutes soaking, plus 30 minutes cooking (15 minutes active)
Serves 4

I am grateful to my lovely friend Ashwini Sidhaye Gole, who is originally from Delhi and who first brought this delicious dish to our table. It's a traditional dish served in most Indian homes, although I omit the whole jalapeño pepper or red chili common in its preparation. Poblano pepper is much milder! This dish can also be made substituting quinoa for rice.

1 cup uncooked white basmati rice
1 large leek bulb plus an inch of the light-green shank
1 thin slice of poblano pepper, minced or whole
1 tablespoon ghee or coconut oil
½ teaspoon black mustard seeds
½ teaspoon cumin seeds
2 to 3 curry leaves (that's leaves, not powder!)
2 cups water
½ to 1 teaspoon Light Grey Celtic Sea Salt
½ cup raw cashews
½ cup freshly chopped cilantro

AYURVEDIC NOTE

The mustard seeds, poblano pepper, and cashews are all mildly heating, and the leeks only mildly so, making this dish fine for everyone on occasion.

P Omit the poblano pepper or use it whole just to season the pot, removing the pepper before adding water. Reduce cashews to ¼ cup.

1. Soak the rice for 30 minutes prior to cooking or overnight, to clear any potential arsenic residue. Rinse and strain the rice. Slice the leek. Slice poblano pepper.

2. Heat the ghee or oil in a 2-quart saucepan on medium heat. When the oil is hot, add the mustard seeds, and cover until the seeds pop like popcorn. Remove the pot from the heat source. Add the cumin seeds, and let them sizzle and become fragrant. Add the curry leaves, and cover the pot, as the oil may splatter. Uncover and add leeks. Reduce heat to low. If using poblano pepper, add the whole slice (for a milder flavor), or mince it first for more intensity. Sauté about 5 minutes until the leeks turn golden. Remove the poblano pepper slice for a milder flavor; leave in, if you prefer.

3. Add the rice to the leeks (and poblano) and stir to coat the grains with ghee. Add the water and salt. Bring to a boil; then reduce the heat, and cover the pot. Chop the cashews and add them to the pot. Cook for 20 minutes or until all the water is evaporated.

4. Serve topped with fresh cilantro.

HOLIDAY DRESSING

Preparation Time: About 2½ hours (1½ hours active)
Serves 8 to 12

Just because vegetarians give up the turkey doesn't mean that they're any less attached to American holiday food traditions. This is a recipe for traditional dressing, as stuffing is called when it's cooked outside a bird. The distinct flavors of holiday dressing—parsley, sage, rosemary, and thyme—are what make Thanksgiving taste like Thanksgiving, along with cinnamon, nutmeg, and cloves! (See the Pumpkin Pudding on page 246.)

10 to 12 cups of bread (pages 67, 68, 71)
2 cups chopped onion
4 stalks celery
10 large fresh sage leaves, chopped (or 2 teaspoons dried)
2 tablespoons chopped fresh oregano (or 2 teaspoons dried)
2 tablespoons fresh thyme leaves (or 2 teaspoons dried)
1 tablespoon fresh chopped rosemary (or 1 teaspoon dried)
10 tablespoons ghee or unsalted butter, plus 1 teaspoon for greasing the baking dish
5 large fresh curry leaves (optional—leaves, not powder!)
1 pinch asafetida (optional)
½ teaspoon ground cumin
½ teaspoon ground coriander
8 ounces shiitake mushrooms
1½ to 2½ cups Easy Vegetable Soup Stock (page 90)
1 tablespoon Bragg Liquid Aminos
¼ cup fresh flat-leaf parsley
1 cup chopped walnuts
2 to 3 teaspoons Light Grey Celtic Sea Salt

COOK'S TIP: 1. Use 1 loaf of Gluten-Free Whole Grain Bread (page 68), Our Daily Bread (page 67), or a double corn bread recipe (page 71). **2.** This dressing is a little soft in the middle and crisp on the outside. If you prefer a dressing that's crisp all the way through, limit stock to 1½ cups.

AYURVEDIC NOTE
Yeasted bread as well as mushrooms will increase *vata*, but the ghee or butter as well as the spices help *vata* stay in balance. Any bread and ghee (or butter) all increase *kapha*, but it's the holiday, so enjoy yourself a little!

P Omit walnuts and reduce amount of ghee or butter by 3 tablespoons.

K Use half the ghee or butter for a drier dressing.

1. If you have time to start the day before, bake the corn bread or slice the loaf bread and let it dry out overnight uncovered on a rack. Otherwise, bake the pieces on a baking sheet for about 10 minutes at 300°F. Hand-tear or cut the bread into ½- to ¾-inch pieces, and place them in a large mixing bowl.

2. Chop onions and celery. Also mince sage, oregano, thyme, and rosemary, and set aside.

3. Heat the ghee or butter in a large sauté pan on medium heat. Once the ghee is somewhat hot, add the curry leaves, and cover the pan briefly in case the oil splatters.

4. Add onions to the pan and cook about 15 minutes on medium heat, or until the onions start to turn uniformly golden. Add the cumin and coriander, and stir. Add the celery, cover, and cook another 10 minutes. Add the asafetida, sage, oregano, thyme, and rosemary, and stir. Let the herbs sauté about 1 minute.

5. While the vegetables sauté, clean and chop the mushrooms. If you have a food processor, put all the mushrooms in the bowl and pulse several times until the mushrooms are minced. After the fresh herbs have cooked for a minute, add the mushrooms to the pan, along with 1½ cups of the soup stock and the Bragg's. Cover the pan and simmer about 10 minutes, stirring occasionally.

6. While the mushrooms simmer, preheat the oven to 400°F, and lightly grease a 9 x 13 or 10-inch round baking dish with a little ghee or butter. Chop the parsley and walnuts.

7. To complete the dressing: Add the cooked vegetable mixture to the bowl of bread pieces. Add parsley, walnuts, and salt. (**Note:** If you are using a boxed or canned stock that is already salted, taste first, and add salt 1 teaspoon at a time as needed.) Stir with a large spoon or spatula, and mix well. If the mixture seems dry, add more stock, up to 2½ cups total liquid. The dressing should be quite moist before it is baked.

8. Transfer the dressing mixture to the baking dish and cover with foil. Bake covered for 30 minutes. Remove the foil and bake another 30 to 40 minutes, or until the top is brown and crisp, to caramelize the onions. (**Note:** If you prepare the dressing the day before, bake 1 hour covered and another 20 to 30 minutes uncovered until the top is browned.) Keep in a warm oven until serving.

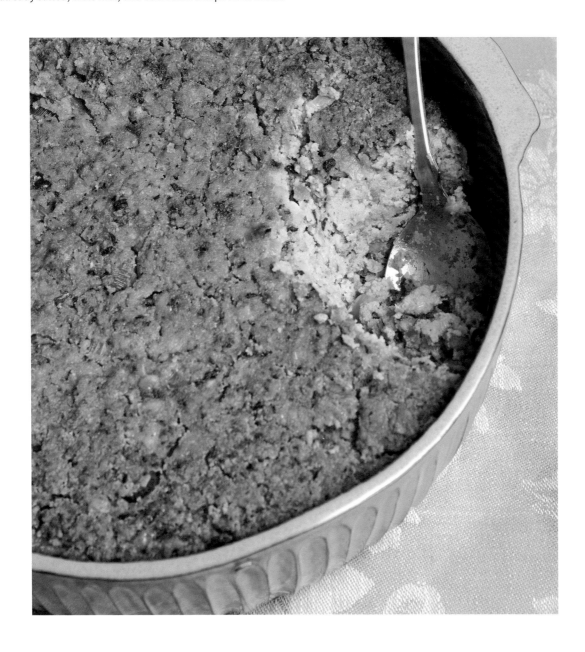

OLD-FASHIONED BAKED BEANS

Preparation Time: 3 to 5 hours (1 hour active)
Serves 8 to 12

Oh, how I love baked beans! One friend was so enthusiastic about this dish that he hounded me to package it and sell it—not quite the Ayurvedic paradigm of fresh food! This sweet-and-sour sauce can also be used on occasion as a high-calorie marinade for grilled vegetables or tofu.

3 cups dry Great Northern beans or navy beans
8 to 9 cups water

FOR THE SAUCE:
2 cups chopped Vidalia or yellow onions
3 tablespoons ghee, coconut oil, or olive oil,
**   plus 1 teaspoon to oil the baking dish**
⅛ teaspoon asafetida
1 thin round slice of poblano pepper
5 curry leaves
2 large heirloom tomatoes, chopped and seeded
2 tablespoons Bragg Liquid Aminos
3 teaspoons ground cumin
3 teaspoons ground coriander
2 teaspoons yellow mustard powder
2 cloves garlic, chopped or pressed
4 to 5 teaspoons Light Grey Celtic Sea Salt
¼ cup coconut sugar
½ cup unsulphured molasses
2 to 3 cups reserved cooking water from the beans

COOK'S TIP: Beans will take varying amounts of time to bake until tender, depending on their quality and age.

AYURVEDIC NOTE

White beans are good for *kapha* and *pitta*, although they are especially difficult to digest for people with *vata* problems. Soaking the beans overnight makes them easier to digest. *Vata* and *kapha* are supported by the asafetida, garlic, mustard, and onions, though the mustard increases *pitta*, and the molasses will increase both *pitta* and *kapha*. Tomatoes increase all *doshas*, particularly *pitta*, which is balanced somewhat by the cumin and coconut sugar. I know, it's starting to sound complicated! What to do? Follow the directions below, based on your type, and save this dish for an occasional treat!

(P) Reduce garlic to 1 clove; omit mustard or reduce to ½ teaspoon.

(K) Reduce molasses to ¼ cup. Double and mince the poblano pepper, and leave the pepper in the sauce.

MENU SUGGESTION

Serve with foods that are easy to digest and pacifying to *vata* and *pitta*, such as Sweet Potato Salad (page 220), Quick Sautéed Asparagus (page 173), and Simple Summer Squash (page 193). Also serve with Summertime Tea (page 85), or peppermint tea to pacify *pitta* and aid digestion.

1. Soak the beans in cold water overnight. Rinse the beans a few times and place them in a 6-quart soup pot, cover with water, and bring to a boil. Reduce heat to medium-low and simmer covered for about an hour, until the beans become just tender. Occasionally lift the lid and skim the froth to keep the pot from boiling over. Do not overcook. Strain the beans, saving 3 cups of the liquid. Return the beans to the pot.

2. Make the sauce: Chop the onion and slice the poblano. Heat the ghee or oil in a large sauté pan or separate soup pot on medium heat. When the ghee is hot, add the asafetida and the single slice of poblano pepper. Add the curry leaves and cover immediately in case the leaves pop. Remove the lid and add onions to the oil, sautéing the onions until they turn golden.

3. While the onions sauté, prepare the tomatoes by cutting them in half. Squeeze each half through a strainer over a bowl to retain the tomato juice. Shake the pulp to discard the seeds; then chop the remaining pulp.

4. Pour tomato juice and the Bragg's into the sauté pan and stir into the onions. Add the cumin, coriander, and mustard powder, and stir well. Add the chopped tomato, garlic, and 4 teaspoons salt, and stir. Cover and simmer on medium-low heat for 15 minutes or until the chopped tomato is tender. Uncover and, if you like a more refined dish, remove the tomato skins that float to the surface. Also remove the poblano slice at this time.

5. While the sauce is cooking, grease a 3-quart, 9 x 13 glass baking dish. Ideally, preheat the oven to 300°F to slow bake the beans for 4 hours. Otherwise, preheat the oven to 350°F, and plan to bake them for at least 2 hours or until the beans are quite tender.

6. To complete the sauce, add coconut sugar, molasses, and 2 cups of the reserved cooking water from the beans. (Refrigerate the remaining cup.) Pour the sauce over the beans and stir well. Transfer the beans and sauce to the baking dish, and bake them uncovered according to the instructions in step 5. After two hours, taste the beans, and add more salt if you wish. Also, if the beans start to look dry, add more of the cooking water from the beans. The beans will be finished when they are very tender and the top is browned.

Muslim Prayer

This traditional invocation, or dua, *is said before meals. Anyone who reads or speaks this* dua *receives blessings for the food they are about to eat.*

Bismillahi wa 'ala baraka-tillah.
With Allah's name and upon the blessings granted by
Allah (do we eat).

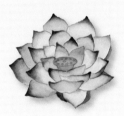

REFRIED BEANS

Preparation Time: 8 hours soaking, plus 1½ to 2 hours cooking (30 minutes active)
Serves 8

I started my exploration of vegetarian food when I was a senior at the University of South Carolina. Near the campus was a vegetarian co-op and small restaurant called 221 Pickens, which was co-owned by a friendly and energetic cook, Frank Lee. I have fond memories of Frank's yummy burritos and chalupas, made with refried beans and piled high with fresh lettuce, tomatoes, and sprouts. This recipe is my tribute to that wonderful dish. I left South Carolina and didn't see Frank for more than thirty years. Recently, my husband and I found Frank at the chic Charleston restaurant, Slightly North of Broad, where I was happy to find him as executive chef and a guiding force in the Low Country's culinary renaissance.

2 cups dried pinto beans
5 cups water
1 large onion
2 cloves garlic, pressed
1 to 2 teaspoons finely diced poblano pepper
2 tablespoons olive oil
1 pinch asafetida
1 teaspoon cumin
1 teaspoon coriander
1 teaspoon fresh ginger
1 to 2 teaspoons Fine Ground Celtic Sea Salt

AYURVEDIC NOTE

Like most legumes, pinto beans are difficult for most people to digest because they increase *vata*, but they are made more tolerable by soaking them overnight. Adding the heating spices of asafetida, garlic, and ginger along with the heat of the onion and poblano pepper also helps balance *vata*, as will ensuring that the beans are not served too dry.

 You may want to omit poblano pepper if you suffer from arthritis.

P Use 1 clove garlic, and olive or coconut oil.

MENU SUGGESTION

Serve as a side dish with grains and easy-to-digest vegetables such as Simple Summer Squash (page 193). Or serve as a base to a Mexican-style entrée such as Sweet Potato Burritos (page 145).

1. Soak beans overnight. Rinse them a few times until the rinsing water is clear.

In a Pressure Cooker: Place the beans in the pot with cold water. Seal the pressure cooker and place it on high heat until it reaches maximum pressure according to the manufacturer's directions. Turn off the heat on a gas stove; on an electric stove, gently move the pot to a cool spot on the stove and allow the pressure to release as the pot cools, about 15 minutes. Finally, open the cooker when it's safe according to the manufacturer's directions. When the cooker is opened, the beans should be tender. If they're still a bit tough, continue to cook them on medium heat, covered but without the seal.

In a Stainless Steel Soup Pot: Bring the beans to a boil in the cold water. Reduce the heat to medium or medium-low, and simmer the beans, covered, 1 to 2 hours (depending on your altitude and humidity and on how long the beans have been stored). As the beans cook, stir them occasionally. Cook until they are fully tender.

2. While the beans are cooking, chop the onion, peel and chop the garlic, and dice a thin round slice of poblano pepper. Heat the oil in a large sauté pan on medium heat. When the oil is hot, add the asafetida to the pan. Add the onions and poblano pepper, and sauté until the onions turn golden. Add the cumin and coriander, and reduce heat to medium-low. Continue to cook the onions slowly, about 15 or 20 minutes, stirring often until their edges start to brown and they caramelize. Add the garlic and ginger, and stir for 30 seconds. Remove from heat.

3. When the beans are tender, drain them, saving 1½ cups of the liquid. Return the beans to their cooking pot. Add salt and mash the beans with a potato masher. Transfer the mashed beans to the sauté pan with the onion mixture and ½ cup of the saved cooking water. Refry the beans on medium heat for about 5 minutes, stirring well to combine the beans with the onions and spices. If the beans look dry, add more of the saved cooking water. The beans should be slightly moist but not runny.

QUICK TOFU

Preparation Time: 30 minutes pressing (optional), plus 12 minutes cooking
Serves 4 to 6

This tofu dish is even quicker to make than the last one. It's perfect on its own or as a side dish for any menu when you want additional protein. It's ideal to press the tofu first, but when I'm hungry NOW, I put it right on the pan, and presto, I have some quick protein! You can make this with one or two spices, whatever your taste buds are calling for.

1 16-ounce cake of extra-firm tofu

2 teaspoons olive oil or ghee

1 tablespoon Bragg Liquid Aminos

½ teaspoon onion powder, mild paprika, or any favorite spice

AYURVEDIC NOTE

All spices are energizing for *kapha* and (with two exceptions) calming to *vata*. Excessive cayenne pepper or paprika can be drying, which will increase *vata*. If you have *pitta* problems, it's best to avoid the strongly heating spices. Bragg's, a flavoring agent, will increase *pitta* and *kapha*, so use sparingly.

K Add a dash of cayenne pepper or red pepper flakes.

1. Press tofu for 30 minutes, if time permits (directions page 170). Cut tofu into 8 planks. Preheat a ceramic nonstick sauté pan on medium heat, and oil the pan.

2. Combine the Bragg's and spice in a small spouted measuring cup.

3. Place the tofu planks on the hot oiled pan. Pour the mixture over the tofu planks and cook for 5 minutes on each side until the tofu browns. Serve immediately.

SAVORY TOFU

Preparation Time: 30 minutes pressing (optional), plus 10 to 30 minutes cooking (10 minutes active)
Serves 4 to 6

I have two super easy ways to approach tofu. With either dish, you can brown the tofu in a ceramic nonstick sauté pan or put it on an indoor or outdoor grill.

1 16-ounce cake of extra-firm tofu
2 tablespoons Bragg Liquid Aminos
1 tablespoon olive oil
1 teaspoon ground cumin
1 teaspoon ground coriander
1 teaspoon freshly grated ginger
1 clove garlic, pressed
1 teaspoon balsamic vinegar
1 teaspoon maple syrup (optional)

COOKS TIP: 1. Press the tofu in advance to increase the tofu's ability to absorb a marinade and hold its shape well. **2.** You can use any combination of favorite herbs and spices. Try dried basil and oregano. Omit either garlic or ginger, keeping one as an aid to digestion. Add a pinch of cayenne. Create your own mixture!

AYURVEDIC NOTE

Ginger and garlic help pacify the *vata*-producing quality of tofu as does the salty Bragg's. Cumin and coriander aid digestion. Vinegar increases *pitta*, but is fine for most people in this small quantity.

P Reduce or omit garlic. Only use 1 tablespoon of Bragg's. You may want to omit vinegar.

K Omit maple syrup.

1. Press the tofu block by placing the tofu block on a heavy dinner plate; then cover the block with a second plate. Place a heavy object such as a cookbook on the plate. Let the tofu rest for 20 to 30 minutes. After pressing and pouring off the water, cut the tofu into 6 or 8 planks. Pour half of the Bragg's over the tofu.

2. Whisk the remaining ingredients (including the second tablespoon of Bragg's) in a small dish until they form a paste.

Use a basting brush to apply the paste to the tofu. Cook in a preheated ceramic nonstick sauté or on a grill pan on medium heat until the tofu starts to brown, 5 to 7 minutes on each side. If you don't have enough stove-top space when cooking a multi-dish meal, you can bake this tofu dish for 30 minutes at 400°F.

NUT-BUTTER SAUCE

Preparation Time: About 10 minutes
Makes about 1 cup

Initially, I devised this as a marinade for tofu, but I've also found it to be utterly delicious—and extremely useful—as a sauce over grilled, sautéed, or steamed vegetables. This sauce can be made successfully with your favorite spread, mine being almond butter.

½ cup almond, cashew, peanut, or sunflower butter
1 teaspoon freshly grated ginger
1 cup washed cilantro
1 tablespoon Bragg Liquid Aminos, or more, to taste
½ to 1 cup water, depending on preferred consistency

AYURVEDIC NOTE
This sauce is slightly heating because of the nut butter and ginger, so it is excellent for fall and winter months. It will increase *pitta* conditions because it is heating and oily, and the oily quality also increases *kapha*. Of the nut butters, almond butter is the least aggravating to *pitta*.

V Add 1 clove pressed garlic if you like.

P Double cilantro.

K Add 1 clove pressed garlic if you like.

1. Put all the ingredients in a blender or food processer, and pulse several times until well blended.

2. Pour over steamed vegetables or cooked tofu, or add to a stir-fry during the last couple of minutes so that the sauce is heated before serving.

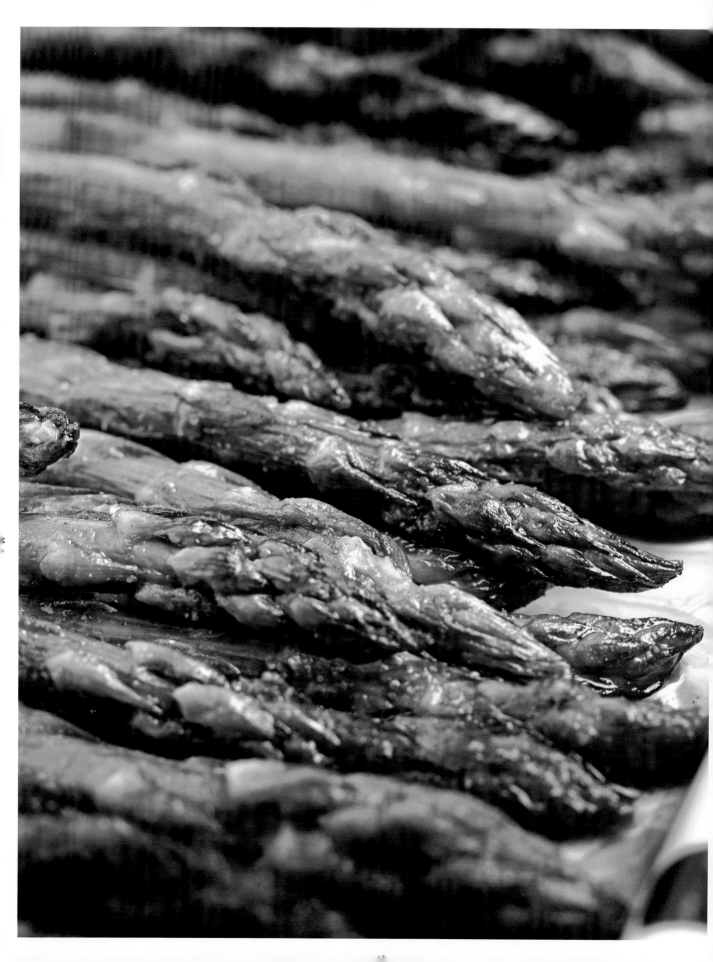

QUICK SAUTÉED ASPARAGUS

Preparation Time: About 10 minutes (5 minutes active)
Serves 4

This is my favorite quick side dish to accompany almost any menu. It comes in especially handy when I'm making a complex and time-consuming main dish and I need an easy recipe to complete the meal.

1 pound asparagus
2 tablespoons ghee or coconut oil
1 teaspoon ground coriander
1 teaspoon ground cumin
1 to 2 tablespoons Bragg Liquid Aminos

SHOPPING TIP: When shopping for asparagus, I choose spears that are as thin as possible. I like the taste, they cook more quickly, and more of the spear is edible. However, our longtime family friend and great cook, Peggy Crowley, used to swear that the thick spears have all the taste. As my mother says, "To each his own." You may want to experiment with both and decide for yourself.

AYURVEDIC NOTE

This version of asparagus is good for all *doshas* and can be served year-round, although it is best eaten in season, which is spring.

 Use only 1 tablespoon Bragg Liquid Aminos.

1. Rinse the asparagus in water. Break and throw away the woody lower quarter or third of each asparagus spear.

2. Heat the ghee or oil in a large sauté pan on medium-high heat. When the oil is hot but not smoking, sprinkle the pan with coriander and cumin, add the asparagus, and splash with Bragg's. Cover the pan and cook for 2 to 3 minutes on medium-high to sear the spices. Remove spears from the pan when the asparagus are tender when pierced with a fork or skewer. With thicker spears, continue cooking on medium-low another 3 to 4 minutes, until tender. Taste and add more Bragg's as needed.

Asparagus Tip

When you bring home asparagus from the store, break off the woody lower quarter of each spear by hand, or cut the lower extremities with a knife and throw them away. (Some people will scrape the tough skins at the bottom of thick spears with a potato peeler, which is great for reducing wastefulness if you have the time to expend the effort.) Rinse the remaining stalks and place them in a wide-mouthed jar or tall glass with about 1 inch of water in the bottom of the container. Store them upright in the refrigerator, and cover with a plastic bag. They will remain fresh enough to eat for up to three days.

ROASTED BEET CHIPS

Preparation Time: About 35 minutes (10 minutes active)
Serves 4

I was forty-something when I first ate fresh beets. Before this, I'd had only canned beets at my mother's table—which is why I didn't much care for beets—but fresh beets are another food altogether. Serve the beets plain as a side dish or over red leaf lettuce, which makes an elegant salad. Slice them extra thin and roast them until they are crisp, and they almost pass for a potato chip–like snack.

4 small or 3 medium- to large-sized beets, no greens
1 tablespoon olive or sunflower oil
1 tablespoon fresh thyme (or 1 teaspoon dried)
¼ teaspoon Fine Ground Celtic Sea Salt
1 teaspoon sesame seeds (optional)
1 teaspoon coconut sugar (optional)

COOK'S TIP: Beets can be very sweet, but sometimes you can get a bitter batch, and these beets increase *vata*. For this reason, you may want to add a little coconut sugar with the herbs and salt.

AYURVEDIC NOTE
Cooked beets are fine for all *doshas*. If you make them too crisp, they will provoke *vata*, even though they are delicious! Sesame products rank in the USDA's list of most common food allergens, so avoid if necessary.

 Use sunflower oil instead of olive oil.

1. Preheat the oven to 425°F. Cover a cookie sheet with parchment paper.

2. Scrub and slice the beets as thinly as possible in a food processor or with a very sharp knife.

3. Combine all the other ingredients except the sesame seeds in a medium-sized mixing bowl. Add the beet slices to the bowl and toss them so they are covered with the oil and spices.

4. Place the slices on the parchment sheet in a single layer. Sprinkle with sesame seeds. Bake for 15 to 30 minutes, depending on their thickness, until the beets are tender when pierced with a fork and their edges just start to blacken. They'll be a little crispy and caramelized.

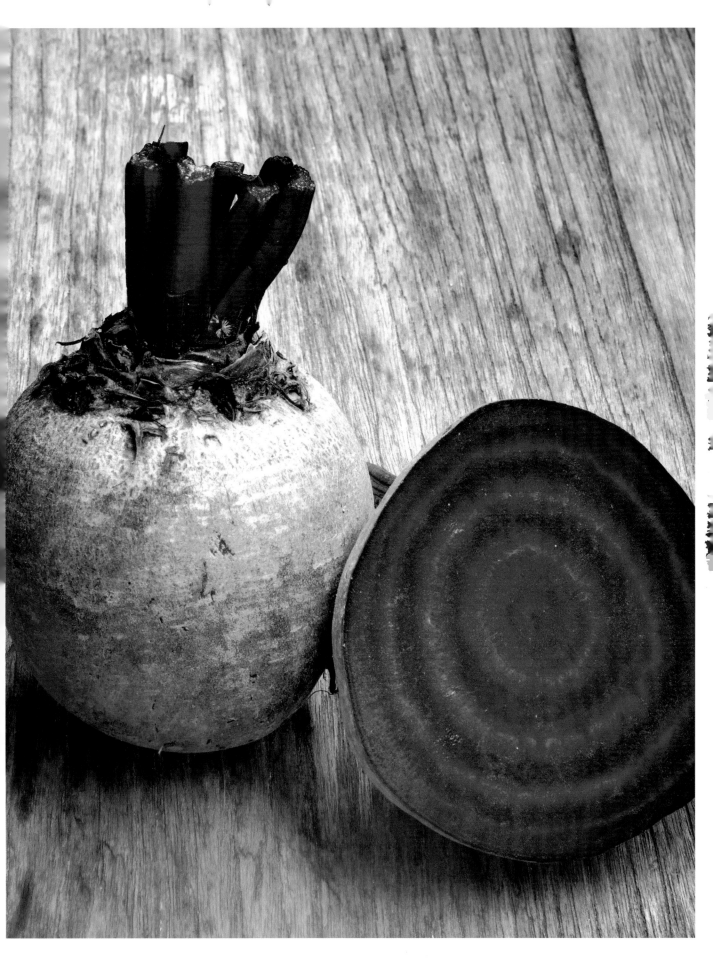

BROCCOLI WITH CARAMELIZED ONION MASALA

Preparation Time: About 1 hour
Serves 6 to 8

This is a special occasion broccoli dish, perfect for company when you hope to impress!

1 medium onion
1½ tablespoons plus 1 teaspoon ghee or coconut oil
1 small or medium tomato
1 garlic clove, pressed or whole
1 teaspoon freshly grated ginger
1 teaspoon ground cumin
½ cup unsweetened dried coconut
½ teaspoon Light Grey Celtic Sea Salt
1 tablespoon coconut sugar
1 tablespoon Bragg Liquid Aminos
1 cup water
3 to 4 stalks broccoli plus florets

FOR THE *TARKA*:
1 tablespoon ghee or coconut oil
½ teaspoon black mustard seeds
½ teaspoon cumin seeds
1 pinch asafetida (optional)
3 large or 5 medium curry leaves (that's leaves, not powder!)
¼ teaspoon ground turmeric
¼ teaspoon garam masala
1 teaspoon ground coriander

AYURVEDIC NOTE

Broccoli is excellent for *pitta* and *kapha* but will increase *vata,* which is calmed by the ghee or oil as well as the heating spices, particularly asafetida, garlic, ginger, and garam masala. Tomato increases all the *doshas,* particularly *pitta,* which is balanced by cumin, coriander, and coconut.

 Reduce garam masala to ⅛ teaspoon.

1. Chop the onion. Heat the 1½ tablespoons of ghee or oil in a large sauté pan on medium heat. Add the onion and cook until brown and crispy—but not black. Remove the sautéed onion with a slotted spoon and drain on a plate covered with a paper towel.

2. Chop the tomato, peel the garlic clove, and peel and grate the ginger. Heat 1 tablespoon of ghee or oil in a 3-quart or larger pot on medium-low heat. Add ground cumin to the pan and stir for about 10 seconds. Add dried coconut and stir for another 10 seconds. Add the diced tomato, salt, coconut sugar, Bragg's, and water. Add the garlic and ginger to the pot. Cover and simmer on medium-low for about 15 minutes or until the tomato is well cooked.

3. While the sauce is simmering, chop off and discard the bottom ½ to 1 inch of the broccoli stalks, peel the remaining stalks, and slice into rounds. Also separate the florets into bite-sized pieces. Place a steamer basket into a pot with 2 to 3 cups of water, enough to bring to a boil without submerging the broccoli. Add the broccoli to the steamer, bring to a boil, and cover the pot. Steam the broccoli for 7 to 10 minutes or until it is just tender. While the broccoli is steaming, create an ice bath in a bowl of water. Remove broccoli from the pot and put it into the ice bath to stop the cooking process. Strain and set the broccoli aside in a mixing bowl.

4. Return to the tomato sauce: Once the tomatoes are tender, transfer the caramelized onions to the pot. Purée the tomato sauce and onions using a handheld immersion blender. Or, once the mixture is cooled, purée it in a blender or food processor; then return the puréed sauce to the pan to stay warm.

5. Create the *tarka*: Heat the ghee or oil in the sauté pan on medium heat. Add the mustard seeds and cover, as they will pop like popcorn. When the seeds finish popping, turn the heat off and remove the pan from the heat source. Add the cumin seeds, and let them sizzle and become fragrant. Add the asafetida and curry leaves; cover immediately for a few seconds, as the curry leaves may splatter. Add turmeric, garam masala, and coriander, and stir for a few seconds.

6. Add the *tarka* to the tomato sauce and stir. Let the sauce simmer with the spices for a couple of minutes. Then pour the sauce over the broccoli. Serve as a side dish or over basmati rice or quinoa.

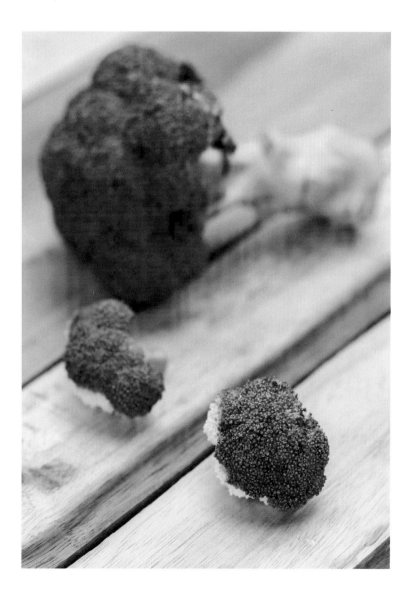

NOT-YOUR-MOTHER'S BROCCOLI CASSEROLE

Preparation Time: About 1¼ hours (45 minutes active)
Serves 10 to 12

Craving something cheesy? Try this variation of a pure Southern comfort-food casserole that my friend Marie Pardue Iddings brought to a vegetarian potluck. If you've given up dairy, as I have in recent years, you can still create a delicious casserole experience with coconut or almond yogurt.

2 cups uncooked quinoa

3 cups water

½ teaspoon Fine Ground Celtic Sea Salt

6 fresh broccoli stalks with florets

10 to 12 shiitake or mini portobello mushrooms

1 medium yellow onion, chopped fine

1 teaspoon minced poblano pepper (optional)

2 tablespoons ghee or coconut oil, plus 1 teaspoon to grease the casserole dish

10 ounces goat Cheddar cheese or 1¼ cups plain vegan yogurt

2 teaspoons freshly grated ginger

Large handful of fresh basil (or 2 teaspoons dried)

2 cups Easy Vegetable Soup Stock (page 90)

½ cup pine nuts or chopped walnuts, pecans, or pistachios

Freshly grated black pepper

FOR THE TOPPING (OPTIONAL):

1 cup fine almond flour

¼ teaspoon Fine Ground Celtic Sea Salt

¼ cup chilled ghee or coconut oil

1 tablespoon coconut sugar (optional)

2 to 3 tablespoons ice water

AYURVEDIC NOTE

Broccoli is excellent for *pitta* and *kapha,* as it is astringent, although it increases *vata* for the same reasons. Mushrooms also increase *vata.* These are balanced by the basmati rice and the heating ingredients: onion, poblano pepper, and ginger as well as by milk and cheese. The dairy will increase *kapha* (mucus formation), which is mitigated somewhat by using ginger. Cheese also increases *pitta,* but it is acceptable on occasion. Coconut milk yogurt is preferable to cheese.

(P) Omit poblano pepper. Use vegan yogurt instead of cheese, or reduce amount of cheese.

(K) Use almond yogurt (not coconut) instead of cheese. Omit breadcrumb topping.

(S) Omit poblano pepper.

1. Cook the quinoa with water and salt by bringing it to a boil; then reduce the heat and simmer on medium-low heat until all the water is absorbed. While the quinoa is cooking, prepare the broccoli. Chop off the bottom inch of the stalks, peel the remaining stalks, and chop into rounds about ⅛-inch thick. Separate the heads into bite-sized florets.

2. Clean and slice the mushrooms. Mince the onion and poblano pepper. Heat the ghee or oil in a 6-quart soup pot or Dutch oven on medium heat. Sauté the onion and pepper 15 minutes or until the onion turns golden and starts to brown. Add the mushrooms and broccoli, cover the pot, and cook for another 10 minutes.

3. Preheat the oven to 350°F. If using cheese, grate it now and set aside ½ cup. Grate the ginger, and chop the basil.

4. In a separate saucepan, heat the stock on medium with all but ½ cup of the cheese. (If you're replacing cheese with yogurt, combine all of the yogurt with the stock.) Add the ginger, and basil, stirring constantly until all the cheese melts. Pour the sauce over the vegetables. Add cooked rice, salt, and nuts. Stir well and taste. Add more salt if needed.

5. If not using a Dutch oven, grease a 3-quart casserole dish, and pour the mixture into the dish. If you wish, sprinkle ½ cup of cheese on the top.

6. If using the topping: Combine the ingredients in a food processor, starting with 2 tablespoons of ice water. Pulse a few times until the flour forms crumbles. Add more water if necessary. Sprinkle the crumbles over the cheese.

7. Bake the dish uncovered for 15 to 20 minutes until the topping has lightly browned or the cheese is melted.

BRUSSELS SPROUTS

Preparation Time: About 30 minutes
Serves 4 to 5

Brussels sprouts look just like baby cabbages and are, indeed, members of the cruciferous family. You can buy Brussels sprouts on the stalk at farmers' markets in the autumn and winter months. They tend to be less bitter when they're fresh on the stalk, and they are still quite inexpensive. When buying Brussels sprouts from a bin, select those that are smallest.

3 shallots or 1 small onion

1 tablespoon olive or coconut oil
1 pinch asafetida (optional)
16 to 20 small Brussels sprouts or the entire bunch on a stalk
1 teaspoon ground cumin
½ teaspoon ground turmeric
1 teaspoon ground coriander
1 teaspoon coconut sugar (optional)
¼ cup water
1 teaspoon freshly ground ginger
1 clove garlic, pressed (optional)
1 teaspoon Fine Ground Celtic Sea Salt
A few drops of balsamic vinegar or a splash of fresh lime juice

AYURVEDIC NOTE

Brussels sprouts, like their kin in the cabbage family, will increase *vata*, which is why I add the touch of asafetida along with the cumin, coriander, turmeric, ginger, and garlic—all digestive aids. Vinegar increases *pitta*, but a few drops should be fine, unless you follow an anti-candida diet.

(V) Use the optional asafetida and/or garlic.

(K) Use the optional garlic, if you like.

1. Dice the shallots or onion. Pull the Brussels sprouts off the stalk and remove any stems. Remove any yellow leaves. Cut an X in the root bottoms.

2. In a large sauté pan, heat oil on medium heat. When the oil is warm, add the asafetida and shallots. Cook until the shallots turn uniformly golden and start to brown, 10 to 15 minutes.

3. Reduce heat to medium-low. Add the cumin, turmeric, coriander, and stir. Add ¼ cup water, coconut sugar, and salt. Add the Brussels sprouts, stir, and let them simmer for 8 to 10 minutes, or until they are just tender. Do not overcook.

4. Add the ginger, optional garlic, and stir. Drizzle with a small amount of good balsamic vinegar or a little fresh lime juice, to taste. Serve immediately.

QUICK STOVE-TOP MAPLE CARROTS

Preparation Time: About 15 minutes
Serves 4 to 6

Need a quick side dish? Look no further.

8 medium carrots
2 teaspoons ghee or unsalted butter
2 tablespoons pure maple syrup
½ teaspoon Fine Ground Celtic Sea Salt
2 tablespoons fresh dill or 2 teaspoons dried
Splash of fresh lime (optional)

AYURVEDIC NOTE

Raw carrots can increase *pitta*, but when cooked, they are sweet and tender, making them fine for all *doshas*.

K Omit maple syrup. If you must add a sweetener, add 1 teaspoon coconut sugar, which is said to have a lower glycemic index than maple, or a pinch of stevia.

1. Scrub the carrots with a vegetable brush, and slice them into ¼-inch-thick rounds.

2. Heat the ghee or butter in a medium-sized saucepan on medium-low heat. Add the carrots, maple syrup, and salt. Cover and cook on medium-low 10 minutes or until the carrots are tender. Stir occasionally.

3. While the carrots are cooking, snip the dill with scissors or pull the fronds off with your hands. Add dill to the carrots and, if you'd like a dish that is both sweet and sour, serve with a splash of lime.

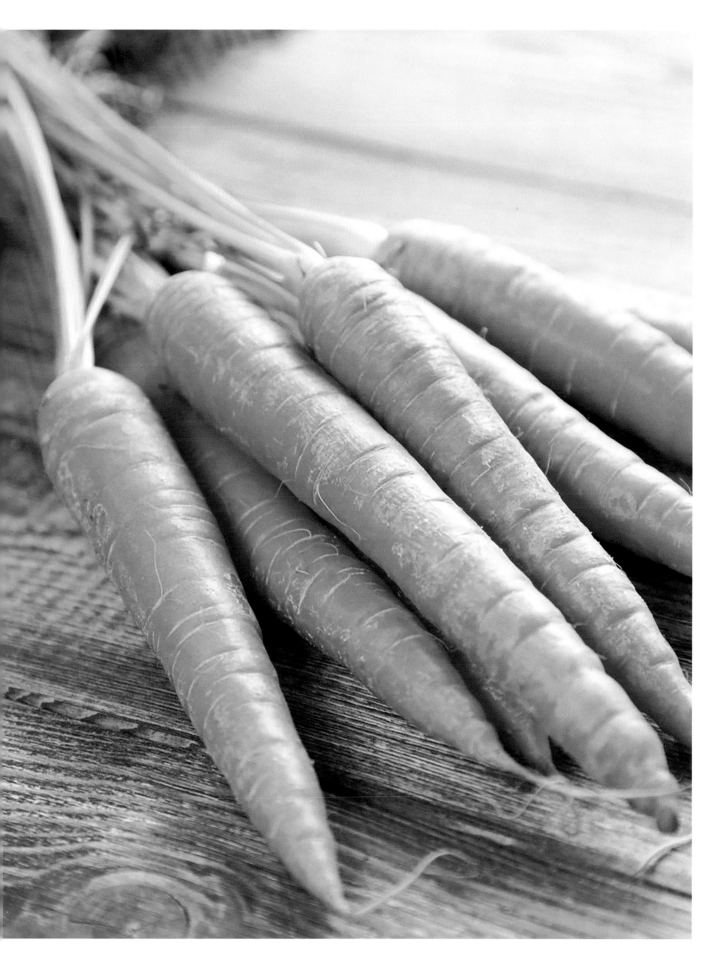

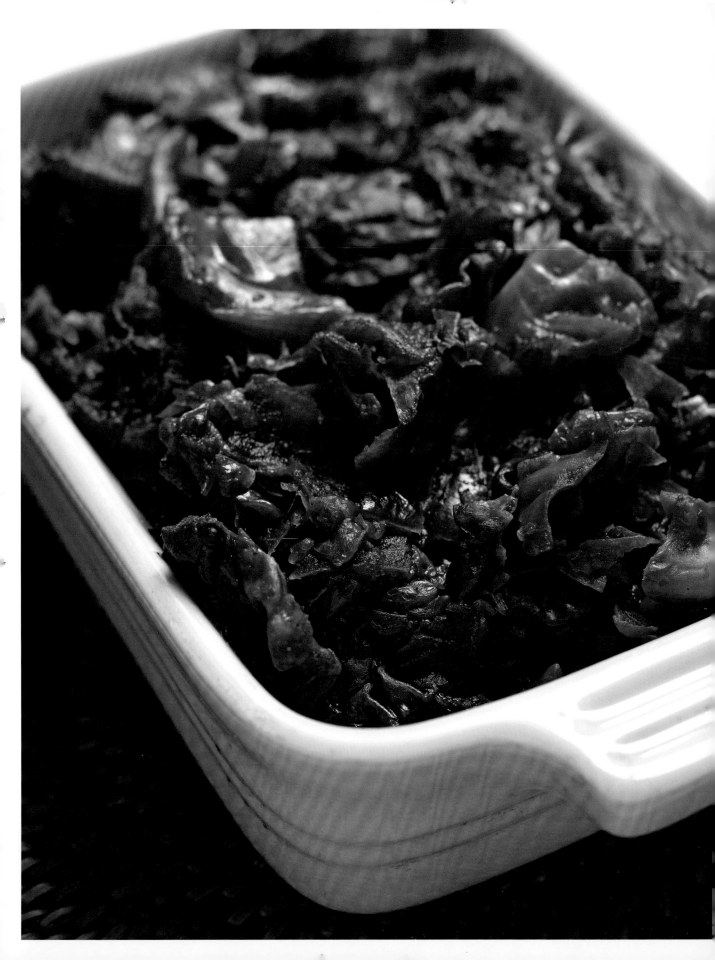

SAUTÉED RED CABBAGE

Preparation Time: About 45 minutes
Serves 6 to 8

I used to think I didn't like cabbage until I tasted a cabbage dish so delectable that I had to ask for the chef's secret. The chef was my friend, the late Gino Izetta, who was raised in Italy and was a successful chef in New York and, later, Raleigh. Happy to oblige, he shared that his "secret ingredient" for this dish was ketchup! He also used balsamic vinegar and garlic—very Italian! I decided to veer in a different direction by adding a mélange of spices to aid digestion, but I did my best to mimic Gino's inspired treatment of braised cabbage.

1 medium onion
2 tablespoons ghee or olive oil
½ teaspoon black mustard seeds
1 to 2 pinches asafetida
3 curry leaves (optional)
1 small to medium head of red cabbage (4 to 6 cups cut)
1 teaspoon ground cumin
1 teaspoon ground coriander
½ to 1 cup water
1 tablespoon coconut sugar (optional)
1 teaspoon Light Grey Celtic Sea Salt
2 tablespoons Bragg Liquid Aminos
2 teaspoons freshly grated ginger
2 to 3 teaspoons fresh lime juice

COOK'S TIP: Since every head of cabbage is a different size, taste the dish to see if it needs more salt, additional ginger, or another squeeze of ketchup to give the dish enough flavor.

AYURVEDIC NOTE

I experience cabbage as one of the more *vata-*increasing vegetables on the planet, which is why I start and finish with some heating spices, including asafetida, mustard seeds, and ginger.

V Add 1 to 2 cloves pressed garlic if you like.

P Omit ketchup, if you'd like to be a purist.

K Omit coconut sugar and cut ketchup in half.

1. Chop onion and set aside.

2. Heat ghee or oil in a large sauté pan on medium heat. When the ghee is hot, add mustard seeds, and cover until the seeds pop like popcorn. When the seeds finish popping, add a good-sized pinch of asafetida as well as curry leaves, and quickly cover for several seconds, as the leaves may pop. Add the chopped onion and sauté until the onion is uniformly golden and has begun to brown, at least 15 minutes.

3. While onion is sautéing, chop the cabbage with a large knife, first into 1-inch-thick circles (the full diameter of the cabbage); then cut these circles into strips, and cut each strip into several bite-sized chunks.

4. When the onion has just started to brown, add cumin and coriander to the pan, and stir for about 10 seconds. Add the cabbage with ¼ cup water, coconut sugar, salt and Bragg's. Stir well and cover. Peel and grate the ginger, add it to the pan, stir, and re-cover. Continue to cook on medium heat, stirring frequently. You may need to add more water if the cabbage starts to stick. Cook 20 to 30 minutes until the cabbage is completely tender. Add lime juice to taste. Stir and serve.

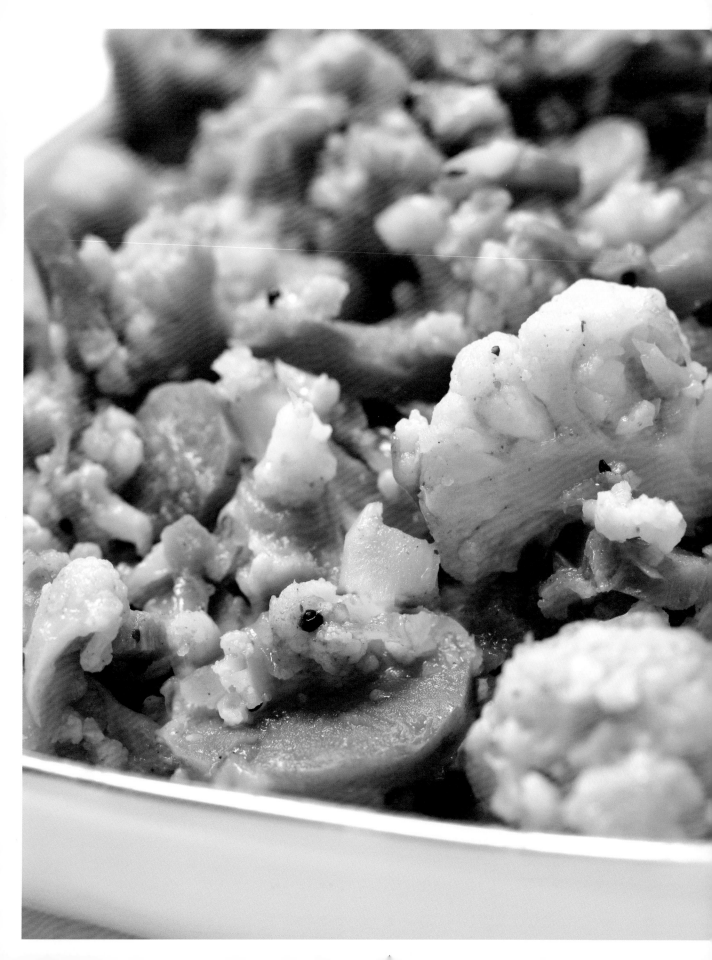

SAVORY CAULIFLOWER AND CARROTS

Preparation Time: About 45 minutes

Serves 4 to 6

Put a plate of plain steamed cauliflower in front of me, and I'll pass. But when it's gussied up enough with the right spices, I've learned to enjoy cauliflower as much as any other vegetable. If you're wary of curries, I hope you'll give this one a try. It has curry flavor without the heat!

1 medium onion

4 medium carrots

2 tablespoons ghee

½ teaspoon black mustard seeds

1 pinch asafetida (optional)

1 teaspoon ground turmeric

1 teaspoon ground cumin

1 teaspoon ground coriander

½ cup water

1 medium or large head cauliflower (3 to 4 cups of florets)

1 tablespoons Bragg Liquid Aminos

1 heaping teaspoon of freshly grated ginger

Salt, to taste

2 teaspoons sesame seeds (optional)

COOK'S TIP: 1. To deepen and sweeten the cauliflower flavor, roast it with a little oil at 425°F about 30 minutes prior to adding to the pan of onions and carrots. Continue to cook the cauliflower with the onions and carrots until all the vegetables are completely tender. **2.** If you have a large amount of cauliflower and would like more gravy to serve over rice, add another ½ cup of water.

AYURVEDIC NOTE

Cauliflower is excellent for *pitta* and *kapha* but will increase *vata*. Cooked carrots are good for all *doshas*, and the heat of mustard seeds, asafetida, and ginger all mitigate cauliflower's *vata* quality.

V Add more ginger.

K Cut the amount of ghee in half. Add 1 or 2 pinches of cayenne pepper, if you don't suffer from *vata* and *pitta* problems.

1. Peel and dice the onion. Scrub and slice the carrots into rounds about ⅛-inch thick.

2. In a large sauté pan or medium-sized soup pot, heat ghee on medium heat. When the ghee is hot, add mustard seeds, and cover, as they will pop like popcorn. Once they finish popping, reduce heat to medium-low, and add the asafetida and diced onion. Sauté until the onion turns uniformly golden, about 10 minutes. Reduce heat to medium-low and continue cooking the onion for another 10 minutes or more so the onion continues to brown and sweeten.

3. Add the turmeric, cumin, and coriander, and stir for about 10 seconds. Add the sliced carrots and ½ cup water, and cover for about 5 minutes.

4. While the carrots are cooking, wash and separate the cauliflower. Add the cauliflower florets to the pan along with Bragg's, and stir. Re-cover the pan, and reduce heat to medium-low, cooking for 10 to 15 minutes, stirring occasionally, until the cauliflower is completely tender.

5. Once the cauliflower is tender, add the grated ginger to the pan, and stir. Add salt, if needed. Then sprinkle the dish with sesame seeds, and serve.

ELEGANT GREEN BEANS

Preparation Time: 30 to 45 minutes (10 to 20 minutes active)
Serves 6

This is one of my favorite recipes! I make it weekly because it's easy, yummy, and complements most any dish. When my husband and I are invited to a potluck, friends often request these elegant green beans. And you'll always find them on the menu at our house on Thanksgiving and Christmas!

4 to 5 cups green beans
2 tablespoons ghee, olive oil, or coconut oil
1 medium leek bulb plus an inch of the light-green shank
2 teaspoons dried basil
1 heaping teaspoon freshly grated ginger
2 tablespoons Bragg Liquid Aminos
2 to 3 teaspoons fresh lime juice (optional)

TIME-SAVER: The trick to making fresh green bean dishes when you come home from work is to snap the beans the night before. This makes cooking time a snap! Make it a 10-minute party around the table with your kids, or snap them while watching your favorite family movie! Faster still, just snap off the ends, and let your family practice the elegant skills of using a fork and knife! Or, you can buy fresh packaged beans, but eat them the same day as your purchase for maximum freshness. Whole Foods now carries bags of fresh, organic green beans with the stems cut off.

AYURVEDIC NOTE

Green beans are fine for all *doshas*, as are basil and ginger in moderation. The ginger and lime also aid digestion. Leeks are the least heating in the onion family, so I find that I can enjoy this recipe in the heat of summer without increasing *pitta*.

P Reduce ginger and lime. Use coconut oil in summer.

K Use sunflower oil rather than using olive or coconut oil.

1. Prepare the beans by snapping off the ends, and, if you wish, snap into bite-sized pieces. Clean and slice the leeks.

2. Heat the cooking oil in a large sauté pan or soup pot on medium. When the oil is hot, add leeks and sauté them 5 to 7 minutes or until they turn golden. Stir occasionally as leeks can burn easily.

3. While the leeks sauté, rinse the green beans in water a few times and strain, leaving a little water on them. When the leeks have turned golden, add the beans on top. Do not stir, so the leeks can cook a little longer. Add basil and 2 tablespoons of Bragg's to the pan, still without stirring. Cover and simmer on medium heat for about 15 minutes without stirring.

4. Peel and grate the ginger, and add it to the pan. Now you can stir. Reduce heat to medium-low, and re-cover the pot. Continue to cook 5 to 10 more minutes, if needed, until the beans are tender. If the vegetables seem to be sticking, add a tablespoon or two of water. Before serving, taste and add more Bragg's or salt, if needed. If you like, add some freshly squeezed lime juice, stir, and serve.

GUJARATI GREEN BEANS

Preparation Time: 30 to 45 minutes (15 to 30 minutes active)
Serves 6 to 8

I learned to make this dish from Alpa Bhatt, an Ayurvedic physician who grew up in the Gujarati city of Baroda. Gujarat, India's westernmost state, has as the signature flavors of its curries the sweet and sour accents of unrefined sugar and lime. The combination is exquisite.

4 cups green beans
1 small onion
2 tablespoons ghee or coconut oil
½ teaspoon ground cumin
½ teaspoon mild curry powder
½ teaspoon ground coriander
1 teaspoon freshly grated ginger
1 cup water
1 tablespoon coconut sugar
1 to 2 teaspoons Fine Ground Celtic Sea Salt
Juice of 1 lime

AYURVEDIC NOTE

Although green beans are typically good for all *doshas*, this particular recipe is somewhat heating because of the curry powder, making it ideal for *kapha* types. I avoid this dish in the heat of summer because the curry increases *pitta*.

V Reduce curry powder to ¼ or ⅛ teaspoon—or omit. If omitting, increase cumin and coriander to 1 teaspoon each, and add 1 teaspoon ground turmeric.

P Reduce curry powder to ⅛ teaspoon—or omit. If omitting, increase cumin and coriander to 1 teaspoon each, and add 1 teaspoon ground turmeric.

1. Prepare the beans by breaking off the ends, and if you wish, break them again into halves or thirds for bite-sized pieces. Rinse the beans well in water and drain.

2. Chop the onion. Heat the ghee or oil in a large sauté pan or small soup pot on medium heat. Add the onion and sauté for 8 to 10 minutes, stirring occasionally, until the onion turns golden and starts to brown.

3. While the onion is cooking, grate the ginger. Bring the water to a boil in a small saucepan. Add the sugar to the water so that it will dissolve, along with the ginger and salt.

4. Once the onion has started to brown, add the cumin, curry powder, and coriander and stir. Now add the green beans to the onion along with the sugar-water mixture. Cover the pan and reduce the heat to medium-low. Simmer for 15 minutes or until the beans are tender. Squeeze on fresh lime juice and toss before serving.

HASH BROWNS

Preparation Time: About 45 minutes
Serves 4

My sweet father, Reuben Cagan—called Rube by his friends and Rubynu by his mother—made wonderful fried potatoes. The only time Daddy was in the kitchen was on a vacation day or a Saturday or Sunday morning when he wasn't playing golf. He would make brunch for us, and he always started by frying a chopped onion with potatoes and spices. In another pan he would make what he called a machel (which must be pronounced with a guttural Yiddish accent), a messy scrambled-egg dish that graciously took in whatever vegetables happened to be in the refrigerator. Over the years, I have brought Ayurvedic influences to bear on my father's fried potatoes, a dish I occasionally serve for dinner, though I prefer sweet potatoes instead of white.

2 large sweet potatoes (or 3 to 4 Yukon Gold potatoes)
1 medium onion
3 to 4 tablespoons ghee or olive oil
5 large curry leaves (optional—leaves, not powder!)
1 teaspoon ground cumin
1 teaspoon ground coriander
1 teaspoon mild paprika
½ teaspoon dried oregano
1 teaspoon freshly grated ginger
1 to 1½ teaspoons Fine Ground Celtic Sea Salt
Freshly ground pepper to taste

COOK'S TIP: Try cooking this recipe in an enamel or cast-iron pan, as the potatoes will be less likely to stick. Start with 2 tablespoons of ghee or oil in these nonstick pans. You will need at least 3 tablespoons using a stainless steel pan, although a little sticking to the pan is fine—just scrape up the sticking potatoes and stir them into the dish.

AYURVEDIC NOTE
Sweet potatoes are grounding for *vata*, while white potatoes are pacifying to *pitta*, and when eaten dry, they will also pacify *kapha*. Because white potatoes are astringent, dry, and cooling, they increase *vata*, and like all nightshades, they may aggravate arthritis. The onions and spices pacify all *doshas* if the onions are cooked until sweet.

V Double the ginger.

P Reduce paprika to ½ teaspoon and increase ginger.

K Increase ginger and double paprika, if you wish.

1. If you wish, peel potatoes and set aside in a bowl of water. Peel and chop the onion.

2. Heat ghee or oil on medium in a large sauté pan that has a cover. When the oil is hot, add the curry leaves, and cover immediately as the leaves may pop. Add the onion, stir, and sauté for about 10 minutes until the onion is uniformly golden and the edges start to turn brown.

3. While the onion cooks, chop the potatoes into ½-inch cubes. When the onion is golden, add the potatoes to the pan. Add cumin, coriander, paprika, and oregano, stir and cover. Continue cooking on medium heat about 30 minutes or until the potatoes are tender and evenly browned. Stir frequently. If the potatoes seem to be sticking, add another tablespoon or two of ghee or oil. Don't worry when the onions start to blacken, as they will taste delicious!

4. Grate ginger and, once the potatoes are tender, add it to the pan along with 1 teaspoon salt. Add more salt, if needed, and pepper to taste.

SAUTÉED OKRA

Preparation Time: About 30 minutes (15 minutes active)
Serves 4

Fried okra is a Southern staple that I tasted in my youth but did not enjoy. Then I ate a sautéed version of this vegetable at an Indian restaurant, and I loved it! The Hindi word for okra is bhindi, *and the recipe below is a foolproof approach to what's known in India as* Bhindi Masala.

1 medium leek bulb plus an inch of the light-green shank
4 cups fresh okra
2 tablespoons ghee or sunflower oil
1 pinch asafetida (optional)
1 teaspoon ground cumin
1 teaspoon ground turmeric
1 teaspoon ground coriander
1 to 2 tablespoons Bragg Liquid Aminos

AYURVEDIC NOTE

Okra is fine for many people, but it will increase *vata* unless the okra is cooked until well done. Cooking okra in oil or ghee mitigates the roughness of the pods, and the spices all aid digestion. Avoid eating under-ripe okra, which is sometimes packaged prematurely when sold in grocery stores, and will be difficult to digest. If the okra crackles when cut or feels like paper under your knife, in my mind it's not dinner-worthy.

 Add 1 to 2 teaspoons of grated fresh ginger.

1. Clean and slice the leek and set aside. Rinse the okra in a colander; pat dry. Chop off both ends of the okra and slice the vegetable into small or medium rounds.

2. Heat the ghee or oil on medium-low heat. Add the leek and sauté 5 to 7 minutes or until golden. Add the asafetida, cumin, turmeric, and coriander, and stir.

3. Add okra to the sauté pan. Add Bragg's. Stir and cover. Reduce heat to medium-low and sauté 20 to 30 minutes, stirring occasionally, until the okra is tender. If the okra seems to be sticking, add 1 tablespoon of water, and re-cover.

MASHED POTATOES WITH BROWNED ONIONS

Preparation Time: About 35 minutes
Serves 4

If you surveyed a large sampling of Americans, my guess is that mashed potatoes would make the top ten list of favorite comfort foods. Being a Jewish American Princess by birth, I have created my own hybrid version of this popular dish. I'm told that my father's lovely mother, Ida Menduik Cohen, made mashed potatoes with onions browned in chicken fat. Oy! Chicken fat was all the rage among the Eastern European Jews who packed into America's cities during the late nineteenth and early twentieth centuries, and all four of my grandparents were Russian Jews. I've created a more modern, healthful version of Grandma Ida's mashed potatoes and added a couple of Indian spices for surprise and balance. All the same, for this satisfying dish I credit both my Grandma Ida, because she brought this recipe with her when she immigrated to the United States in January 1920, and my mother, Bonnie, because she carried on my father's family tradition.

3 large or 4 medium Yukon Gold potatoes
1 medium to large onion
3 tablespoons ghee or olive oil
½ teaspoon black mustard seeds (optional)
1 pinch asafetida (optional)
¾ to 1 teaspoon Fine Ground Celtic Sea Salt
Freshly ground black pepper to taste

COOK'S TIP: Ghee will tolerate medium to high heat for some time without burning, making it ideal for popping mustard seeds and browning the onions.

TIME-SAVER: You can also prepare the potatoes in a pressure cooker, following your cooker's directions.

AYURVEDIC NOTE
White potatoes are excellent for *pitta* and *kapha* but increase *vata* because they are astringent, dry, and cooling. The ghee and heating qualities of onions, asafetida, black mustard seeds, and black pepper are balancing for potatoes, making this dish fine when eaten on occasion. If you are diabetic or insulin resistant, however, it is best to avoid white potatoes.

V Add 1 to 2 cloves pressed garlic if you like. Avoid white potatoes if you have arthritis.

K Reduce ghee to 1 tablespoon.

1. Peel the potatoes (or not, if organic), cut them into quarters, and place them in a 3-quart or larger pot. Cover potatoes with water, cover the pot, and bring to a boil. Once the water is boiling, reduce heat to medium, and continue cooking until the potatoes are completely tender, about 20 minutes.

2. While the potatoes are cooking, chop the onion. Heat 1 tablespoon of ghee or oil in a medium sauté pan on medium heat. When the ghee is hot, add the mustard seeds to the pan and cover it, as the seeds will pop like popcorn. When the seeds finish popping, add the asafetida and chopped onion. Cook the onion until quite brown but not burned, stirring occasionally.

3. When the potatoes are tender, strain them while retaining about 1 cup of the cooking water. Mash the potatoes in their cooking pot, either by hand or with an electric mixer, adding in 2 more tablespoons ghee, salt, and some of the cooking water. Start with ½ cup of the water, and mix well, adding more of the water until you reach the consistency you prefer. The potatoes should not be dry. Stir in the browned onions. Taste and add salt if you wish. Serve with freshly ground black pepper.

Avoid Combining Milk and Potatoes

The popular American tradition of whipping white potatoes with milk, cream, and/or cheese does not get a seal of approval from Ayurvedic experts. This food combination—white potatoes and most forms of dairy—lead to the development of toxins in the GI tract. Instead of milk, I mash the potatoes in some of their own cooking water along with ghee, and I think you'll find this dish is still quite creamy. If you want an even creamier texture, you can also mash the potatoes with coconut or almond milk.

Although ghee is derived from dairy, the milk solids that cause gastric problems have been removed. Ghee is, in fact, balancing for white potatoes because white potatoes are quite dry and need the lubrication of a fat, such as ghee, to mitigate their *vata*-increasing effect.

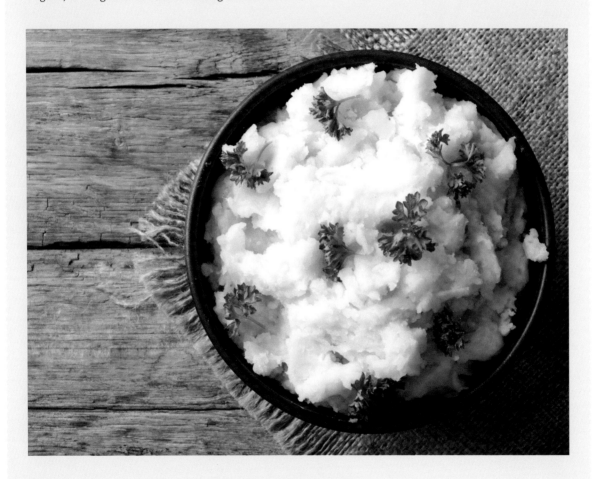

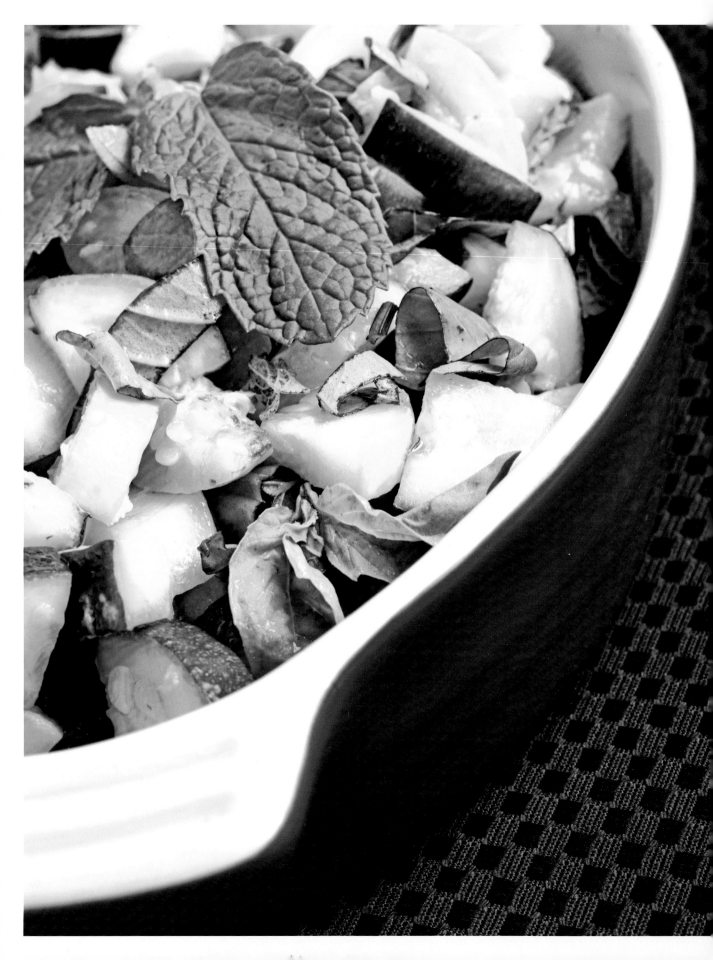

SIMPLE SUMMER SQUASH

Preparation Time: About 20 minutes
Serves 4

With zucchini and yellow squash so abundant in the summer, I like mixing them in this easy recipe. Thanks to my friend Janis Pettit for the idea of adding fresh mint and basil for a taste of summer.

2 tablespoons olive oil or ghee
1 small clove garlic
2 large zucchini
2 large yellow squash
2 tablespoons fresh basil (or 1 teaspoon dried)
2 tablespoons fresh mint (or 1 teaspoon dried)
½ teaspoon fine ground mineral salt such as Himalayan

GRILLING OPTION: Cut the squashes into long ¼-inch-thick slices. Marinate the vegetables in the oil and garlic, and grill them for 5 to 6 minutes each side on medium heat. Add basil and mint after you turn the squash to grill the second side.

AYURVEDIC NOTE

Zucchini and summer squash are excellent for *pitta* and *vata*; however, they will increase *kapha* because they are so watery. Slightly cooling, these squashes are a great summertime dish.

 Add black pepper.

1. Slice the zucchini and yellow squash into rounds ¼- to ½-inch thick; then quarter the rounds. Chop the herbs.

2. Heat the oil or ghee in a large sauté pan on medium-high heat. (If you use a larger pan, you may need a little more oil.) When the oil is hot, add the squash and garlic. Cook covered for about 2 minutes, to sear and steam the squash. Then reduce the heat, uncover the pan, add the herbs, and cook for another 5 to 7 minutes, stirring a few times. Cook until the squash is tender but not mushy. Add salt to taste, and serve.

EASY WINTER SQUASH

Preparation Time: About 1¾ hours (5 to 10 minutes active)
Serves 2

This is another one of those simple-yet-delicious side dishes that bakes all by itself in the oven while the cook lavishes more time and attention on a main dish or more elaborate vegetables.

1 acorn or butternut squash for every two people
1 teaspoon ghee, butter, or coconut oil per person
Dash Fine Ground Celtic Sea Salt per serving
¼ teaspoon vanilla per serving, or more, to taste

COOK'S TIP: To spread the squash further with smaller servings, scoop out all the flesh into a serving bowl after the squashes cool. Mash the flesh with ghee, salt, and vanilla. With this variation, you can also combine 1 large butternut squash with 1 large acorn squash.

AYURVEDIC NOTE

All squashes are very easy to digest and are especially good for *vata* and *pitta* types. People with *kapha* problems may want to eat this dish in moderation.

 Omit ghee or coconut oil.

MENU SUGGESTION

The sweet flavor of the squash combined with the spices balances a menu with sour, astringent, or pungent flavors. Use on a vegetable plate with greens and/or cruciferous vegetables: broccoli, Brussels sprouts, cabbage, and cauliflower, or serve as a side to Asparagus Soup (page 92).

1. Preheat the oven to 450°F. Line a baking sheet or baking dish with parchment paper. Cut each acorn squash in half around the middle, and remove their stalks. Cut each butternut squash in half lengthwise. Remove and discard the strings and seeds.

2. Place each half on a baking sheet with the flesh side down, and cover with foil. Bake about 1 to 1½ hours, until the squash is completely tender. So it will be easy to digest, the squash should be cooked so that it is as soft as baby food. Remove the squash from the oven and let cool about 5 minutes.

3. Before serving, turn the squash over so its cut side is up, and add to each a small dollop of ghee, butter, or coconut oil, followed by the salt and vanilla. When you begin to eat, mash the squash and ghee mixture like a mashed potato.

WILTED BABY SPINACH WITH SUNFLOWER SEED BUTTER

Preparation Time: 10 minutes

Serves 2 to 3

This is a quick-and-easy side dish that, because of its delicious sauce, dazzles all the same.

FOR THE SAUCE:

3 tablespoons sunflower butter

1 tablespoon Bragg Liquid Aminos

1 teaspoon freshly grated ginger

⅓ cup water

FOR THE SPINACH:

1 tablespoon ghee or olive oil

1 tablespoon water

1 pound baby spinach

1 tablespoon sunflower seeds

SHOPPING TIP: You can buy sunflower seed butter in health food stores and online, or you can easily make your own (page 74).

AYURVEDIC NOTE

Cooked spinach and sunflower seeds are excellent for all *doshas* in moderation. Bragg Liquid Aminos, being very salty, can increase *pitta* but is also fine in moderation.

P Reduce Bragg's or replace with 1 teaspoon Fine Ground Celtic Sea Salt.

1. Whisk all the ingredients for the sauce together in a bowl or large measuring cup.

2. Heat the ghee or oil in a large sauté pan (5 to 5½ quarts) on medium heat. Add spinach and a tablespoon of water. Cover and steam 5 minutes until all the spinach is wilted.

3. Reduce heat to medium-low. Pour sauce over the spinach, stir, and re-cover until the sauce is heated through, 2 to 3 minutes. Taste and add salt, if needed. Sprinkle with sunflower seeds. Serve immediately.

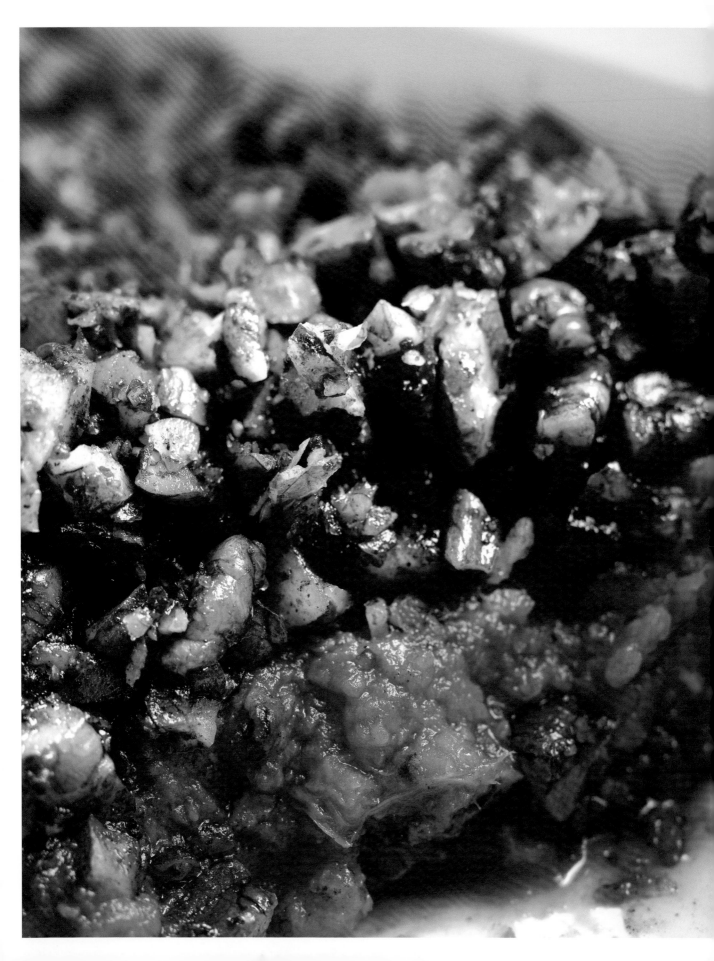

HOLIDAY SWEET POTATOES WITH GLAZED PECAN TOPPING

Preparation Time: About 3 hours (30 minutes active)
Serves 12 to 16

When I became a vegetarian, I still kept faith with a traditional Thanksgiving through the pleasures of side dishes and a pumpkin dessert. My stepdaughter, Celeste, convinced me to increase the pecans from ½ pound (my original recipe) to 1½ pounds (the recipe below). She was right. The new version is infinitely more delicious!

6 to 8 large sweet potatoes
1 to 1½ teaspoons Fine Ground Celtic Sea Salt
2 to 2½ tablespoons ghee or unsalted butter

FOR THE TOPPING:
1 to 1½ pounds whole shelled pecans, chopped
5 to 7 tablespoons ghee or unsalted butter
1 to 2 teaspoons Fine Ground Celtic Sea Salt
2½ to 3½ teaspoons ground cinnamon
3 to 6 tablespoons coconut sugar

COOK'S TIP: 1. The salt, cinnamon, and sugar amounts are given in ranges that accommodate the range of pecans. Add more to taste. **2.** This dish can be prepared the day before and refrigerated. Reheat covered for 40 minutes to heat all the way through, and then heat uncovered for 10 more minutes. **3.** You can make extra pecan topping, and set it aside to top special occasion pancakes!

AYURVEDIC NOTE

Everyone can savor this dish as a holiday treat. Sweet potatoes are excellent for pacifying *vata* and *pitta*. The nut topping will increase *kapha* and *pitta*, though I find that nuts are not a problem when I eat them in moderation. If you have *kapha* problems, go easy on this dish because all of the ingredients increase *kapha*!

P Reduce pecans and spices by half.

K Cut the amount of ghee or butter in half.

1. Preheat the oven to 450°F. Line a heavy cookie sheet with aluminum foil. Pierce each potato a few times with a fork or sharp knife; then wrap each potato in tinfoil. Place them on the cookie sheet and bake for about 90 minutes, until the potatoes are very soft. When the potatoes are completely tender, remove them from the oven, and let them cool for about an hour until they can be handled easily. If you're working on other projects, you can also let them cool in the oven after you turn it off.

2. While the potatoes are cooling, grease a 2½- to 3-quart casserole dish and prepare the topping.

3. For the topping: Melt the ghee or butter in a large skillet on medium. Add 1 teaspoon of the salt, the cinnamon, and 3 tablespoons of the coconut sugar to the ghee. Stir. Add the nuts, and stir for about a minute or until the nuts are well coated. Taste and add more sweetener, cinnamon, and salt to your liking. Set the pan aside to cool.

4. Preheat the oven to 350°F. Once the potatoes have cooled, unwrap them and place them in a large mixing bowl. Pinch the end of each potato and pull the skins off. Add salt and ghee or butter. Purée the potatoes with an electric mixer or mash by hand. Transfer the puréed potatoes to the casserole dish. Spoon the pecan mixture on top. Cover the dish and bake for 15 minutes. Uncover and bake 10 minutes more.

OVEN-BAKED SWEET POTATO CHIPS

Preparation Time: About 25 minutes (10 minutes active)
Serves 3

If you crave French fries but want to avoid their side effects, try this baked version with either sweet potatoes or (if you must) white.

1 large sweet potato
1 tablespoon sunflower or olive oil
¼ to ½ teaspoon Fine Ground Celtic Sea Salt
1 teaspoon ground cumin
1 teaspoon ground coriander

AYURVEDIC NOTE
Sweet potatoes are good for *vata* and *pitta* but will increase *kapha*. Sweet potatoes are balancing for blood sugar when eaten in moderation.

K Add ½ teaspoon paprika or a dash of cayenne to the spice mixture.

1. Preheat the oven to 450°F. Line a baking sheet with parchment paper.

2. Scrub the potato. If it's not organic, peel it since the peels may have a chemical residue. Slice the potato into rounds, as thin as you can slice them.

3. Combine the oil with the spices in a large mixing bowl. Toss the potato slices in the oil and spice mixture, transfer them to the baking sheet, and move the sheet to the oven. Bake 13 to 15 minutes, depending on the thickness, until the potatoes are tender and a little crisp.

ROASTED VEGGIES

Preparation Time: About 1 hour (30 minutes active)

Serves 4 to 6

Roasting vegetables in a hot oven is a lovely way to warm your house on a cold winter's day!

4 large carrots

1 large onion

1 large parsnip

2 cups cubed butternut squash

¼ cup olive or sunflower oil

1 teaspoon Fine Ground Celtic Sea Salt

½ to 1 teaspoon sweet paprika

2 teaspoons fresh rosemary or dried tarragon

AYURVEDIC NOTE

These vegetables can be eaten in moderation by everyone, although sweet paprika is too hot for anyone who is sensitive to peppers. Onions, when cooked until they caramelize, transform from hot to slightly sweet, making them fine for everyone.

V Reduce paprika to ¼ teaspoon.

P Omit paprika or reduce to ¼ teaspoon.

K Use sunflower oil instead of olive oil.

1. Preheat the oven to 400°F.

2. Wash carrots with a vegetable brush. Peel the parsnip. Cut both into 2-inch-long chunks. Peel the butternut squash, remove seeds, and cut into 1-inch cubes. Chop the onion into quarters.

3. In a large mixing bowl, assemble the oil, salt, and spices. Add the vegetables to the bowl and stir well to coat.

4. Line two baking sheets with parchment paper. Spoon the vegetables onto the sheets, separating the squash onto a separate sheet. Bake the squash about 30 minutes and remove from the oven once it pierces easily with a fork. Let the remaining vegetables bake another 10 minutes or so or until they are also tender. Serve immediately.

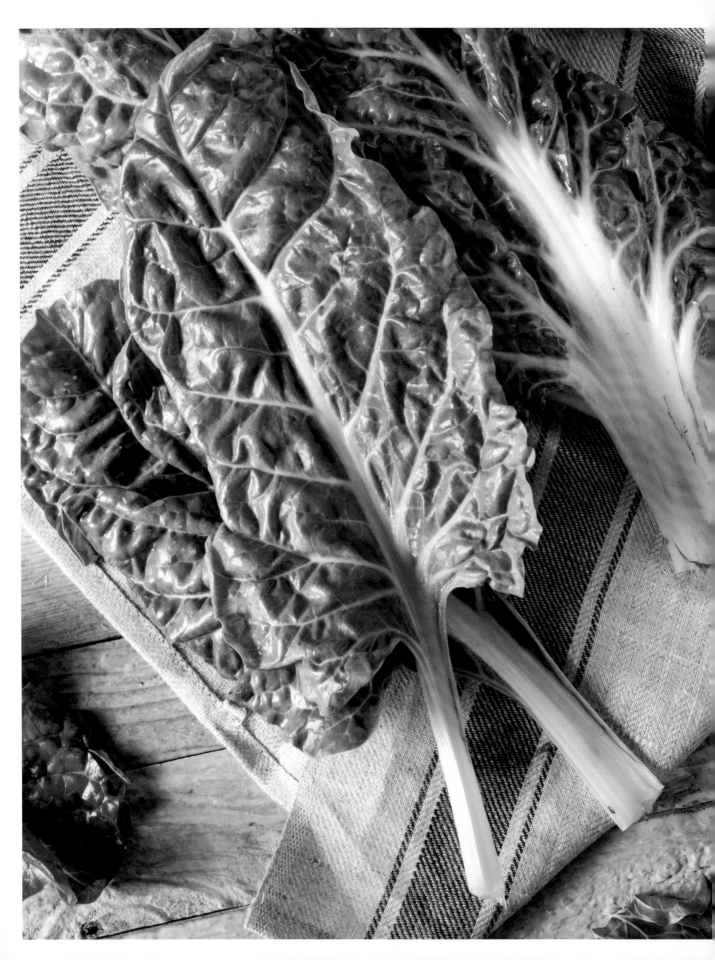

SMOKY SWISS CHARD

Preparation Time: About 20 minutes (10 minutes active)
Serves 2 to 3

I know that kale is all the rage, but I much prefer Swiss chard because it's less bitter and it cooks so quickly. Chard also has more fiber and protein than kale and is equally rich in antioxidants.

2 pounds green, red, or mixed chard
1 tablespoon ghee or coconut oil
1 teaspoon freshly grated ginger
1 teaspoon smoked salt
1 to 2 tablespoons pure maple or coconut syrup
½ cup chopped almonds, walnuts, or pistachios

COOK'S TIP: 1. Although chard picked from the garden may last in the refrigerator for a few days, it spoils quickly if you're buying it in the grocery store. It's best to cook chard within 24 hours. **2.** Try Artisan Salt Company's Salish Smoked Salt (Coarse Grain). **3.** You can also use this recipe for prewashed and precut kale.

AYURVEDIC NOTE

Chard is slightly astringent, so it may increase *vata*, although it is fine for *pitta* and *kapha*. The sweetener is good for *vata* and *pitta*. Real maple syrup is said to be strengthening when eaten in moderation.

V Add extra ginger.

K Omit or decrease syrup.

1. Soak the chard in the sink or large bowl of water to remove any residual soil. Spin the greens in a lettuce spinner or pat them dry. Chop off the hard center stems and slice them as you would celery. Stack the leaves on top of each other. Slice the leaves vertically down the middle; then slice the two strips horizontally into several two-inch sections.

2. Heat the ghee or oil in a large sauté pan on medium. When the oil is warm, add the salt to the oil with the sliced stems. Cover for 5 minutes. Add the chard leaves and ginger, and stir. Drizzle the greens with maple syrup. Cover the pan and cook for 5 to 10 minutes until all the leaves are wilted and tender. Sauté uncovered another 5 minutes if necessary to cook off any natural liquids. While the chard is cooking, chop nuts to add to the dish, if you'd like.

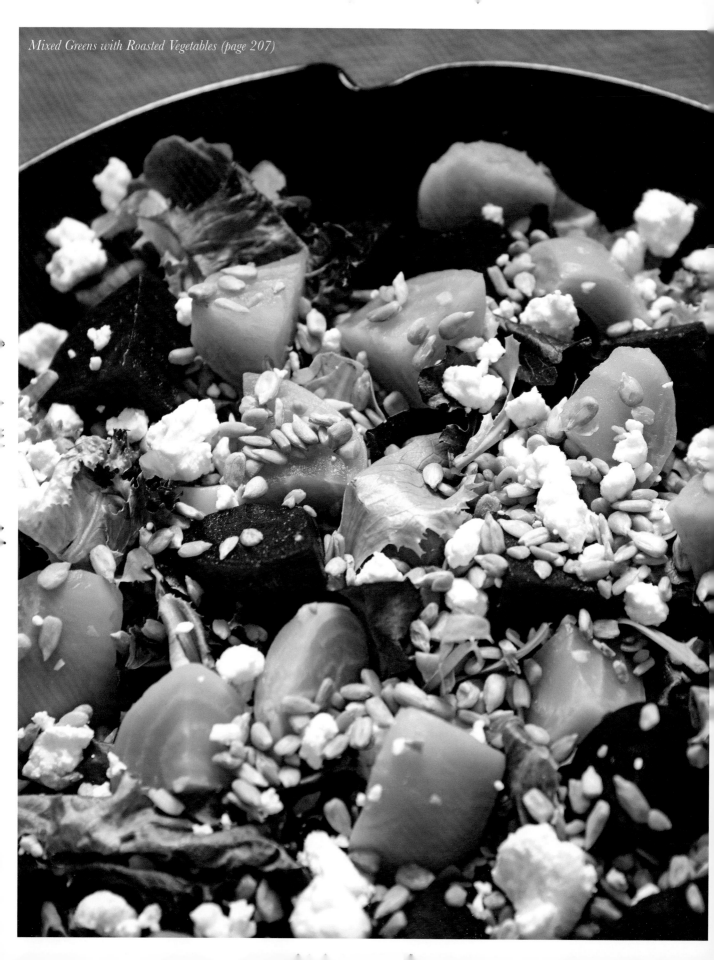

Mixed Greens with Roasted Vegetables (page 207)

CHAPTER 10.

Salads

Out of love the earth brings forth nectarian food.

⌐ Swami Muktananda

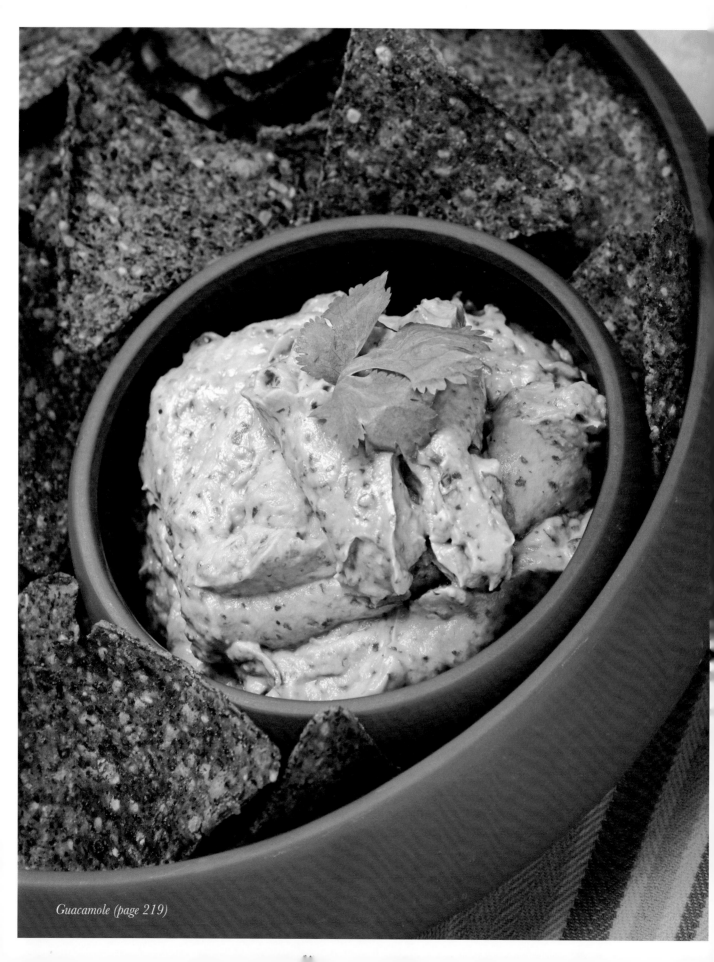

Guacamole (page 219)

An Ayurvedic Guide to Salad

On a sultry summer day there is no better relief for cooks and diners than salad. Salads not only provide respite from a hot stove, they also can help cool the metabolism. Lettuce and other salad favorites, such as cucumbers and sprouts, are naturally cooling.

Traditional Ayurvedic practitioners generally do not recommend raw-food salads and caution against eating them daily since raw foods take considerably longer to digest than cooked foods. Because raw-food salads are generally light and cooling, they tend to increase *vata* and *kapha*. (For more information about raw foods, see pages 41–42.) I do take this guidance to heart—yet I also want the flexibility a range of foods gives me. So, I've developed some salad recipes that fit within Ayurveda's parameters of healthy eating.

The key is to start with the less crispy varieties of lettuce, which are easier to digest for most people because they are less likely to increase *vata*. I often use a butterhead lettuce such as Boston or Bibb, which have soft, sweet-tasting leaves, or a leaf lettuce such as red-leaf, or a mesclun mix. If you're eating a crisp lettuce such as romaine or iceberg, you can balance it in part with an oily dressing and a dose of heating spices like fresh ginger or garlic. If you add roasted vegetables or cooked grains to your salad, you have an altogether healthy appetizer or entrée.

Notice how you feel a few to several hours after you eat a salad. If you experience an increase in *vata* symptoms (page 22), you may want to avoid the crisp types of lettuce and raw vegetables. You can also experiment with eating salads less frequently or avoiding them altogether during cooler months, when *vata* is naturally higher.

For the dressing, olive oil is my favorite base, and I also like to add a little heating spice or condiment such as ginger, mustard, or tahini. This is an excellent way to address any *vata* problems. Balsamic vinegar also does the trick for adding heat to the balance. A little balsamic can be good once in a while, as it kindles *agni*, the digestive fire, and this is especially helpful when you're eating raw vegetables. Either vinegar or mustard on a regular basis, however, is not advised for people with *pitta* problems, and vinegar is not advised for anyone on a candida diet. With this in mind, I've developed some dressings that do not rely on either vinegar or prepared mustard for flavor.

Tomato lovers will notice the absence of these gorgeous fruits in the *Sacred & Delicious* salad recipes. My intention is to provide delectable salad options for people who need to avoid tomatoes because of health problems associated with nightshades (page 142).

It is best to serve salads at room temperature rather than cold from the refrigerator. And, in the preparation, I like to soak the greens in water unless I buy the prewashed boxed greens.

SIMPLE GREEN SALAD

Preparation Time: About 10 minutes
Serves 4 (modest portions)

You're invited to a potluck with little time to prepare? You'll still delight the party with this simple salad.

5 ounces mixed salad greens (about 8 cups)
¼ cup fresh basil leaves
1 small to medium cucumber
1 ripe avocado
1 cup fresh sprouts
¼ to ½ cup sunflower or pumpkin seeds

AYURVEDIC NOTE

This salad is excellent for *pitta* as it is cooling. For the same reason, lettuce is slightly aggravating to *vata*, but here it's balanced by oily dressing and avocado. Cucumbers are easier to digest once the seeds are removed. Avocado and most salad dressings increase *kapha* and so should be eaten in moderation by anyone with *kapha* problems.

(V) Omit the cucumber.

(K) Omit the cucumber or avocado.

SERVING SUGGESTION

Serve with Ginger Dressing (page 210), Lime Vinaigrette (page 210), or Tahini Dressing (page 212).

1. Use a bag or box of prewashed greens. Or hand-tear a head of washed lettuce into a large serving bowl.

2. Chop the fresh basil leaves, and toss with the greens.

3. Slice the cucumber in half, lengthwise. Scrape out seeds with a teaspoon, and cut cucumber into half-round slices.

4. Peel and chop the avocado.

5. Toss together the first four ingredients. Just before serving, dress with your favorite salad dressing. Top the salad with sprouts, seeds, and (if you wish) croutons.

MIXED GREENS WITH ROASTED VEGETABLES

Preparation Time: About 1¼ hours (15 minutes active)
Serves 4

You can use one or a combination of any of these vegetables, or try others you may prefer.

½ cup pecan, walnut, or pistachio pieces
1 large red bell pepper, 4 medium-sized beets or carrots, or a cup of roasted butternut squash cubes
4 to 6 cups of combined red leaf, arugula, and Bibb lettuce
4 to 8 ounces goat or goat feta cheese (optional)

AYURVEDIC NOTE
This salad is fine for everyone in moderation, though it is best to avoid cheese if you're suffering from a cold, cough, or congestion—all signs of excess *kapha*.

P Reduce or avoid the nuts.

K Omit or decrease the goat cheese. Roast the nuts for 5 to 10 minutes (in a 350°F oven) so they are a bit dried.

SERVING SUGGESTION
Serve with Ginger Dressing (page 210), Lime Vinaigrette (page 210), or Tahini Dressing (page 212).

1. Roast the vegetables (page 199), and when they're cool enough to handle, slice them for the salad.

2. Place salad greens in a large serving bowl.

3. Add the vegetables, nuts, and goat cheese to the greens. Toss and serve with your favorite salad dressing.

(RECIPE PHOTO ON PAGE 202)

MEDITERRANEAN ROOT VEGETABLES AND GREENS

Preparation Time: About 30 minutes
Serves 4 to 6

My thanks to Sal Corbo, one of the best cooks I know, for sharing this recipe he created one evening for friends.

FOR THE SALAD:

1 or 2 large carrots
1 medium or large white turnip
1 cup mung bean sprouts
3 or 4 cups mesclun or other washed greens
6 fresh mint leaves

FOR THE VINAIGRETTE:

1 tablespoon fresh lemon juice
2 tablespoons fresh lime juice
1 teaspoon ground mustard
1 teaspoon paprika
1 tablespoon honey or coconut sugar
¼ teaspoon Fine Ground Celtic Sea Salt
Dash black pepper
½ cup olive oil

AYURVEDIC NOTE

This is a perfect dish for many people who crave salads year-round, as the vinaigrette ingredients are heating and provide a good balance for cool fall and winter months. Turnips, which are pungent and dry, increase *pitta* as well as *vata*. The vinaigrette's oil and spices pacify *vata*, while mint leaves and sprouts help balance *pitta*.

(V) Replace the turnips with parsnips, and blanch them for 2 minutes.

(P) Omit the lemon and replace with lime. Reduce the mustard to ½ teaspoon.

(S) Omit the lemon and replace with lime. Reduce the mustard to ½ teaspoon.

1. Bring water to boil in a 3-quart (or larger) pot.

2. Cut the carrots and white turnip into pieces ⅛ inch by ⅛ inch by 1½ inches.

3. Blanch the turnips, sprouts, and carrots by submerging each batch briefly in boiling salted water. (Blanch white vegetables first and carrots last. Blanch times for each are as follows: mung sprouts, 15 seconds; white turnip, 1 minute; carrot, 2 minutes.) Remove each from boiling water, and immediately submerge in ice water to stop them from cooking further. Drain. Place in a bowl, cover, and refrigerate.

4. Make the vinaigrette: Squeeze the lemon and lime juices into a bowl. Mix in the mustard powder, paprika, sweetener, salt, and black pepper. As you whisk vigorously, add about a tablespoon of oil, then add remaining oil in a slow stream while whisking.

5. Pour enough of the vinaigrette over the vegetables to coat them. Cover the bowl and let the vegetables marinate for an hour, either in the refrigerator or at room temperature. Mix them occasionally.

6. Place the mesclun in a bowl large enough to hold all ingredients. Add the vegetables, their vinaigrette, chopped mint, salt, and pepper. Toss until evenly mixed. Add additional vinaigrette if desired. Serve immediately.

SALAD BAR ENTRÉE

Preparation Time: 15 minutes to 1 hour
Serves 4 to 6

During the summer I often make a few of the veggies listed below and pile them on a plate of greens for lunch or dinner. Sometimes I set up a buffet of these items when serving guests, letting them choose their own salad toppings. On the hottest of days, when I don't want to even think about turning on a stove, I might buy a few takeout deli items like the ones below to add to salad greens, or I use my leftovers from the night before when pulling together lunch at home. Here are some ideas for salad toppings that are both tasty and filling.

1 bunch red leaf lettuce, washed
1 5-ounce box of mixed salad greens, washed
2 cups of arugula, escarole, endive, or radicchio to add pungent or bitter flavors
Grilled or roasted asparagus
1 to 2 ripe avocados, sliced
2 roasted bell peppers, sliced
4 zucchini or yellow crookneck squash, sliced and grilled
Beet salad (page 213)
Roasted or steamed beets (page 174)
12 to 15 pitted kalamata olives
1 large cucumber, seeded and chopped
½ cup fresh basil, mint, or cilantro, chopped
Wild or black rice (page 162)
Cooked chickpea, kidney, or black beans
½ cup chopped almonds, walnuts, pecans, pistachios, pumpkin seeds, or sunflower seeds
Grilled or baked tofu cubes (page 170)
Hard-boiled eggs, crumbled or sliced
¼ to ½ cup goat feta cheese (see Ayurvedic Note)

AYURVEDIC NOTE

If you do not plan to use the tofu, eggs, or beans, then you could add goat feta cheese. If combined with the tofu, eggs, or beans, the cheese would be difficult to digest and might create toxins in the digestive track.

1. Grill asparagus or summer squash or both, with a little oil and salt.

2. Combine the leaf lettuce with mixed greens.

3. Add the assorted toppings to salad, and finish with your favorite dressing.

GINGER DRESSING

Preparation Time: About 10 minutes
Serves 4 to 5

I've always loved the ginger dressings served in Thai restaurants, and this inspired me to come up with my own version.

1 small rib celery or fennel
2 teaspoons freshly grated ginger
1 tablespoon ketchup
1 tablespoon coconut sugar
1 to 2 teaspoons fresh lime juice
2 tablespoons Bragg Liquid Aminos
½ cup olive or sunflower oil

COOK'S TIP: This dressing will last up to three days when refrigerated.

AYURVEDIC NOTE
This dressing is excellent for balancing *vata*. Since ketchup is tomato-based and contains vinegar, it will increase *pitta*, but should be fine for most people when eaten on occasion. Sunflower oil used in salad dressing is fine for all *doshas* in moderation; olive oil increases *kapha*.

 Use sunflower oil.

1. Wash the celery or fennel, and place in a blender.

2. Leaving the celery or fennel in the food processor, add the other ingredients, and purée.

LIME VINAIGRETTE

Preparation Time: 3 minutes
Serve 4 to 6

This light vinaigrette is my favorite dressing! It's quick, simple, and a perfect complement to every salad. It's also great for dressing beans, tofu, or steamed vegetables.

½ cup olive oil
3 to 4 teaspoons fresh lime juice
2 to 3 tablespoons Bragg Liquid Aminos

COOK'S TIP: This dressing will last up to three days when refrigerated.

AYURVEDIC NOTE
This dressing is good for balancing *vata* and is fine for most *pitta* types. All oil-based dressings are best eaten in moderation by anyone with *kapha* problems, but olive oil increases *kapha* more than some other oils.

K Reduce the amount of oil by half and/or replace the olive oil with sunflower oil.

1. Combine all ingredients in a bowl or 1-cup measuring cup. Start with smaller amounts of lime and Bragg's.

2. Whisk briskly and add more lime or Bragg's to taste. Serve immediately. (Whisking emulsifies the dressing, but the components will separate if the dressing sits for more than a few minutes.)

Zen Buddhist Recitations
Before and After Meals

This Zen Buddhist prayer is known as
"The Five Contemplations."

This food is the gift of the whole universe—the earth,
the sky, and much hard work.

May we be aware of the quality of our deeds and live in
a way that makes us worthy to receive this meal.

May we practice mindfulness to transform our greed,
hatred, and ignorance.

May we take in only foods which nourish us and
bring us health.

In gratitude, we accept this food so we may realize
the path of practice—of love, compassion and peace
for the benefit of all beings.

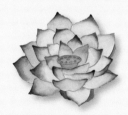

TAHINI DRESSING

Preparation Time: 10 minutes or less

Serves 4 to 6

I know it's bragging, but I can't resist saying that I've watched dinner guests eat this dressing with a spoon! If you like tahini, this dressing is equally interesting poured over steamed vegetables or tofu for a quick side dish. Try over carrots and broccoli, pour over sautéed spinach or kale, or use this dressing as a dipping sauce for a steamed artichoke.

1 cup tightly packed cilantro or fresh basil

½ cup tahini

½ cup water

2 teaspoons fresh lime juice

1 to 2 tablespoons Bragg Liquid Aminos

1 tablespoon coconut sugar

1 to 2 teaspoons freshly grated ginger or 1 clove garlic

COOK'S TIP: This dressing lasts for no more than a day because cilantro and basil spoil quickly.

AYURVEDIC NOTE

Tahini will increase *pitta*, but here it is balanced nicely by the fresh cilantro. Because of the tahini, this dressing is good for balancing the coolness of lettuce as well as other cooling vegetables, such as broccoli, cauliflower, and spinach. Avoid tahini if you are suffering from a cold, cough, or allergies.

(P) Avoid or reduce garlic.

(S) Avoid garlic. Use cilantro or mint instead of basil.

1. If your cilantro is not already cleaned, soak it in water to clean completely. Shake off excess water and cut the amount you will need.

2. Combine all ingredients in a food processor or blender. Add lime, Bragg's, and ginger to taste.

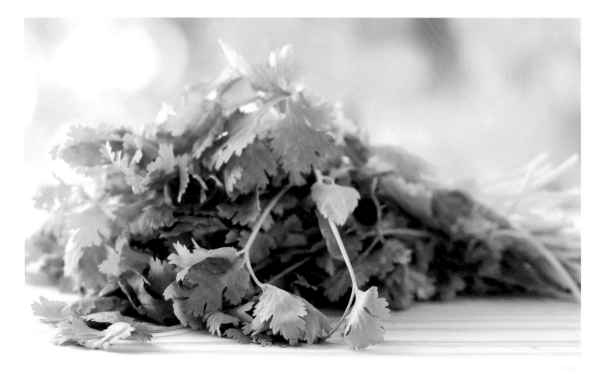

BEET SALAD WITH VINAIGRETTE

Preparation Time: 1 to 1½ hours
Serves 4

Fresh beets are a nutritious delicacy and worth a little time to bring to the table! Roasting beets may be necessary for the connoisseur, but I like them steamed just as well—and steaming cooks them a little faster.

3 to 4 medium beets
1 teaspoon fresh dill or a handful of chopped cilantro
2 teaspoons sesame seeds (optional)

FOR THE VINAIGRETTE:
1½ to 2 tablespoons olive oil
1 to 2 teaspoons fresh lime juice
½ teaspoon Fine Ground Celtic Sea Salt
1 teaspoon coconut sugar (optional)

AYURVEDIC NOTE
Cooked beets are excellent for all *doshas*.

K Replace the olive oil with high oleic sunflower oil.

1. Scrub the beets well, cut in half or quarters, and roast or steam them.

To steam the beets: Place them in a steamer above 1 or 2 inches of water. Cover and bring to a gentle boil. Cook about 45 minutes until the beets are completely tender and can be pierced with a fork or paring knife. Let cool 15 minutes or more before rubbing off the skins.

To roast the beets: Preheat the oven to 400°F. Scrub the beets with a vegetable brush. Place them in a baking pan filled with about an inch of water, and cover the pan with aluminum foil. Bake 45 minutes to 1 hour, until the beets are tender and easily pierced with a fork or paring knife. Remove from the oven, and let the beets cool for 15 minutes or longer before rubbing off the skins with your hands.

2. Chop the beets into cubes, or grate them, either in a food processor or by hand. Transfer the grated beets to a mixing bowl.

3. In a separate bowl or measuring cup, combine the ingredients for the dressing, including a little sugar if the beets taste bitter, and whisk well. Pour the dressing over the beets. Add fresh dill or cilantro and stir. Add more lime and salt, to taste. Sprinkle sesame seeds on top if you like, and serve this as a side dish or over salad greens.

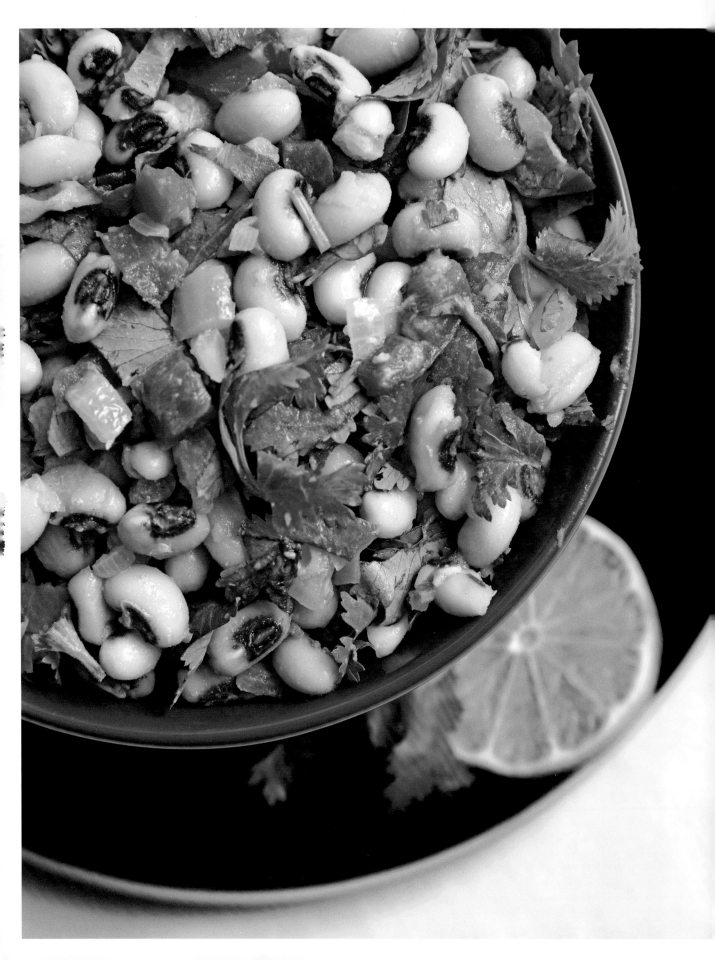

BLACK-EYED PEA SALAD

Preparation Time: 1 to 8 hours soaking, plus 45 minutes cooking (15 minutes active)
Serves 12

I created this distinctly Southern dish for my blog, but it was such a hit I decided to add the recipe to this book before it went to press! Black-eyed peas, also known as cowpeas, are softer than most beans. As long as you can soak them an hour or two, they will cook quickly. If you want to let them soak for eight hours while you're at work, that's fine, too.

1½ cups dried black-eyed peas
4 cups water
1 teaspoon Light Grey Celtic Sea Salt
1 fresh bay leaf
Bulb of one medium to large leek
1 small red pepper
2 tablespoons olive oil
½ teaspoon ground cumin
½ teaspoon ground coriander
1 teaspoon balsamic vinegar
2 to 3 teaspoons fresh lime juice
1 large clove garlic, pressed
1 teaspoon freshly grated ginger
½ cup tightly packed chopped fresh cilantro (or basil)
½ to 1 teaspoon Fine Ground Celtic Sea Salt
Black pepper to taste (optional)

AYURVEDIC NOTE

Black-eyed peas are the easiest beans for *vata* to digest, though they still benefit by the addition of ginger, garlic, and asafetida. Red pepper can aggravate arthritis, but may be OK in small quantities. Lime pacifies the peas' *vata* quality without aggravating *pitta*. The vinegar aids digestion but will increase *pitta*, which is cooled by cilantro. *Kapha* types can enjoy black-eyed peas regularly.

(V) Omit or decrease amount of red pepper. Add extra ginger. Cook vegetables with 1 pinch of asafetida.

(P) Replace garlic with more ginger. Omit vinegar.

(K) Add a dash of cayenne, if you like.

1. Soak the beans for at least 1 hour before cooking and up to 8 hours.

2. When ready to cook, rinse the peas under cold water several times. Strain the peas and transfer them to a 6-quart soup pot. Add water, Grey Celtic Sea Salt, and a bay leaf, and bring to a boil. Reduce heat to medium, and simmer covered for 25 to 30 minutes. Be careful not to overcook the peas or they will get mushy, but they should be tender when pierced with a fork. Once tender, strain them and transfer to a large mixing bowl to cool.

3. While the peas are cooking, wash the leek and red pepper, and dry them. Slice the leek and finely dice the red pepper.

Heat a medium-sized sauté pan on medium heat with oil. When the oil is moderately hot, add leeks and red pepper. Sauté the vegetables until the leeks turn golden, about 5 minutes. Add cumin and coriander, and stir. Set aside until the peas have been strained; then spoon the vegetable mixture into the peas.

4. Combine the vinegar, 2 teaspoons lime juice, garlic, and ginger in a small bowl or measuring cup. Whisk together, and pour over the peas and vegetable mixture. Finish the salad with cilantro (or basil), and add Fine Ground Celtic Sea Salt and more lime, to taste. Serve the salad at room temperature or slightly chilled.

SALAD SIDES

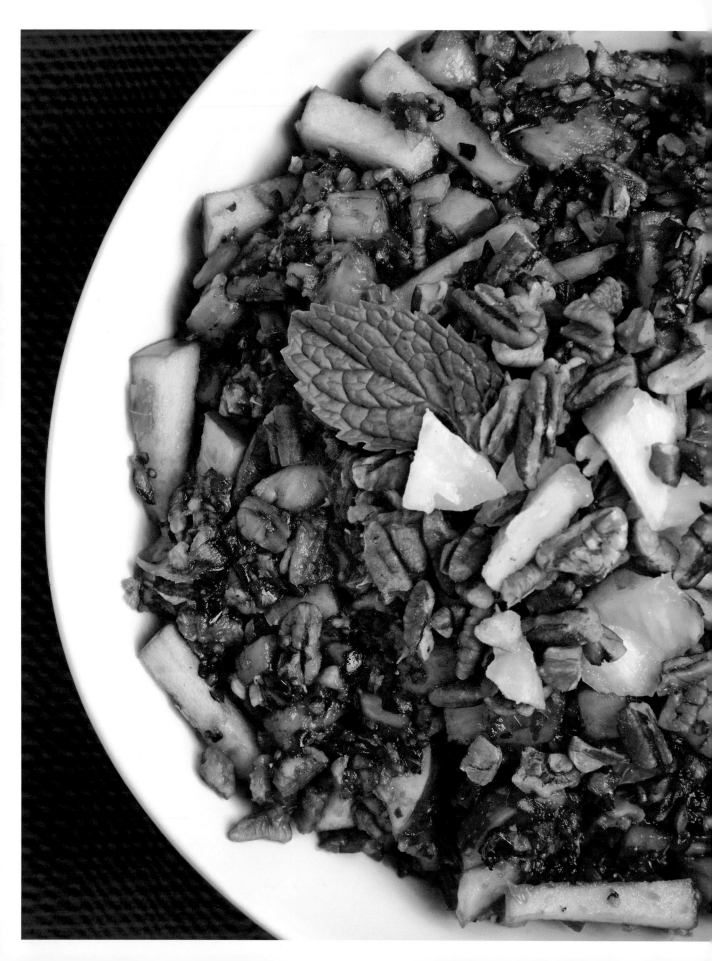

FRESH CRANBERRY SALAD

Preparation Time: 30 minutes or less

Serves 12

I adapted this easy recipe from one my brother shared with me. He and his friends credit the dish to Andrea Amburgey's Aunt Louise. I discarded the original Jell-O foundation and made the dish less sweet—but it's still sweet enough, even for the holidays!

8- to 12-ounce bag of fresh cranberries
½ pound pecans
1 peeled orange
1 to 2 cups fresh pineapple chunks
1 small red apple, cored
½ cup coconut sugar

AYURVEDIC NOTE

This is a special occasion dish that doesn't conform to Ayurveda's preference for cooked food. The sweet fruits and sugar balance the sour cranberries. If you have delicate digestion, it's best to eat this dish as an appetizer or dessert, either a half hour or hour before or after your holiday meal.

(V) Add 1 to 2 teaspoons of fresh, minced ginger.

(K) Omit the sugar or decrease it by at least half.

(W) Add 1 to 2 teaspoons of fresh ginger.

1. Grind the cranberries and orange in a food processor or blender, and place the mixture in a mixing bowl. Chop the nuts and add to the bowl.

2. Chop the pineapple and apple (by hand) and add them to the bowl. Add sugar and mix gently with a spatula or wooden spoon. Refrigerate until thirty minutes before serving. At that time take the bowl out of the fridge so it can warm to room temperature.

VERSATILE GRAIN SALAD WITH VEGETABLES

Preparation Time: 45 minutes to 1 hour

Serves 4 to 6

I created this salad for long travel days when I don't want to worry about airport food. It's easy to pack in a to-go container, and it's filling enough to help me avoid eating junk. It's also a lovely summer dish.

1½ cups quinoa or millet

2 tablespoons extra virgin olive oil

1 teaspoon freshly ground ginger

1 clove garlic (optional)

1 small sweet potato

2 cups asparagus or zucchini, chopped, or 1 cup each

1 tablespoon Bragg Liquid Aminos

2 to 4 teaspoons fresh lime juice

1 teaspoon fresh oregano or ¼ teaspoon dried

2 tablespoons fresh basil, chopped, or 2 teaspoons dried

½ cup chopped almonds, walnuts, pecans, or pistachios

½ to 1 cup chopped kalamata olives

Salt and pepper, to taste

COOK'S TIP: You can substitute the grain with your favorite pasta.

AYURVEDIC NOTE

Millet is easier to digest than quinoa, which can be difficult to digest for *vata* types. I add sweet potatoes, zucchini, garlic, and olives, which are balancing for *vata*. Asparagus is fine for all *doshas*. Nuts provide some needed protein for the road.

V Millet or rice preferred to quinoa.

P Omit the garlic.

K Omit the zucchini and use fewer olives.

1. Cook the quinoa (directions on page 161) or millet (directions on page 160).

2. While the grain is cooking, prepare the vegetables. Fill a pot with about 2 inches of water. Place a steamer basket inside, cover the pot, and bring the water to a boil. Chop the sweet potato into ½-inch cubes, and add them to the steamer. (You don't need to peel the potato if it's organic.) Cover the pot and steam the potatoes for 7 minutes or until they are tender.

3. Peel and grate the ginger. Chop the garlic and prepare the asparagus and/or zucchini. Heat the oil in a medium sauté pan on medium heat. Add the garlic and sliced green vegetables. Add the Bragg's and cover, cooking for 6 to 8 minutes, until all the vegetables are just tender.

4. Transfer all of the vegetables and cooked grain to a large mixing bowl. Add 2 teaspoons lime, oregano, basil, nuts, and olives. Stir gently to mix, adding salt, pepper, and more lime to taste.

GUACAMOLE

Preparation Time: About 10 minutes
Serves 4 to 6

One of my very favorite foods is guacamole, although many restaurants serve a version with so much garlic, tomato, and raw onion that I leave the table with a case of heartburn. Try this cooler version, and you may be able to give up your stock of antacids!

3 to 4 ripe Hass avocados
1 small clove garlic (optional)
1 bunch fresh cilantro (about 1 cup tightly packed)
½ teaspoon Fine Ground Celtic Sea Salt
1 to 2 teaspoons fresh lime, to taste

AYURVEDIC NOTE
Avocados lower *vata* and *pitta* but increase *kapha*. This recipe is fine for most people when eaten in moderation. If your *pitta* is very high, you might want to reduce the garlic and go easy on the lime.

(V) Add 1 additional clove of garlic.

(P) Reduce the garlic by half.

(K) Add 1 additional clove of garlic.

(S) Reduce the garlic by half.

(W) Add 1 additional clove of pressed garlic.

1. Peel the avocados, remove the pits, and cut avocados into chunks. Place the cut fruit into the bowl of a food processor or a mixing bowl.

2. Press the clove of garlic into the bowl, using a whole clove or half, to taste.

3. Soak the bunch of cilantro in a bowl or sink of cold water to remove any dirt. Throw the whole bunch into the food processor or finely chop enough leaves for the mixture.

4. Add the salt and lime juice. If using a food processor, press the pulse button several times. You can serve this guacamole a little bit chunky or purée it until it's smooth. You can also mash it with a potato masher, stirring in cilantro after mashing. Taste, and adjust with extra salt or another splash of lime.

(RECIPE PHOTO ON PAGE 204)

SWEET POTATO SALAD

Preparation Time: About 40 minutes
Serves 4 to 6

When making a potato salad, I like to substitute sweet potatoes for white. The outcome is healthier yet I find it equally satisfying and quintessentially picnic-worthy.

2 large sweet potatoes
1 leek or large shallot
1 large or 2 small stalks fennel or celery
½ cup diced red pepper (optional)
2 tablespoons extra-virgin olive oil
½ teaspoon ground cumin
½ teaspoon ground coriander
1 to 2 teaspoons prepared brown mustard
2 to 3 teaspoons fresh lime juice
½ to 1 teaspoon Fine Ground Celtic Sea Salt
½ cup chopped cilantro

COOK'S TIP: If you don't have fresh fennel, you can use a stalk of celery, but the fennel gives the dish a unique flavor. You can save the bulb for a side dish or include it in soup or stew.

AYURVEDIC NOTE

This salad is fine for everyone in moderation. Sweet potatoes are great for pacifying *vata* and *pitta* but will increase *kapha*, which is balanced somewhat by the mustard. Raw veggies will increase *vata*, and raw leeks will increase *pitta*, which is why they are slightly cooked in this recipe.

 Omit or decrease the mustard by half.

1. Wash and scrub the potatoes, or peel them if they are not organic. Cut them into bite-sized pieces, and place them in a steamer over 1 or 2 inches of boiling water. Cover the pot and steam the potatoes 10 to 12 minutes until the pieces are just tender but not mushy. Carefully transfer the potatoes to a mixing bowl and let them cool.

2. While the potatoes are cooking, slice the leek (or shallot), fennel, and red pepper. Heat 1 tablespoon of the oil in a medium skillet on medium heat, and add the cumin and coriander. Stir for 10 seconds. Add the leek or shallot and sauté for 2 minutes; then add the other veggies and sauté 5 minutes more. Remove from the heat and let cool.

3. Put the remaining tablespoon of oil into a small measuring cup with a spout. Add the mustard, lime juice, and salt (start with smaller quantities), and whisk. When the potatoes have cooled, add veggie mixture to the potatoes. Pour the mustard mixture over the potatoes and veggies. Add the cilantro and gently stir to blend all the ingredients. Taste, and adjust salt, lime, and mustard as needed. Serve at room temperature.

WILD RICE SALAD WITH WINTER SQUASH

Preparation Time: About 1¼ hours
Serves 4

1 cup wild or black rice
1 small butternut squash
2 cups water or soup stock (page 90)
1 teaspoon Fine Ground Celtic Sea Salt, divided
1 tablespoon walnut oil
1 teaspoon balsamic vinegar
¼ to ½ cup shelled pistachio nuts
½ tablespoon rosemary

COOK'S TIP: This salad would also be delicious with black rice, which can be cooked with the same amount of liquid.

AYURVEDIC NOTE

This dish is fine for everyone on occasion. However, if wild rice is undercooked, it is rubbery and hard, which will increase *vata*.

V Add roasted garlic.

P Omit the vinegar.

K Add roasted garlic.

1. Bring the water and ¾ teaspoon salt to a boil in a 3-cup saucepan. (Omit the salt if cooking with salted stock.) Add the wild rice and reduce heat to medium-low. Simmer about 45 minutes, until the grains have puffed up and the rice is tender, not chewy.

2. Bake the butternut squash: Preheat oven to 375°F. Peel squash and cut in half. Scoop out seeds. Cut squash into strips and then into bite-sized cubes. Place squash cubes on a baking sheet covered with parchment paper. Bake for 30 minutes or until the squash cubes are just tender. Remove from the oven and set aside.

3. Toast the pistachio nuts in the oven on 350°F for 5 to 10 minutes until the nuts are slightly browned. Chop the rosemary.

4. When the liquid has been absorbed into the rice, add the walnut oil, vinegar, roasted squash, nuts, and rosemary. Toss and add salt, to taste. Serve as a side dish or on a bed of romaine lettuce or mixed greens.

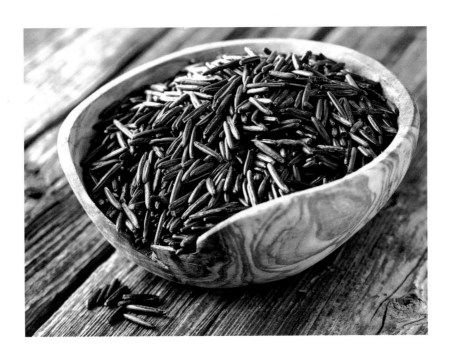

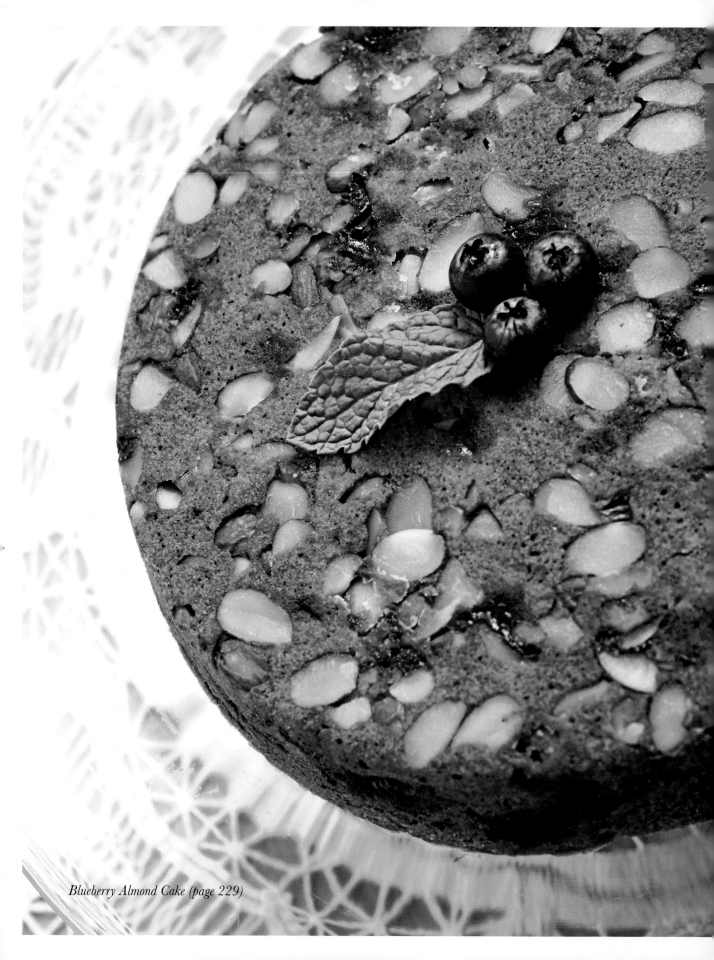

Blueberry Almond Cake (page 229)

CHAPTER 11.

Desserts

To sit down at a table with freshly baked bread
and a steaming bowl of soup filled with gorgeous vegetables!
Oh, what abundance! What heavenly smells! What joy!
And who can deny himself the pleasure of a bissel *dessert?*
This pleasure is no sin! In fact, it's so very close to God.
And that's why we say a blessing before a meal and give thanks afterward.

⌐ Rabbi Zalman Schachter-Shalomi

Ayurveda and the Pleasure Principle

Cakes and Fruit Desserts

Frostings and Toppings

Vegan Cookies

Puddings with Vegan Options

Food Notes

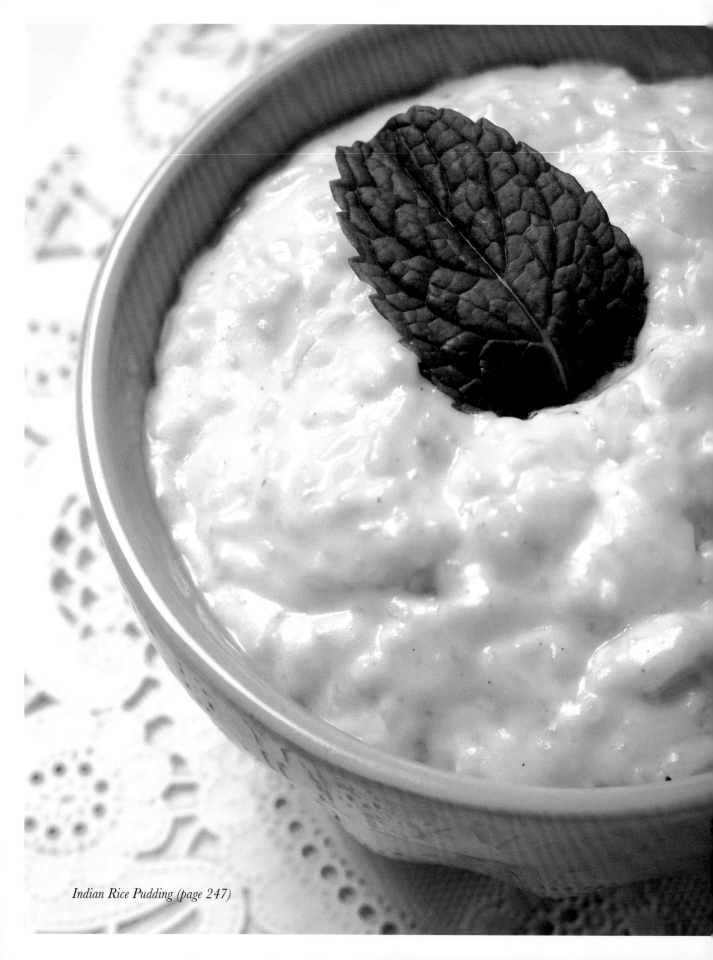

Indian Rice Pudding (page 247)

Ayurveda and the Pleasure Principle

Without a doubt, a little dessert is part of a sublime life. I am not one to deny myself this pleasure from time to time, but you may have guessed that desserts as we know them in the Western world have no real place in Ayurveda. You're probably familiar with the ones I mean, most notably a five-inch-high piece of cake called Death by Chocolate. Think about it! But a few bites of something light and sugary from time to time—that's a bit of heaven. As the great Rabbi Zalman Schachter-Shalomi said, "Who can deny himself the pleasure of a *bissel* dessert?" *Bissel* is Yiddish for "a little bit," and this is supremely wise advice.

Eating sweets in moderation was the norm across cultures for most of history, from the dainty tea cakes of Great Britain and the early American colonies to the bite-sized sweets of India and across Asia. A traditional Ayurvedic meal might include two or three mouthfuls of something sweet once or twice a week. This sweet is served as a small portion alongside the rest of the meal. It might be *khir*, Indian Rice Pudding (page 247) or a *laddu* (a small ball of sweetened dough). Once again "mouthful" is the operative word here. No ice cream by the pint after dinner—and I speak from guilty experience!

At the end of sacred events in India, and Vedic-style rituals performed worldwide, participants are offered *prasad*, blessed food. The *prasad* is just one bite—perhaps a piece of succulent fruit or a sugary *laddu*. This food has been ritually offered to God before it is handed to everyone as a parting gift. I've experienced leaving many such events with a luscious morsel of *prasad* on my tongue. Just one bite, yet it is a container that seems to hold within it all the grace experienced in worship. My husband and I carried this tradition into our wedding. After we exchanged vows and rings, we each offered *prasad* to the other. It was a small piece of dark chocolate (my personal favorite!) to symbolize the sweetness and abundance of life and the divine flavor of our destinies being joyfully intertwined.

If we can only learn to treat dessert with this kind of respect and restraint, we can savor each pleasurable mouthful and do no harm! Most people have discovered this for themselves. If you overdo, you live to regret it! But a single bite of a delicious dessert is a choice to savor for a long time to come.

How do you find that perfect sweet spot, if you'll forgive the pun? Remember that positive food choices support your overall well-being. Recognize dessert as a special treat to celebrate life, and remember moderation.

A Guide to Moderation

As with all food, the key to making dessert a guilt-free pleasure is to eat sweets in moderation. For me, "moderation" means the special occasions rule. I serve a sweet last course in our home for celebratory events but not as an everyday or even weekly occurrence. As Michael Pollan puts it, "There is nothing wrong with special occasion foods, as long as every day is not a special occasion." I enjoy offering dessert when we invite guests to dinner for the first time. I love pampering my family with a birthday cake or Thanksgiving pie. These are *my* special occasions, and they are part of the American experience and culinary culture that won't be denied. And because they are infrequent, they don't fuel my personal health challenges.

That said, I've become increasingly cautious about my sugar intake. For me, even an unrefined sweetener like coconut sugar seems best in modest doses. If you are being careful about blood sugar—if you have energy swings as I do—you'll likely feel better if you forgo a dessert habit.

For anyone who lives with chronic pain or illness, the special occasions rule is likely to be the best route unless you have the self-discipline to forgo desserts altogether. And that I applaud! Doing without sugar and excess fat, of course, gives the body a greater capacity to heal.

If you do eat some sweets, you can determine what your own standard for moderation should be by paying attention to how you feel after you eat dessert—for a couple of hours, even a couple of days. Do you feel speedy from a sugar rush? Do you have trouble sleeping that night? Or do you crash thirty minutes after eating dessert? (If so, you could be hypoglycemic and might want to get your blood tested.) Do you come down with a cold after eating sugar for a few consecutive days? (Sugar can compromise the immune system.) If you have any negative response to sugar, my suggestion is that you eat sugar infrequently. You may also want to switch to stevia, a plant-based sweetener that has no negative impact on blood sugar.

Ultimately, the goal of moderation is to focus your dessert experience on pleasure and to avoid any pain! At any time, it's best to avoid emotional eating. It may be natural for us to crave a little sweet taste to offset the challenges and sorrows that we encounter along life's journey, but when you reach for sugar, try to do so consciously. Then when you experience the rapture of dessert, you can pause to remember your many blessings and give thanks for this moment of absolute pleasure.

About These Desserts

Except for the *khir*, I broke with Ayurvedic tradition when developing recipes for *Sacred & Delicious,* and I did this for one reason: very few Americans will be deterred from eating birthday cake and an occasional brownie or chocolate chip cookie! And when we do, we're doomed to eat overly sweet, refined-everything, toxic desserts—unless someone creates healthier versions of our occasional indulgences. So this is what I set out to do! This means avoiding refined sugar and, for many, also gluten content. **To that end, all of these desserts are gluten-free, and most have vegan options.**

I have taken these desserts to many social events with people who eat all kinds of food and have received consistently high reviews—including the most coveted of all comments: "This can't be gluten-free!" I think it's because I don't scrimp on butter (or for me, ghee) and eggs.

Eggs are not part of Ayurvedic cuisine, but then neither is cake! I prefer to bake cakes with eggs because they help gluten-free flours to hold their form. As important, the protein in eggs is at least a partial balance to the sugar grams in desserts. For these reasons I've used eggs in all but one of the cake recipes and list eggs as an option in the cookies.

Butter is also not in an Ayurvedic diet, except in the form of *ghee*, which is clarified butter (see pages 72–73). In daily cooking I use ghee, and I've settled on ghee for baking, as well. I have to say the outcomes have also been quite delectable. The bonus is that I no longer have *kapha* symptoms from the lactose in butter. Most people who are dairy intolerant can eat food made with ghee because the milk solids have been removed. I still include butter as an optional ingredient because it's less expensive than ghee—unless you make your own.

If you're vegan, substitute equal amounts of oil.

The Sugar Conundrum

As I've said, I gave up refined sugar (white table sugar) long ago. (If you need persuasion, see page 40 for "About Sugar and Other Sweeteners.") In recent years I've settled on unrefined coconut crystals as my sweetener of choice for baking. It bakes well, tastes delicious, and is high in mineral content and amino acids. Most importantly, coconut sugar has a relatively low glycemic index compared to other sugars I've tested. For recipes that are light-colored, I use maple sugar, though I must admit that it's quite expensive. But, then, all unrefined sugars are more expensive than white sugar. It's easier to tolerate the higher price if you prepare desserts only for special occasions.

As a final word of caution on sweeteners, I want to speak directly to anyone who has diabetes, hypoglycemia, or any chronic illness involving blood sugar. Although the Ayurvedic notes at the end of each recipe suggest that people of all *doshas* can eat unrefined sugar and maple syrup with no ill effects if they do so only on occasion, please understand those remarks are not for you—unless you're able to stop after one bite! There is no home-free card here for diabetics and hypoglycemics. If you have a medical issue involving blood sugar, my suggestion is to follow your doctor's nutritional advice with regard to eating any kind of sweetener.

Low- vs. No-Gluten

Although eating gluten-free is imperative for many people, gluten-free baking can still present some health issues. When I made my first stab at creating gluten-free desserts, I used one of the excellent gluten-free mixtures that are now widely sold. The outcomes were the right texture and taste, but I felt I could do better from a nutritional standpoint. These mixtures are highly refined, using ingredients such as tapioca and potato starch along with white rice flour. Run your fingers through these flours and you'll feel it immediately; they are pure carb. So I rewrote and retested all of my dessert recipes, this time combining almond flour with gluten-free oat flour, which both have some protein. In these experiments I found the texture of the Carrot Cake, the Vegan Chocolate Cake, and the Date Nut Bundt Cake still required a measure of refined carbs, but the remaining cakes and cookies work well with the new formula. My tasters were delighted with the results!

One compromise I made was to include xanthan gum. It's difficult to bake a gluten-free cake successfully without it. Xanthan gum is not food per se but a substance, which is concocted in a lab and derived from corn, dairy, soy, and sometimes wheat. For a while, I resisted using it. Then I was surprised to learn that xanthan gum is used in medicines to lower blood sugar and total cholesterol in people with diabetes. On further reflection, I've decided to accept it as a necessary additive that might have health benefits. I check labels to make sure the xanthan gum I buy is gluten-free.

Christian Blessing

As with all of the traditions cited, there are many
Christian blessings for food. Here is one.

Give us grateful hearts, our Father, for all thy mercies,
and make us mindful of the needs of others; through
Jesus Christ our Lord. Amen.

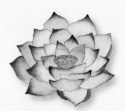

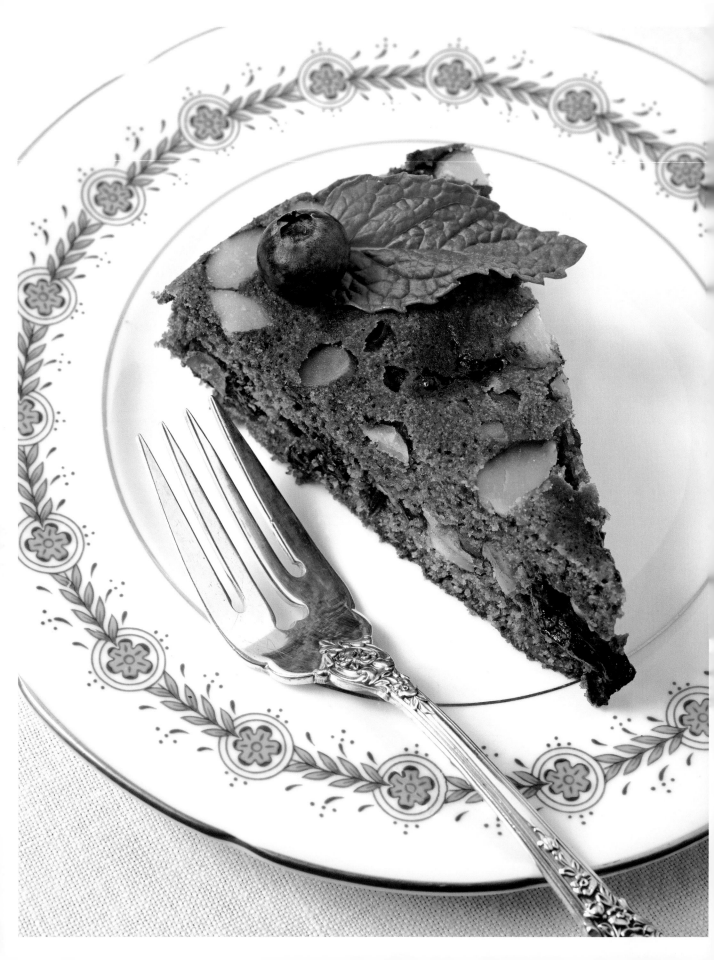

BLUEBERRY ALMOND CAKE

Preparation Time: Roughly 1½ hours (30 minutes active)

Serves 12 to 16

This is a small cake that is delightfully easy to make. It is intentionally moist and just a bit sweet, making it entirely guilt-free!

¾ **cup sifted fine almond flour**

¾ **cup gluten-free oat flour, plus some for dusting the pan**

½ **teaspoon xanthan gum**

1 **teaspoon baking powder**

½ **teaspoon baking soda**

½ **teaspoon Fine Ground Celtic Sea Salt**

1 **teaspoon ground cardamom**

9 **tablespoons ghee, butter, or coconut oil, room temperature, plus some for greasing the pan**

½ **cup coconut sugar**

1 **teaspoon vanilla extract**

3 **large eggs, room temperature**

½ **cup unsweetened almond milk**

¾ **cup sliced almonds**

8 **ounces fresh blueberries (1½ cups), rinsed and strained**

TIME-SAVER: Buy packaged sliced almonds.

AYURVEDIC NOTE

Almond and oat flour are excellent for *vata,* good for pitta, and better for *kapha* than all-carb cakes. Coconut sugar in moderation is fine for *vata* and *pitta.* All sugars increase *kapha.* Sweetened blueberries are fine for all *doshas.*

1. Lightly grease a 9-inch cake pan or an 8-inch square cake pan. Cover the bottom of the pan with parchment paper, and grease the top of the paper. Lightly flour the pan (about 1 teaspoon of flour) and invert it to tap out excess flour. Adjust the oven rack to the lower-middle position, and preheat the oven to 350°F.

2. In a small mixing bowl, combine the flours, xanthan gum, baking powder, baking soda, salt, and cardamom, and blend together with a whisk. Set aside.

3. In a large mixing bowl, briefly cream the ghee, butter, or coconut oil with a whisk or electric mixer. Add the sugar and vanilla, and beat until well combined. Add the eggs and whisk or beat until the eggs are mixed in. Add almond milk and mix again.

4. Fold in the flour mixture with a rubber spatula, and stir until all the ingredients are well mixed. Add ½ cup of the almonds (reserving ¼ cup), and stir. Complete the batter by gently stirring in the blueberries.

5. Sprinkle the reserved almonds into the bottom of the cake pan. Pour the batter on top of the almonds. Bake for 55 to 60 minutes, rotating the pan once halfway through, until a toothpick inserted in the middle comes out almost clean. Transfer the pan to a wire rack, and let the cake cool in the pan for 10 minutes. Run a knife along the edges of the pan to loosen the cake before inverting the pan onto a rack to continue cooling. Peel off the parchment paper. Let cool at least an hour before slicing.

CARROT CAKE

Preparation Time: 4 hours (1 hour active)

Serves 12 to 16

When I began experimenting with gluten-free flours, I learned the hard way that a carrot cake requires at least some high-carb flour to build a proper texture. As a sweetener, I offer maple sugar as the first option for bakers who prefer a lighter-colored cake—the traditional carrot-cake look. The darker coconut sugar tastes just as good, has a lower glycemic index, and is less expensive.

4½ tightly packed cups of grated carrots (1 pound)

1½ cups sifted fine almond flour

1½ cups King Arthur Gluten-Free All-Purpose Flour

2 teaspoons baking powder

1 teaspoon baking soda

¾ teaspoon xanthan gum

1 teaspoon Fine Ground Celtic Sea Salt

1 tablespoon ground cinnamon

½ teaspoon ground nutmeg

4 large eggs, room temperature

2 cups maple or coconut sugar

½ cup plus 2 tablespoons sunflower or walnut oil, plus some for oiling the pan(s)

¼ cup plain unsweetened almond milk

2 teaspoons vanilla extract

BAKER'S TIP: This cake can be baked in two 9-inch cake pans (40 to 45 minutes), three 9-inch pans for skinny layers (30 to 35 minutes), or in a 9 x 13 pan (45 to 50 minutes).

AYURVEDIC NOTE

Almond flour, which is excellent for *vata* and fine for *pitta,* helps balance the recipe's carb load for *kapha.* Maple sugar, considered strengthening, and coconut sugar are fine for *vata* and *pitta* in moderation. All sugars increase *kapha,* as will flour and nut flour. Eggs partially offset the sugar and carbs. Cooked carrots are excellent for all *doshas.*

1. Lightly oil cake pan(s). Cover the bottom with parchment paper, and oil the top of the paper. Lightly flour (about 1 teaspoon of flour for each pan) and invert to tap out excess flour.

2. Scrub the carrots and grate them in a food processor or by hand. Measure out 4½ cups and set aside. Adjust the oven rack to the lower-middle position, and preheat the oven to 350°F.

3. In a medium mixing bowl, sift the almond flour. Remeasure and transfer 1½ sifted cups to a second mixing bowl. Add King Arthur flour, baking powder, baking soda, xanthan gum, salt, cinnamon, and nutmeg to the flour, and combine with a whisk.

4. In a separate mixing bowl, whisk the eggs or beat them with an electric mixer on a moderate speed. Add sugar and mix again. Add oil, vanilla, and almond milk, and beat briefly until well combined. Fold in flour mixture with a rubber spatula, stirring only until all the ingredients are well mixed. Fold in the carrots until they are completely blended into the batter.

5. Pour the batter into the prepared pans in equal amounts and bake for the amount of time specified in the Baker's Tip or until a toothpick inserted in the middle comes out clean. A few crumbs are OK. If using the 9-inch cake pans, place the cake pans on wire racks for 10 minutes after baking. Run a knife along the edges of each pan to loosen the cake before inverting each pan onto a rack to continue cooling. Remove the parchment paper.

If using a 9 x 13 pan, pour all of the batter into the pan. After baking, leave the cake in the pan on a wire rack for about two hours until the cake is completely cooled. Once the cake has cooled, run a knife along the edge to loosen the cake from the pan. Invert the pan onto a cake board or serving tray.

6. While the layers are cooling, prepare the frosting (page 237). You can frost the cake once it has reached room temperature, ideally after cooling at least 2 hours. Cover the cake in a domed container but do not refrigerate. The cake will keep for two days unrefrigerated.

DARK CHOCOLATE LAYER CAKE

Preparation Time: 4 hours (1 hour active)
Serves 8 to 12

When it's time to blow out the candles, we all deserve a birthday cake, and sometimes only chocolate will do!

FOR THE CAKE:

4 ounces unsweetened chocolate
1½ cups sifted fine almond flour
1½ cups oat flour, plus some to dust the pans
2 teaspoons baking powder
1 teaspoons baking soda
1½ teaspoons xanthan gum
1 teaspoon Fine Ground Celtic Sea Salt
1 cup ghee, butter, melted coconut oil, or walnut oil, plus some to grease the pans
1½ cups coconut sugar
5 eggs, room temperature
2 teaspoons vanilla extract
1 cup unsweetened almond milk, room temperature

BAKER'S TIP: This cake can be baked in two 9-inch cake pans (32 to 35 minutes), three 9-inch pans for skinny layers (28 to 30 minutes), or in a 9 x 13 pan (about 45 minutes).

AYURVEDIC NOTE

Modern science tells us that dark chocolate is full of antioxidants—yay! Ayurvedic experts also note that chocolate, when eaten in excess, increases all *doshas*. Coconut sugar is OK in moderation for *vata* and *pitta*. All sugars increase *kapha*, which is also increased by ghee or oil. Enjoy this dessert for special occasions!

SERVING SUGGESTION

Enjoy with a cup of chai tea spiced with an extra pinch of cardamom, which is the Ayurvedic antidote to chocolate. Or serve the cake with warm milk or almond milk spiced with cardamom and fresh ginger—yummy!

1. Adjust the oven rack to the lower-middle position, and preheat the oven to 350°F. Lightly grease cake pans with ghee, butter, or oil; then cover the bottom of each pan with parchment paper, and grease the top of the paper. Lightly flour the pans (about 1 teaspoon of flour each) and invert them to tap out excess flour.

2. Melt the chocolate in an uncovered double boiler on low heat or small open saucepan on low heat. (If using a double boiler, place about 1 inch of water in the bottom pan and place the chocolate in the top pan, which is not touching the water.) Bring to a gentle simmer, which will heat the chocolate enough for it to melt. Once the chocolate is melted, remove the insert pan from the double boiler or remove the saucepan from the heat source to allow the mixture to cool.

3. While the chocolate is cooling, place flours in a medium-sized mixing bowl, and stir with a whisk. Gently whisk in baking powder, baking soda, xanthan gum, and salt.

4. In a separate large mixing bowl, use an electric mixer on medium speed to cream the ghee or oil until smooth and aerated, about 2 minutes. Add the coconut sugar, and beat another minute until well combined. (If using oil, simply mix together.) Add the eggs one at a time, beating briefly on low

speed after each addition. Add the vanilla and cooled chocolate, and mix. Alternate folding in the flour mixture and almond milk a little at a time, using a spatula. Mix briefly by hand until the ingredients are well combined and the batter is smooth. Let the batter sit 5 minutes and then stir it again before pouring it into the pans.

5. Pour the batter into the prepared pans in equal amounts and put the pans in the oven. (See Baker's Tip for suggested baking times.) Let the cake pans cool on a wire rack for 10 minutes. Run a knife along the edges of each pan to loosen the cake before inverting each pan onto a rack to continue cooling. Remove the parchment paper.

If using a 9 x 13 pan, leave the cake in the pan for about two hours after it has finished baking, until the cake is completely cooled. Once the cake has cooled, run a knife along the edge to loosen the cake from the pan. Invert the pan onto a serving platter or clean cutting board.

6. Finish the cake with Dark Chocolate Frosting (page 238) or Dark Chocolate Vegan Frosting (page 240). Apply the frosting to the top of each layer and cover the sides. Cover the layered cake in a domed container but do not refrigerate. Keeps for three days.

VEGAN CHOCOLATE SHEET CAKE

Preparation Time: 4 hours (45 minutes active)
Serves 8 to 12

Sometimes I go to an event that I know some vegans will attend, and to honor those friends, I developed this cake. My experience is that even people who are not vegans enjoy it all the same.

2 cups sifted fine almond flour

2 cups King Arthur Gluten-Free All-Purpose Flour, plus 1 tablespoon more to dust the pan

¾ cup unsweetened cocoa powder

2 teaspoons baking powder

2 teaspoons baking soda

2¾ teaspoons xanthan gum

1¼ teaspoons Fine Ground Celtic Sea Salt

2 tablespoons plus 1 teaspoon psyllium husk

1 cup sunflower or almond oil, plus some to grease the pan

2 cups coconut sugar

1 tablespoon vanilla extract

2 cups plus 2 tablespoons plain unsweetened almond milk

AYURVEDIC NOTE

Chocolate, when eaten in excess, increases all *doshas*. Coconut sugar is fine in moderation for *vata* and *pitta*. All sugars and oils increase *kapha*, coconut oil in particular. Enjoy this dessert for special occasions.

1. Adjust the oven rack to the lower-middle position and preheat the oven to 350°F. Lightly grease a 9 x 13 cake pan with a little oil; then cover the bottom of the pan with parchment paper and grease the top of the paper. Lightly flour the pan and invert the pan to tap out excess flour.

2. Whisk the flours in a medium-sized mixing bowl with the cocoa powder, baking powder, baking soda, xanthan gum, salt, and psyllium husk.

3. In a separate large mixing bowl, combine the coconut sugar with the oil, and beat it for a minute with an electric mixer on medium speed to add some air. Add the vanilla and mix briefly. Slowly add flour mixture to the large bowl a little at a time and mix on low speed, alternating with the almond milk, until all the ingredients are well combined and the batter is smooth.

4. Pour the batter into the prepared baking pan and bake 45 to 50 minutes, or until a toothpick inserted in the middle comes out clean or has a few crumbs. You don't want to overbake, as that would make the cake dry. Remove the pan from the oven and place it on a wire rack, allowing the cake to cool in the pan completely, about two hours. Once the cake has cooled, run a knife along the edge to loosen the cake from the pan. Invert the cake onto a clean cutting board or serving tray and remove the parchment.

5. Finish the cake with Dark Chocolate Vegan Frosting (page 240) or with the vegan option of the Cream Cheese Frosting (page 237). You can cover the cake with plastic and frost the next day, but do not refrigerate. It will keep at room temperature for three days.

DATE NUT BUNDT CAKE

Preparation Time: 4 hours (40 minutes active)
Serves 12 to 16

This is a wonderful, moist cake that is not overly sweet and has the health benefits (high fiber and essential minerals) that come with dates. Thanks to Martina Straub for her family recipe, which inspired this rendition.

18 Medjool or 1 pound other dried dates
1¾ cups boiling water
1 teaspoon baking powder
1 teaspoon baking soda
1 cup sifted fine almond flour
1 cup oat flour
1 cup King Arthur Gluten-Free All-Purpose Flour,
    plus 1 tablespoon more to dust the pan
1¼ teaspoon Fine Ground Celtic Sea Salt
¾ teaspoon xanthan gum
⅔ cup ghee or butter, room temperature,
    plus some to grease the pan
1 cup coconut sugar
1½ teaspoons vanilla extract
4 large eggs, room temperature
1½ cups chopped pecans

AYURVEDIC NOTE

Dates are used in Ayurvedic medicine to help rebuild energy for those who have become debilitated. When dates have been soaked in water, they are excellent for *vata* and *pitta*. This dessert will elevate *kapha* but is OK for everyone on occasion.

SERVING SUGGESTION

Although this cake is lovely by itself, you may enjoy serving it with plain (or vegan) cream cheese, or toasted with butter or ghee.

1. Remove date pits and chop the dates into bite-sized chunks. Soak the date chunks in the boiling water with baking powder and baking soda until they cool completely. Do not strain. (You can use room temperature water if you do this step the day before you bake, letting them soak overnight.)

2. Adjust the oven rack to the lower-middle position, and preheat the oven to 350°F. Grease a 10-inch (3-quart) nonstick tube pan or Bundt pan, and lightly dust with flour. Invert the pan over the sink and tap out excess flour.

3. Whisk together the flours, salt and xanthan gum, and set aside.

4. In a separate bowl, use an electric mixer to cream the ghee or butter until smooth. Add the coconut sugar and beat until fluffy, another 2 minutes. Add the vanilla, and mix well. Add the eggs one by one, beating briefly after each addition.

5. Using a spatula and adding just a bit at a time, fold the flour mixture and the date mixture into the butter/sugar mixture in alternating rounds. Then fold in chopped pecans, and pour batter into the pan.

6. Bake 60 to 65 minutes. Test with a toothpick inserted in the center, which should come out with no batter residue and showing a few crumbs. Let the cake cool about 2 hours in the pan; then invert the pan onto a rack and let the cake cool completely before slicing. Cover the cake in a domed container but do not refrigerate. It keeps for three days at room temperature.

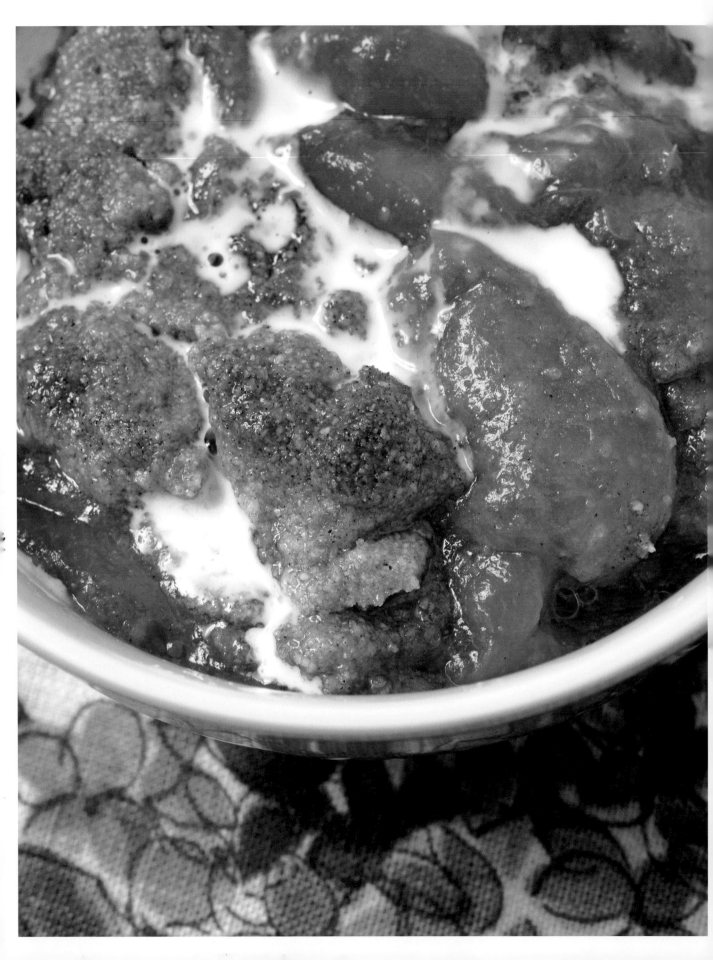

PEACH COBBLER

Preparation Time: 1½ hours (45 minutes active)
Serves 8 to 12

You know it's summer in the Deep South when the peaches start to ripen. Come late June or early July when Tom and I drive to the Carolina beaches, we always stop at the roadside stands to pick up a basket of the fresh peaches that are coming right out of the orchards. I wait a day or two until the peaches are perfectly ripe, and then . . . the bliss of Peach Cobbler! Cobbler is so much easier to make than pie if you don't like rolling a crust. You can use more or fewer peaches, depending on your budget and how thick you like your cobbler. The almond flour works perfectly, either for crumbles or for a biscuit-like crust.

FOR THE FILLING:
8 to 10 cups of fresh peach slices (12 to 14 large peaches)
1 cup coconut sugar
2 teaspoons vanilla extract
¼ cup arrowroot
Ghee, butter, or coconut oil to grease the baking dish

FOR THE TOPPING:
2 cups fine almond flour
½ teaspoon Fine Ground Celtic Sea Salt
2 teaspoons baking powder
¾ cup maple crystals or coconut sugar
1½ teaspoons cinnamon
½ cup cold unsalted ghee, butter, or coconut oil
¼ cup ice water

BAKER'S TIP: Sift the flour for a finer texture.

AYURVEDIC NOTE
Cooked peaches are excellent for *vata* and *kapha*, but when they are tart, peaches will aggravate *pitta*, which is pacified by ghee and sugar. The ghee and sugar will increase *kapha*. If you serve this with coconut ice cream, as I like to do, that's more of a problem for *kapha*!

K Reduce sugar by half.

1. For the filling: Peel the peaches. Halve each peach, remove the pit and slice each half into six or eight thin wedges. Place the cut peaches in a large mixing bowl. Add coconut sugar and vanilla. Toss gently to mix. Cover and let rest at room temperature for 30 minutes.

2. Adjust oven rack to lower-middle position, preheat oven to 425°F, and grease a 3-quart (9 x 13) baking dish. Place the water and ghee for the topping in the refrigerator to chill.

3. While the peaches are resting, start the topping: Place a dough paddle in the bowl of a food processor and set the processor on the dough setting. Place the flour, salt, baking powder, cinnamon, and all but 1 tablespoon of the maple crystals (or coconut sugar) into the bowl of the processor. Pulse two to three times. (If you don't own a processor, you can make this dough in a mixing bowl. Mix the dry ingredients together with a whisk; use a dough cutter when adding the ghee and water in step 5.)

4. After 30 minutes, strain the liquid from the peaches into a bowl, discarding all but ½ cup, and set the peaches aside in their mixing bowl. Transfer the peach juice to a saucepan, and add the arrowroot while the juice is still at room temperature. Whisk to smooth out any lumps. Bring the juice mixture to a gentle boil on medium heat, whisking constantly for about 5 minutes or until the mixture starts to thicken. Stir the thickened mixture back into the fruit. Spoon the peaches with their thickened liquid into the baking dish and bake for 10 minutes.

5. While the peaches are baking, finish the topping. Add the ghee or butter to the almond flour and pulse a few times. Add 2 tablespoons of ice water and pulse just a few times until the flour forms crumbles. If you prefer a biscuit-style crust, add a full quarter cup of water and pulse until it becomes a dough.

6. Remove the baking dish from the oven and scatter the crumbles over the peaches or drop tablespoons of the dough across the peaches in staggered rows, so they are not too close to each other. Sprinkle the last tablespoon of maple sugar across the topping. Bake for 20 to 25 minutes, until the topping has lightly browned and the peaches are bubbling. Let cool for 10 minutes and serve. Top with vanilla or coconut ice cream, if you wish.

About Fruit Desserts

There are various schools of Ayurveda, which began as an oral tradition and was passed down from master to disciple throughout India over the millennia. Some surviving traditions suggest not eating fruit with any other kind of food. These traditions say that the fruit ferments in the stomach when combined with other food. I have, however, heard one Ayurvedic expert give permission for peach pie or cobbler, saying that improper food combining is less of a problem when foods are cooked together. The reason: when cooked together these foods begin to take on each other's qualities.

This is especially true when foods share what in Ayurveda is called *vipak*, the aftertaste. Because the aftertastes of both peaches and almond flour are sweet, their comingling in this recipe is easier on digetsion.

All I can say is, "Yay!"

The best bet for anyone with delicate digestion is to wait until 30 minutes to 1 hour after your meal to partake of this fruit dessert. This would avoid combining the peaches with the rest of your food.

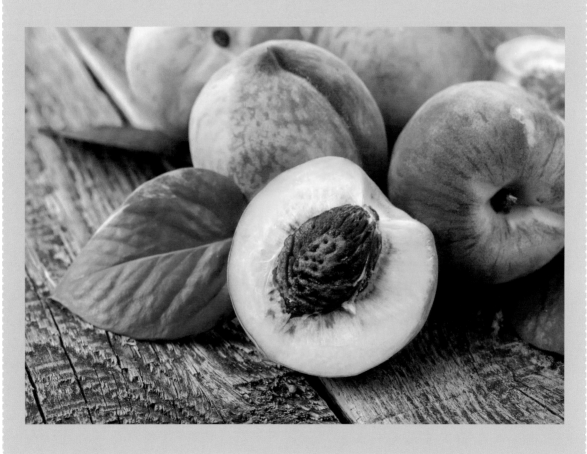

CREAM CHEESE FROSTING

Preparation Time: About 10 minutes
Enough for one 9-inch double- or triple-layer cake or a 9 x 13 sheet cake

This frosting is quite versatile and can be used on many types of cake or cupcakes.

16 ounces cream cheese, room temperature

1 cup ghee, or unsalted butter (2 sticks), room temperature

4 teaspoons vanilla extract

⅔ cup maple syrup or coconut nectar, plus optional
    2 tablespoons

⅛ teaspoon Fine Ground Celtic Sea Salt

1½ cups chopped pecans or walnuts

VEGAN OPTION: Replace the cream cheese and ghee with 24 ounces of either Kite Hill Cream Cheese Style Spread (made from artisan almond milk) or less expensive dairy-free brands such as Tofuti or Daiya.

AYURVEDIC NOTE

Dairy cream cheese increases *pitta* and *kapha*. Although nuts increase *kapha* and *pitta*, one piece of cake will have a small quantity, which is fine for most people. Maple syrup is strengthening to the body and is fine for all *doshas* on occasion.

1. Place the cream cheese, ghee (or butter), vanilla, ⅔ cup maple syrup (or coconut nectar), and salt into a stainless steel bowl and beat with a mixer until the frosting is smooth and starts to form peaks like whipped cream. If it's still lumpy or not sweet enough to your taste, add 2 more tablespoons of maple syrup.

2. Set aside 2 tablespoons of the chopped nuts. Fold the remaining nuts into the frosting with a spatula, mixing it gently but well.

3. Once you have finished frosting the cake, sprinkle the remaining 2 tablespoons of nuts over the top.

DARK CHOCOLATE FROSTING

Preparation Time: About 15 minutes

Makes enough for a 9-inch double- or triple-layer cake or a 9 x 13 sheet cake

If you wish, use standard confectioner's sugar. If you prefer unrefined sugars and you own a Vitamix, you can powder your own with this winning combination! (There may be another professional-grade blender that will powder sugar, but I haven't come across it yet.)

4 tablespoons ghee or unsalted butter

4 ounces unsweetened chocolate

1½ cups coconut sugar*

1½ cups maple sugar*

⅛ teaspoon of Fine Ground Celtic Sea Salt

¼ cup whole milk or half-and-half

1 teaspoon vanilla extract

¼ cup chopped walnuts or pecans (optional)

* Substitute 2½ cups standard confectioner's sugar for the coconut and maple sugar, if preferred.

COOK'S TIP: Three cups of these unrefined sugars will become about 2½ cups once powdered. Most store-bought cakes have frosting that is far too sweet for my taste, but if you like that model of sweetness, you will want to increase the amount of sugar called for in this recipe: start with 3 cups standard confectioner's sugar, or a total of 3½ cups of unrefined sugars, before processing in the Vitamix. Add an additional 2 tablespoons of almond milk, and more if necessary.

AYURVEDIC NOTE

Chocolate increases all *doshas*, particularly *vata* and *pitta*, which are pacified by milk. Maple and coconut sugar increase *kapha*, as does milk or half-and-half. Enjoy this on special occasions!

1. Slowly heat the ghee (or butter) and chocolate in an uncovered double boiler on medium heat, or use a small saucepan on low heat, stirring constantly, until the chocolate melts completely. Remove the insert pan from the double boiler to allow the mixture to cool, or remove the saucepan from the heat source.

2. While the chocolate mixture cools, briefly process the coconut sugar and maple sugar in the Vitamix.

3. Place the sugar in a mixing bowl. Add the milk (or half-and-half), vanilla, and salt. Blend well with an electric mixer. Pour the chocolate mixture over the sugar mixture, and beat well until creamy and spreadable.

FROSTINGS AND TOPPINGS

In Search of a Healthier Frosting

Because I wanted to create a healthier chocolate cake, I spent years experimenting with countless sugar alternatives—especially for the frosting. I wanted to avoid the highly processed confectioners' sugar, which is the vital ingredient of most frostings, because refined sugar is highly inflammatory and increases all *doshas*. For one reason or another, I was disappointed with every taste test until it occurred to me to create my own powdered sweetening with unrefined sugars. I found that the Vitamix works beautifully for this. I haven't investigated the efficacy of other blenders, but if you own one, I suggest that you give it a try.

The two chocolate frosting recipes I've created use a combination of coconut sugar and maple sugar. The frosting is sweet enough and not at all gritty when processed in this high-powered machine. Maple sugar by itself is delicious, though quite expensive. Coconut sugar performing solo is not, in my opinion, quite as tasty or refined. My solution is to combine them and lower the cost. If you buy a small bag of the expensive maple product, you can save half for a future cake. And in my local store, coconut sugar is only $1 more than organic powdered sugar.

If you only bake a cake with frosting a few times a year, you may prefer to relax your dietary concerns and use the least expensive option, which is standard confectioners' sugar.

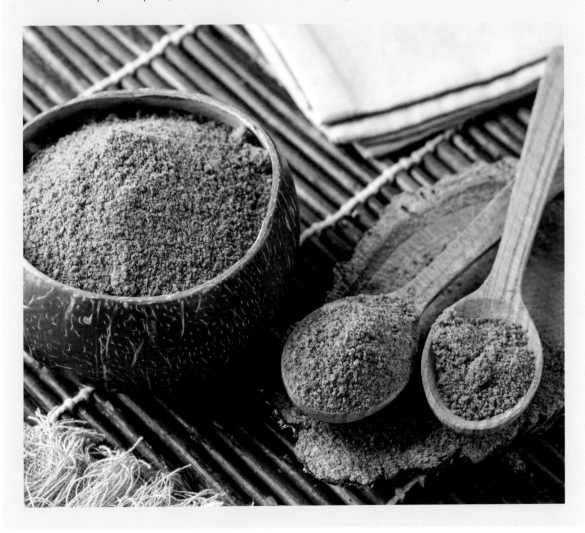

DARK CHOCOLATE VEGAN FROSTING

Preparation Time: About 15 minutes
Makes enough for a 9-inch double- or triple-layer cake or a 9 x 13 sheet cake

If you wish, use standard confectioner's sugar. For those who prefer unrefined sugars, I suggest powdering them with a Vitamix.

3 tablespoons coconut oil
4 ounces unsweetened chocolate
1½ cups coconut sugar*
1½ cups maple sugar*
⅛ teaspoon of Fine Ground Celtic Sea Salt
¼ cup almond milk, or coconut cream, room temperature
1 teaspoon vanilla extract
¼ cup chopped walnuts or pecans (optional)

*** Substitute 2½ cups standard confectioner's sugar for the coconut and maple sugar, if preferred.**

COOK'S TIP: Three cups of these unrefined sugars will become about 2½ cups once powdered. Most store-bought cakes have frosting that is far too sweet for my taste, but if you like that model of sweetness, you will want to increase the amount of sugar called for in my recipe: start with 3 cups standard confectioner's sugar or a total of 3½ cups of unrefined sugars before processing them. Add 2 tablespoons more almond milk, and more if necessary.

AYURVEDIC NOTE
Chocolate increases all *doshas*, particularly *vata* and *pitta*, which are pacified a bit by the coconut oil. Maple and coconut sugar increase *kapha*, as does coconut oil. *Kapha* never has a break when it comes to dessert!

1. Slowly heat the coconut oil and chocolate in an uncovered double boiler on medium heat, or use a small saucepan on low heat, stirring constantly, until the chocolate melts completely. Then remove the insert pan from the double boiler or remove the saucepan from the heat source.

2. While the chocolate mixture cools, briefly process the coconut sugar and maple sugar in the Vitamix.

3. Place the sugars in a mixing bowl. Add the salt, almond milk or coconut cream, and vanilla. Blend well with an electric mixer. Pour the chocolate mixture over the almond milk mixture and beat well until creamy and spreadable.

WHIPPED CREAM

Preparation Time: 5 minutes (but note chilling time needed)
Makes enough for a dollop of cream for 6 to 8

Once again, I cannot say this recipe is inspired by Ayurveda, but it is inspired by American tradition!

1 cup heavy cream or coconut cream
1 teaspoon vanilla extract
1 to 2 tablespoons real maple syrup or coconut nectar

AYURVEDIC NOTE
Although dairy cream is pacifying for *vata*, the fat in cream will increase *pita* and *kapha*. Maple syrup strengthens the constitution when used in moderation, although all sweets increase *kapha*.

1. Store the dairy cream and maple syrup (or coconut nectar) in the refrigerator so both are cold for preparation. (If using coconut cream, do not refrigerate it.) Place a stainless steel mixing bowl and stainless steel beaters in the refrigerator at least 30 minutes prior to preparing.

2. Pour the chilled cream (or coconut cream) and syrup (or nectar) into the chilled bowl. Add the vanilla. Beat for two minutes with an electric mixer and taste for sweetness. If you like a truly sweet topping, add more syrup. Continue to beat until peaks form and serve over your favorite desserts.

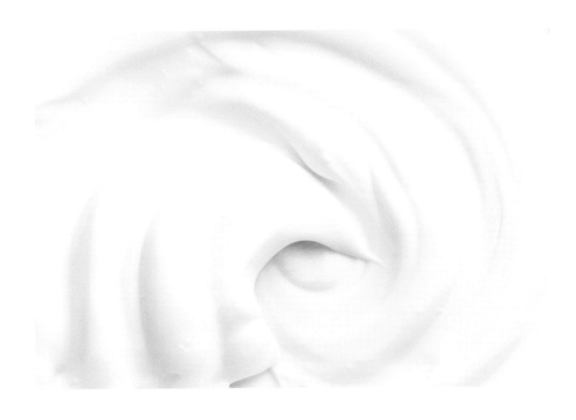

CARDAMOM ROSE COOKIES

Preparation Time: About 1½ hours (45 minutes active)
Makes 2 dozen small cookies

I took this concept from my husband and translated it into a gluten-free recipe. Being the family's resident cookie monster, Tom was the first in our household to start developing healthier cookie recipes to satisfy his occasional sweet tooth!

6 tablespoons ghee, butter, or coconut oil
15 cardamom pods (or 1 teaspoon ground cardamom)
1 cup fine almond flour
1 cup oat flour
¾ teaspoon xanthan gum
1 teaspoon baking soda
¾ teaspoon Fine Ground Celtic Sea Salt
1½ teaspoons psyllium husk, whole flakes
1 cup maple or coconut sugar
¼ cup unsweetened almond milk, room temperature
2 teaspoons rosewater

AYURVEDIC NOTE
Cardamom is slightly heating, which is balanced by cooling rosewater, making these cookies good for a year-round treat. Cardamom also helps balance *kapha*, which is increased by the flours, sugar, and fat.

BAKER'S TIP: 1. If you like the taste of cardamom, it's worth the trouble to grind your own seeds, as cardamom fresh from the pod has a much stronger flavor—and, in most cases, a markedly different flavor from any prepared powder you can buy in a store. For a milder taste, use half the amount. **2.** Use maple sugar if you want the cookies to look like traditional sugar cookies. **3.** If you prefer crisp cookies, reduce almond milk to 3 tablespoons.

1. Melt the ghee, butter, or coconut oil in a saucepan on low heat. Remove from heat to cool to room temperature.

2. If using cardamom pods, break them open and extract the black seeds. Pound the seeds with a mortar and pestle until you have a fine and fragrant gray powder.

3. In a medium-sized bowl, whisk together the flours, cardamom powder, xanthan gum, baking soda, salt, and psyllium husk.

4. Remeasure the melted fat into a separate mixing bowl, and return any excess to its container. Add the sugar to the melted fat and whisk until smooth. Add almond milk and rosewater. Mix well. Add the flour mixture, and mix well with a spatula. Be sure to mash any almond flour clumps. Cover the dough and chill it in the refrigerator for 30 minutes or longer.

5. When ready to prepare the cookies, preheat the oven to 350°F, and line a cookie sheet with parchment. Use a small scoop or measuring tablespoon to gather dough and drop 12 balls onto the parchment, leaving space between the cookies to spread. Bake for 13 to 14 minutes, until slightly browned. The edges will have begun to set, but the centers will still be soft. Let the cookies cool for 5 minutes on the baking sheet; then transfer the baked cookies on their parchment sheet to a rack to continue cooling. Keep the cookies in an airtight container for up to 3 days.

FRESH GINGER COOKIES

Preparation Time: About 1½ hours (45 minutes active)
Makes 2 dozen small cookies

Continuing the quest for healthier desserts, I dreamed up these cookies for the cold winter months.

6 tablespoons ghee, unsalted butter, or coconut oil
1 cup fine almond flour
1 cup oat flour
¾ teaspoon xanthan gum
1 teaspoon baking soda
¾ teaspoon Fine Ground Celtic Sea Salt
1½ teaspoons psyllium husk, whole flakes
1 cup coconut sugar
2 teaspoons vanilla extract
2 tablespoons unsweetened almond milk, room temperature
2 tablespoons freshly grated ginger

AYURVEDIC NOTE

Almond is an excellent gluten-free flour for *vata* and *pitta*. Flours and sweeteners of any kind increase *kapha*, which is balanced by the ginger. Ginger pacifies *vata* and *kapha* and is fine for *pitta* in moderation.

1. Melt the ghee, butter, or coconut oil in a saucepan on low heat. Remove from heat to cool to room temperature.

2. In a medium-sized bowl, whisk together the flours, xanthan gum, baking soda, salt, and psyllium husk.

3. Remeasure the melted fat into a separate mixing bowl, and return any excess to its container. Add the sugar to the melted fat and whisk until smooth. Stir in the vanilla, almond milk, grated ginger, and psyllium husk. Add the flour mixture, and mix well. Cover the dough and chill it in the refrigerator for 30 minutes or longer.

4. When ready to prepare the cookies, preheat oven to 350°F, and line a cookie sheet with parchment. Use a small scoop or measuring tablespoon to gather dough and drop 12 balls onto the parchment, leaving space between the cookies so they can spread. Bake for 13 to 14 minutes, until slightly browned. The edges will have begun to set, but the centers will still be soft. Let the cookies cool for 5 minutes on the baking sheet and transfer the baked cookies on their parchment sheet to a rack to continue cooling. Keep the cookies in an airtight container for up to 3 days.

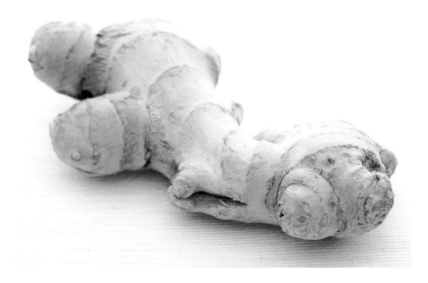

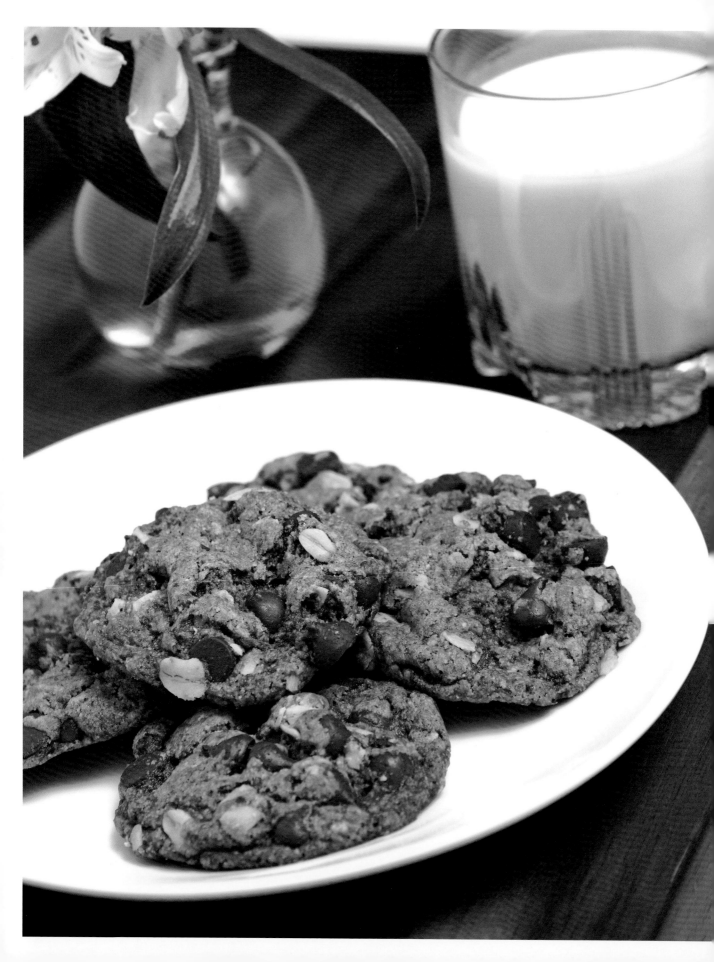

OMG OATMEAL CHOCOLATE CHIP COOKIES

Preparation Time: About 1½ hours (20 minutes active)
Makes about 2 dozen cookies

Nothing pleases better than a batch of not-so-sinful chocolate chip cookies. There is one requirement—they have to be yummy, even when they're gluten-free!

6 tablespoons ghee, butter, or coconut oil
⅔ cup fine almond flour
½ cup oat flour
¾ teaspoon xanthan gum
1 teaspoon baking soda
¾ teaspoon Fine Ground Celtic Sea Salt
1½ teaspoons psyllium husks (whole flakes)
1 cup coconut sugar
3 tablespoons warmed water
1 teaspoon vanilla extract
½ cup rolled oats
1 cup chocolate chips
½ cup chopped pecans (optional)

BAKER'S TIP: 1. Be sure to use whole psyllium husks (the flakes!), not psyllium powder, or your cookies will be hard as rocks. **2.** If you would like added protein with the sugar, you can replace psyllium husks and water with 1 egg. **3.** Take special care to measure everything precisely, and use every drop of the fat and water (or egg) as directed, or the cookies will be dry. **4.** You can use semi-sweet chocolate chips, although I prefer the 65 or 70 percent cocoa chips, which contain less refined sugar. **5.** These are chewy cookies. If you prefer crisp cookies, bake the cookies 2 to 3 minutes longer. **6.** For richer cookies, add 1 additional tablespoon of fat (7 tablespoons total) and refrigerate the baked cookies when storing. **7.** If you love cardamom, try this with ½ teaspoon ground cardamom. This spice is said by Ayurvedic experts to balance chocolate.

AYURVEDIC NOTE

I use fewer chocolate chips than some recipes because the chocolate and the sugar in the chips will increase all *doshas*. If you opt for eggs and nuts, these increase *pitta*. Finally, I bake cookies until they are brown but still soft and chewy—not hard and crispy, which increases *vata*. Save these cookies for the times when you want to delight your family or the neighborhood kids.

SERVING SUGGESTION

Serve with a cup of chai tea spiced with an extra pinch of cardamom, which is the Ayurvedic antidote to chocolate. Or serve with a cup of hot milk spiced with cardamom . . . yummy!

1. Melt the ghee, butter, or coconut oil in a saucepan on low heat. Remove the pan from the heat source to cool to room temperature.

2. In a medium-sized bowl, whisk together the flours, xanthan gum, baking soda, salt, and psyllium husks, and set aside.

3. Remeasure the melted ghee, butter, or coconut oil into a separate mixing bowl, and return any excess to its container. Add the coconut sugar to the melted fat along with the water and vanilla; whisk together. Add the flour mixture, and mix well with a spatula. Add oats and mix well. Fold in chips (and nuts, if using). Cover and chill the dough in the refrigerator for 30 minutes or longer.

4. When ready to bake, preheat the oven to 350°F. Line a baking sheet with parchment. Use a small scoop or measuring tablespoon to gather one tablespoon of dough per cookie. For perfectly shaped cookies, roll the dough in your hands for a second or two to form a ball. Drop 12 balls on the parchment, leaving about 2 inches between so the cookies can spread. Bake 11 to 13 minutes. The cookies will have started to brown, and the edges will have begun to set; the centers will still be soft. Let the cookies cool for 5 minutes on the baking sheet; then transfer the baked cookies on their parchment sheet to a rack to continue cooling for at least 10 minutes before serving—if you can wait that long! Keep the cookies in an airtight container for up to 3 days.

PUMPKIN PUDDING

Preparation Time: About 2½ hours (30 minutes active)
Serves 6

It's not Thanksgiving without pumpkin desserts, which, as far as I'm concerned, rival all others! This gourmet treat is wonderful in the fall and into the winter, as long as fresh pumpkins are still available.

3 cups puréed pumpkin from 1 small sugar pumpkin (about 2 pounds)

1 cup plus 2 tablespoons half-and-half, whole milk, or coconut cream

½ cup maple syrup or coconut nectar

1 teaspoon vanilla

1 teaspoon ground cinnamon

1 to 1¼ teaspoons ground ginger

¼ teaspoon ground cloves

¼ teaspoon ground nutmeg

½ teaspoon Fine Ground Celtic Sea Salt

2 tablespoons arrowroot

COOK'S TIP: I like a lot of ginger, but you may want to start with 1 teaspoon.

TIME-SAVER: Bake the pumpkin the day before. Let it cool and purée it to cut cooking time to 20 minutes.

AYURVEDIC NOTE

Fresh pumpkin is a wonderful food from the perspective of Ayurveda, as it is so easy to digest and it calms both *vata* and *pitta*. If you tolerate milk well, the dairy is also good for pacifying *vata* and *pitta*, as is maple syrup. The spices support *kapha*, although this dessert is not recommended for *kapha* except for special occasions because of the high-fat dairy. Coconut cream will also increase kapha.

1. Preheat oven to 425°F. Line a large baking dish or cookie sheet with parchment paper. Cut the pumpkin in half and scoop out the seeds and strings, and discard. (Or clean the seeds and roast in the oven.) Place the pumpkin halves flesh down on the paper. Cover with foil and bake for 45 minutes to an hour, until the pumpkin flesh is completely tender when you poke it with a fork. Let it cool 15 minutes or longer. Scoop out the flesh and purée it in a food processor. Check it to make sure there are no lumps, and if you find any, pulse the pumpkin again until it's completely smooth. If the purée is watery, strain first and then measure out 3 cups to set aside for the recipe.

2. When ready to finish the pudding, pour all but a ½ cup of the half-and-half, milk, or vegan milk into a 3-quart stainless steel pot on medium heat for about 5 minutes until it warms up. Stir often so that the milk does not burn. Once warm, remove the pot from the heat source, and add syrup (or coconut nectar) and vanilla. Also add the cinnamon, ginger, cloves, nutmeg, and salt. Stir and set aside.

3. Place arrowroot into a small bowl or measuring cup. Add the ½ cup of cold milk to the bowl a few tablespoons at a time, and whisk after each addition until all lumps are removed. Return the arrowroot mixture to the pot of milk, and return the pot to a burner on medium-low heat. Whisk continually until the milk thickens, about 10 minutes. (**Note:** The pudding will not thicken unless the mixture gets hot, but be vigilant about stirring constantly with the whisk.) Once the milk starts to thicken, stir in pumpkin purée and whisk until well combined.

4. Pour pudding into ramekins, small bowls, or dessert glasses and let cool for at least an hour. If you do not like skin on a pudding, place plastic wrap directly on top of each serving of the pudding. Serve with whipped cream (page 241).

INDIAN RICE PUDDING *(KHIR)*

Preparation Time: About 90 minutes to 2 hours (1 hour constant attention)
Serves 6 to 8

My friend Geetha Hariharan taught me how to make this lovely dish. Geetha learned to make this Indian rice pudding in Delhi, where she lived before moving to the United States with her husband and family. I grew up on the other side of the world, in South Carolina, eating my mother's Jewish rice pudding. Mom's version is exquisite but super rich with eggs and heavy cream. Fortunately, I've grown to love this lighter version, and now I can eat a guilt-free serving—and for a Jewish girl, that's saying something!

1 cup white basmati rice
8 cups whole milk or coconut cream, plus additional
   coconut cream for reconstituting
1 pinch of saffron threads
½ cup maple sugar crystals or rock sugar
12 to 15 cardamom pods or 1 teaspoon ground cardamom
2 tablespoons blanched almonds
¼ teaspoon rosewater

COOK'S TIP: 1. Since the cost of maple sugar can be prohibitive, I've included a less expensive option, rock sugar, which can be purchased at Asian grocers or online. **2.** I much prefer the Chaokoh Classic Gold Coconut Cream purchased online to the coconut milk I've found in grocery stores. **3.** Pudding made with coconut cream will need to be reconstituted after refrigeration. Reheat in a pot with 1 extra cup of the coconut cream for about 15 minutes. Stir often. If you wish, add more sugar, to taste. **4.** I make this dish when I'm cooking a full meal so that I'm always near the stove and can stir the pot frequently.

AYURVEDIC NOTE

Khir, when eaten in moderation, is considered *sattvic* food, meaning it is pure and calming for the mind and emotions. *Khir* is balancing for *vata* and *pitta* disorders. Maple sugar strengthens the constitution. Rock sugar is sometimes used in Ayurvedic medicine to carry nutrients to specific tissues, including the nervous system. Cardamom helps prevent the formation of excess mucous, which is often associated with cow's milk or coconut milk. Digestion of cow's milk is also aided by boiling the milk. Rosewater is a cooling agent and is especially good for people with *pitta* problems. Those with excess *kapha* should avoid *khir*, particularly when suffering from a head cold, bronchitis, or asthma.

1. Soak the rice in water for an hour or more. Rinse the rice in water and strain.

2. Place the rice and milk (or coconut cream) in a heavy stainless steel 6-quart soup pot, uncovered, on medium-low heat. Rub the strands of saffron between your thumb and forefinger to release the saffron's full flavor, and add the spice to the rice and milk mixture. Bring the pot to a gentle boil, stirring every couple of minutes so the milk does not burn. Once the mixture has started to bubble, reduce the heat to medium and continue to stir frequently for 20 to 30 minutes so that the rice doesn't stick to the bottom of the pot.

3. Once the rice is fully cooked (about 45 minutes), reduce the heat to low, add the sugar, and stir.

4. Break open the cardamom pods and grind the small, black seeds to a powder with a mortar and pestle. Add this ground spice to the pot and stir. (You can use commercially ground cardamom, but the freshly ground spice will have a richer flavor.)

5. At this point, the vegan version with coconut milk will be complete. If you're cooking with cow's milk, continue simmering the rice and milk another 30 minutes or longer. As the pudding approaches its completion, the milk will continually form a skin, which you should fold into the mixture while stirring, creating a thick, creamy texture. Continue this process until the pudding approaches the preferred thickness. If a skin is not forming, either cook the pudding longer on low heat or increase the heat level slightly and stir conscientiously. The final texture should be thick and creamy, like a custard.

6. Remove the pot from the heat source. Add the almonds and rosewater, and stir. Pour into a large serving bowl, and let the pudding cool to room temperature. (**Note:** As the pudding cools, it will continue to thicken a little bit more, and you will need to stir the skin that forms into the final version before serving.)

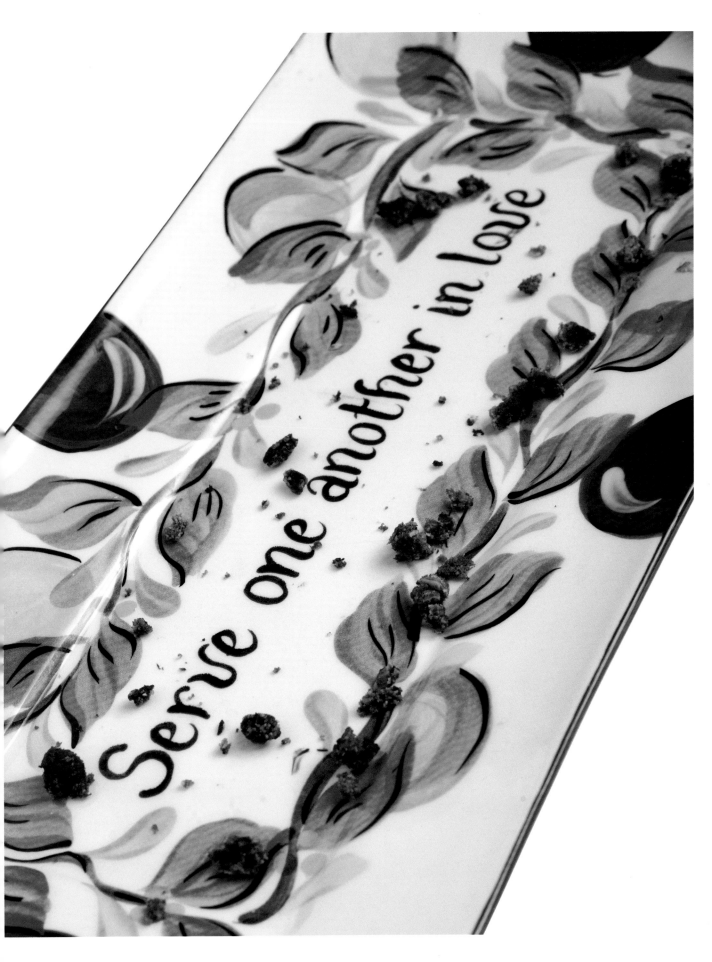

Appreciations

I never dreamed Ayurveda would lead me into the kitchen as a second career, but as I began studying this ancient dietary approach at age forty-three to recover from chronic illness, I began to love cooking! A routine activity that had felt like a chore became exhilarating as I began to explore ways of applying Ayurvedic principles of balance to many of my favorite foods. I started capturing lists of ingredients in a spiral-bound notebook so I'd remember how to make these new dishes, and when friends started asking for recipes, *Sacred & Delicious* emerged like a *spanda,* a divine burst of joy.

It has been an amazing journey of healing and self-discovery, and it would not have happened without the gentle urging of my husband, Tom Mitchell, who inspired me to explore Ayurveda, encouraged my cooking experiments, and coached and refined my understanding of this vibrant approach to wellness and healing. This immensely tender man supported and encouraged me in every conceivable way as I went through the sometimes joyful, sometimes daunting, task of creating a book about a subject for which I have no formal training or expertise beyond my own experience.

In 1998, Tom introduced me to the Ayurvedic Institute in Albuquerque, New Mexico, where I first recognized the power of Ayurveda while recovering from several chronic health problems. It was there, during a gentle detoxification program, that I tasted my first *kitchari.* I will be forever indebted to the institute's founder, Dr. Vasant Lad, who awakened my passion about Ayurveda with his effective and benevolent care that shifted the course of my health.

I never would have met another *vaidya* if not for Tom, who began to study pulse assessment with Dr. Pankaj and Dr. Smita Naram in 2001. So, because of my husband, I've had the opportunity to interview, attend lectures, and spend time with three of the world's most respected contemporary Ayurvedic masters. Whatever knowledge I have of Ayurveda, I have received from these distinguished teachers. Each has generously shared their knowledge with me. Both Dr. Lad and Dr. Smita Naram graciously invested time to support my writing of this book. And I send my special *pranams* to Smita for her gracious validation of my cooking—and for dancing with me in my kitchen!

I am also deeply indebted to Ed Danaher, manager of the Ayurvedic Institute's *panchakarma* department, for explaining Ayurvedic principles and answering my dozens of questions as I developed recipes and wrote the Ayurvedic primer for *Sacred & Delicious*

I send special thanks to Dr. Alpana Bhatt, my first Ayurvedic cooking teacher. Alpa taught me about the healing power of spices, gave me an Indian-style spice box, and taught me how to make an Indian *tarka*: the magical spice mixture that finishes many Indian-style foods. I'm especially grateful to three other Indian sister-friends: Alka Singh,

Geetha Hariharan, and Ashwini Sidhaye Gole, who helped me navigate writing about Indian-style food, taught me particular cooking techniques, and whose dishes inspired some of my own. Others who added to my knowledge of Indian cooking were Smita Shrimanker and Azah Mulchand.

Most of the food in *Sacred & Delicious* does not originate from India, and I happily acknowledge all that I have received from my good friend Dr. Ellen Brock, whose creative and extraordinary cooking most informed my own exploration of vegetarianism. This began in the time we roomed together as seniors at the University of South Carolina. When I was twenty, Ellen taught me to bake bread, use fresh vegetables, make healthy food, and how to cook with unabashed joy.

Ultimately, it took a small army to bring this big book to life, and I want to express my sincere appreciation to all of you for your unique contributions. I have infinite gratitude for my astonishingly proficient editor Margaret Bendet. There are no truer words than "I couldn't have done it without you!" Thank you for being my steadfast partner since 2008, when I first began jotting down notes to unfold my revelatory title, *Sacred & Delicious*. How fortunate I was to find a professional editor who is also steeped in Vedic knowledge. Thank you for your genius with words and the ability to organize my sometimes hodgepodge of ideas into a coherent narrative.

Sacred & Delicious would be incomplete without desserts, and I had hardly baked a thing before embarking on writing this book! For that reason, I am indebted to my friend Martina Straub, who taught me to roll a pie crust, offered a recipe or two, and often served as my baking buddy, mentor, and (on many occasions) confidence booster. She also edited an early draft of the desserts chapter. A big thank you as well to Marie Haulenbeek and Melissa Dittmer, who both offered me invaluable tips on desserts.

For bringing this book into form, I am especially grateful to Brooke Warner, publisher of She Writes Press and a remarkable force in the publishing industry. Thank you so much for trusting and believing in my vision for *Sacred & Delicious*. Thank you, too, for assembling the outstanding professional team that supported this book with skill and patience, especially the project manager Cait Levin, proofreader Pamela Long, and my brilliant designer Tabitha Lahr. Blessings to you, Tabitha, for creating a gorgeous book that many readers will want to curl up with.

The "look" of *Sacred & Delicious* also had a great deal of early support. I am profoundly grateful to Karin Michele Anderson, who blessed this book cover by painting an extraordinarily beautiful image filled with *shakti*—the light of the divine feminine!—and to Ingrid Beckman, who developed early design templates for special sections.

No cookbook is worth its salt without photographs that make your mouth water, and most of these wonderful images were taken by Roger W. Winstead. Ingrid Beckman brought expert styling and sheer delight to each session! A couple more photos were contributed by Jeanne Reinelt and Ann Stratton. Much appreciation to Brook and Tom Ayres, who graciously opened their home to be a photography studio. Thanks also to Anthony Aber, director of career services at The Chef's Academy in Raleigh, who introduced me to Abir Heikal. Both Abir and Alka Singh worked as my able cooking assistants, helping prepare almost forty dishes that were photographed over three weeks.

Also, I send much appreciation to the publicist Ann-Marie Nieves and Nadea Mina of Get Red PR and to my friends Jane Kuhn (for additional public relations support) and Janis Pettit (for marketing coaching). Also pranams to Ingrid Beckman, who designed the *Sacred & Delicious* website and marketing materials. And thanks to Laurie Hirneisen for cheerful administrative support.

I have enormous appreciation for my early readers and proofreaders. First among them was my sweet mother, Bonnie Silver Cagan, who took delight in seeing me blossom as a creative cook and encouraged me at every turn with great generosity. I had never written a recipe before *Sacred & Delicious* started to take form, and it was my mother who gently set me straight on how to do so correctly! Sadly, my father did not live to see what a perfect *balabosta* I have become, as he would have particularly loved my thick soups.

My amazing readers-in-the-trenches were Amy Allen, Karin Anderson, Louise Applebome, Denise Bernier, Ellen

Brock, Gin Burchfield, Paulette Costanza, Allyson Falk, Chris and June Forsyth, Olivia Fried, Linda Lusk, Christine McNally, Duffy Poindexter, and Penny Savage.

I have much appreciation for those who offered recipes that I was able to use as written or adapt to an Ayurvedic or gluten-free approach: Alpa Bhatt, Ellen Brock, Marvin Brown, Bonnie Cagan, Sal Corbo, Ashwini Sidhaye Gole, Marie Pardue Iddings, Jodi Kimmelman, Maureen McNelis, Janis Pettit, and Martina Straub. Special thanks to the chef Sal Corbo, who also helped me perfect the seasoning for the Green Bean and Shiitake Mushroom Soup.

And I send a million thanks to the legions of testers and tasters, family, friends, and colleagues who offered time, recipe testing, and other types of enthusiastic support: Amy Allen, Andrea Amburgey, Karin Michele Anderson, Susan Anzalone, Denise Bernier, Ellen Brock, Marvin Brown, Jennie Boyd Bull, Rick and Victoria Cagan, Peggy Crowley, Sharon Cutler, Melissa Dittmer, Kathee Dowis, Michael Fischman, Wilda Fisher, Elizabeth French, Libby and Graham Gell, Kathy Harkins, Annie Hassell, Marie Haulenbeek, Johanna Hoey, Marie Iddings, Gino Izetta, Michelle Johnson, Jessica Kasinoff, Maggi Kennedy, Cindy Krimmelbein, Margot Knepp, Trish Koontz, Jeanne LaPointe, Linda Lusk, Judy MacHaffie, Rani Margolin, Melanie McGhee, Randa McNamara, Maureen McNelis, Betty Mitchell, Linda Morse, Duffy Poindexter, Jeanne Reinelt, Julie Schmidt, Latha Sabesa, Vicki Sprague Ravenel, Judith Schafman, Candice Stark, Kathy Stewart, Emili Stoll, Brandi Studer, Leslie Todd, Carol Walborn, Lisa Werness, Andrea Williams, Bonnie Wolf, Ginger Yancey, and (last but not least) Karen Ziegler. If I have overlooked anyone, please know that this is not from a lack of gratitude for your contribution.

Thank you to Harold McGee, author of *On Food and Cooking*, for taking the time to answer a first-time author's query about cooking science.

I am also immensely grateful to those who provided prayers and blessings from various cultures: Rabbi Raachel Jurovics, Fiaz Fareed, Michael Fischman, Jack Gladstone, Ammal Mammoud, Stephanie Smith, and Andrew Weiss. Special thanks to Rob Quist for introducing me to Jack Gladstone from the Blackfeet Nation, and deep gratitude to Jack for the privilege of publishing for the first time this prayer given to his family from Chief Bird Rattler (1860-1909). Also thanks to Rabbi Jurovics for connecting me with Rabbi Zalman Schachter-Shalomi—whose encouragement was, indeed, a blessing.

I also have profound gratitude to all my family and my many dear friends who often cheered me on from afar (some by being endlessly enthusiastic about my cooking) and who kept faith with me when other obligations pulled me away from reaching the finish line. I'm especially grateful to my brother, Rick Cagan, for his ongoing support, and to my stepdaughter, Celeste Mitchell, who came into my life a few months after I met her father twenty-five years ago. Celeste was a great tester and taster of desserts!

My life is blessed with the riches of many sister-and-brother friends, and I have eternal gratitude to all of you who have energized me along the way. Afraid that I might miss one, I will not list you by name—but, rather, will blow a kiss to you each. You know who you are; we live in each other's hearts.

And for supporting all of me, body and soul, during this long process, I send my heartfelt thanks to Cathy Bradway, Mary Cochran, Lauren Jubelirer, Steven Marcus, Melanie McGhee, Duffy Poindexter, Bonnie Tomek, and Lisa Werness. I am enormously grateful to each of you for helping me reach my full potential.

Let me end with expressing my appreciation to Sri Sri Ravi Shankar, my husband's guru and my compassionate benefactor. I give thanks daily for your blessings upon our marriage and continual blessings for our health and well-being.

Finally, my deepest gratitude to Gurumayi Chidvilasananda, my beloved meditation Master and spiritual guide. Thank you for awakening in me the recognition of my true Self, for rekindling my joy, and for your daily inspiration on the path of the Heart.

APPENDIX

Some Key Ayurvedic Principles

1. The body has the innate intelligence to heal itself, and the most essential means of its doing so is the ingestion of nurturing food.

2. Food, when used correctly, sustains us and supports healing; food, when misused, will surely make us sick.

3. The more interesting and delicious a food becomes through the informed use of diverse spices, the more nurturing that food is for the body.

4. Ayurveda recognizes the organizing intelligence of the body. These three dynamic principles are called *doshas*: *vata* (air), *pitta* (fire), and *kapha* (earth). Every living being has a unique combination of all three *doshas*, which offer a blueprint for health and an early-detection warning system for disease.

5. What we eat plays a primary role in keeping the three *doshas* in balance, and maintaining balance is essential to good health.

6. By learning the attributes of the *doshas* and the attributes of various foods, you can learn which foods best support your body.

7. To understand how foods and spices affect the *doshas*, consider this fundamental premise: Like increases like; opposites create balance. Stated another way, foods and spices with qualities similar to a *dosha* typically increase or aggravate that dosha; foods and spices with qualities that are the opposite or at least different from a *dosha* typically decrease or pacify that *dosha*.

8. In dealing with dietary changes, moderation is always the key.

9. Good digestion is the secret to sustaining good health. The secret to sustaining good digestion is to support *agni*, the digestive fire, through right diet and lifestyle.

10. The vital rule of digestion: eat only when you are hungry, and stop eating before you are full. Overeating weakens *agni*.

11. Weak *agni* leads to the accumulation of toxins, called *ama*. Toxins are also formed because of eating foods processed or grown with chemicals—chemical preservatives, chemical coloring agents, chemical fertilizers.

12. Pain and disease occur because of weak *agni*, high *ama*, and imbalanced *doshas*. Such conditions can usually be resolved when caught early enough and treated through right diet, supervised detoxification (*panchakarma*), herbal supplements, and a supportive lifestyle.

Sources

Sources referred to in the text, as well as some that influenced my thinking or provided information, are listed below by chapter, generally alphabetized by the name of the author. At times, for the reader's convenience, the sources are grouped by topic. Website URLs are current as of September 2017.

Introduction

The epigraph is from Gurumayi Chidvilasananda, *The Yoga of Discipline* (South Fallsburg, NY: SYDA Foundation, 1996), 135. Reprinted with permission from the SYDA Foundation.

Part One: The Fundamentals

The epigraph is from the author's notes while a guest at a lecture Dr. Vasant Lad gave to the Ayurvedic Studies Level 2 Program at The Ayurvedic Institute in Albuquerque, NM. Printed with permission from The Ayurvedic Institute.

Chapter 1: Principles of Ayurveda

The epigraph is a statement made by Dr. Vasant Lad during a class lecture at The Ayurvedic Institute in 2003. Printed with permission from The Ayurvedic Institute.

The comments attributed to Ed Danaher, director of the *panchakarma* clinic at The Ayurvedic Institute, are from multiple conversations with the author between 2003 and 2011. Printed with permission from The Ayurvedic Institute.

American Cancer Society. "Common Questions about Diet and Cancer." https://www.cancer.org/healthy/eat-healthy-get-active/acs-guidelines-nutrition-physical-activity-cancer-prevention/common-questions.html.

Atreya. *Perfect Balance: Ayurvedic Nutrition for Mind, Body, and Soul.* (New York: Avery, 2001), 21, 83, 84.

Boyles, Salynn. "Study: Acid Reflux on the Rise, Obesity Increase Likely to Blame, Researchers Say." Web MD, December 22, 2011, http://www.webmd.com/heartburn-gerd/news/20111222/study-acid-reflux-prevalence-increasing.

Colbin, Annemarie. *Food and Healing.* (New York: Ballantine, 1996), 284.

Crowe, Dr. Francesca. "Vegetarian Diet Reduces Risk of Heart Disease by a Third." *Medical News Today*, January 31, 2013, http://www.medicalnewstoday.com/articles/255644.php.

Frawley, Dr. David, and Dr. Subhash Ranade. *Ayurveda: Nature's Medicine.* (Twin Lakes, WI: Lotus, 2001), 99, 100.

Joshi, Dr. Sunil V. *Ayurveda & Panchakarma: The Science of Healing and Rejuvenation.* (Twin Lakes, WI: Lotus, 1997), 59, 64, 68, 75. Reproduced with permission from Lotus Press, a division of Lotus Brands, Inc., PO Box 325, Twin Lakes, WI 53181, USA,www.lotuspress.com ©1997 All Rights Reserved.

Lad, Usha, and Dr. Vasant Lad. *Ayurvedic Cooking for Self-Healing*, 2nd ed. (Albuquerque, NM: Ayurvedic Press, 1997), 15–18, 20, 22, 31, 34–37, 209, 215, 232–38. The final reference is to Appendix. C: "Qualities of Food Substances." Here the Lads expand his earlier list of popular foods and discuss how each impacts the *doshas*, including taste, aftertaste, and metabolic effect.

Lad, Dr. Vasant. *Ayurveda: The Science of Self-Healing: A Practical Guide.* (Santa Fe, NM: Sunstone, 1984), 90–99B. Dr. Lad lists foods popular in the West and defines them according to Ayurvedic principles.

Lad, Dr. Vasant. *The Complete Book of Ayurvedic Home Remedies.* (New York: Three Rivers, 1998), 31, 101. Dr. Lad focuses on treating common ailments with traditional Ayurvedic remedies.

Masson, Jeffrey Moussaieff. *The Face on Your Plate: The Truth about Food.* (New York: W.W. Norton, 2009), 34–58.

Maisto, Michelle. "Eating Less Meat Is World's Best Chance for Timely Climate Change, Say Experts." *Forbes*, April 28, 2012, http://www.forbes.com/sites/michellemaisto/2012/04/28/eating-less-meat-is-worlds-best-chance-for-timely-climate-change-say-experts/.

McGee, Harold. *On Food and Cooking: The Science and Lore of the Kitchen.* (New York: Scribner, 2004), 271, 489.

Naram, Dr. Smita. *Secrets of Natural Health.* (Mumbai, India: Ayushakti, 2002), 12, 22, 23.

Physicians Committee for Responsible Medicine. "Vegetarian Foods: Powerful for Health." http://www.pcrm.org/health/diets/vegdiets/vegetarian-foods-powerful-for-health.

Pole, Sebastian. *Ayurvedic Medicine: The Principles of Traditional Practice.* (Philadelphia, PA: Churchill Livingstone Elsevier, 2006), 20, 244.

Scheer, Roddy, and Doug Moss. "How Does Meat in the Diet Take an Environmental Toll?" EarthTalk®, December 28, 2011, http://www.scientificamerican.com/article/meat-and-environment/.

World Health Organization. "A Strategy for Traditional Medicine." *Traditional Medicine.* (Fifty-Sixth World Health Assembly, Report by the Secretariat, March 31, 2003), http://apps.who.int/gb/archive/pdf_files/WHA56/ea5618.=pdf.

Zhao, Yafu, MS, and William Encinosa, PhD. "Statistical Brief no. 44: Gastroesophageal Reflux Disease (GERD) Hospitalizations in 1998 and 2005." The Healthcare Cost and Utilization Project (HCUP), January 2008, http://www .hcup-us.ahrq.gov/reports/statbriefs/sb44.jsp.

Chapter 2: Eating Well in the Modern World

The epigraph was written by Dr. Smita Naram for *Sacred & Delicious* and was shared in a personal letter to the author. Printed with permission from Dr. Smita Naram.

The discussion on fermented foods is, in part, from the author's interviews with Dr. Smita Naram at Ayurshakti Ayurved in Mumbai, India, in December 2005 and is printed by permission from Dr. Smita Naram.

The discussion on fermented foods also stems from the author's interview with Ed Danaher at The Ayurvedic Institute in Albuquerque, NM, on April 24, 2003. Printed by permission from The Ayurvedic Institute.

Chilton, Floyd H., PhD, with Laura Tucker. *Inflammation Nation.* (New York: Fireside, 2005), 7.

Joshi, Dr. Sunil V. *Ayurveda & Panchakarma*, 134, 139.

Lad, Usha, and Dr. Vasant Lad. *Ayurvedic Cooking for Self-Healing*, Appendix: Food Guidelines for Basic Constitutional Types, Condiments.

Neuman, Alfred E. *SearchQuotes*, http://www.searchquotes.com/quotation/We_are_living_in_a_world_today_where_ lemonade_is_made_from_artificial_flavors_and_furniture_polish_i/29801/.

Pollan, Michael. *The Omnivore's Dilemma: A Natural History of Four Meals.* (New York: Penguin, 2006), 113, 179.

Pollan, Michael. *In Defense of Food: An Eater's Manifesto.* (New York: Penguin, 2008), 8, 101–136.

Refined Sugar

Crayhon, Robert, MS CN. *Nutrition Made Simple: A Comprehensive Guide to the Latest Findings in Optimal Nutrition.* (New York: M. Evans, 1996), 56.

Lustig, Robert H.; Laura A. Schmidt; and Claire D. Brindis. "Public Health: The Toxic Truth about Sugar." *Nature: International Weekly Journal of Science*, vol. 482, February 2, 2012. Reprint available: https://uhs.berkeley.edu/sites/ default/files/wellness-toxictruthaboutsugar.pdf.

Yacoubou, Jeanne. "Is Your Sugar Vegan?" *Vegetarian Journal*, no. 4, 2007, 15.

Food Combining

Lad, Usha, and Dr. Vasant Lad. *Ayurvedic Cooking for Self-Healing*, 47.

Minton, Barbara L. "For Digestive Bliss Eat Foods that Don't Fight." *Natural News*, February 17, 2009, http://www .naturalnews.com/025651_food_protein_foods.html#.

Chapter 3: The Essential Ingredient

The epigraph is from Sri Sri Ravi Shankar's talk "Offer Everything," the fifth in a series entitled *The Path of Love*, on Narada's *Bhakti Sutras*. (Santa Barbara: Art of Living Foundation, 1990), tape 5. Printed with permission from the Art of Living Foundation.

The prayer "Annadaata Sukhi Bhavah" is an Indian folk blessing, and the translation is by Sri Sri Ravi Shankar. It is printed with permission from the Art of Living Foundation.

Regarding the impact of food on the *doshas*: Usha and Dr. Vasant Lad's *Ayurvedic Cooking for Self-Healing*, 47.

The discussion on the Buddhist perspective on cooking and mindfulness is from the author's conversations with Andrew JiYu Weiss, a meditation teacher and ordained Zen priest.

Thoughts on the importance of blessing a meal were addressed by Charles Poindexter, a spiritual healer, in a letter to the author.

The significance of the sound *ummmm* was discussed by Dr. Vasant Lad in 2007 in a class at The Ayurvedic Institute. Printed with permission from The Ayurvedic Institute.

Chapter 4: Getting Started

The epigraph is from Dr. Deepak Chopra, Perfect Health: The Complete Mind Body Guide, (New York: Three Rivers Press, revised 2000), 315.

Part Two: The Recipes

The information about the impact of food on the *doshas* found in the author's Ayurvedic Notes following each recipe has been gleaned from Usha and Dr. Vasant Lad's *Ayurvedic Cooking for Self-Healing*, Appendix: Qualities of Food Substances.

Chapter 5: Breakfast, Breads, and Beverages

The epigraph is from the *Prashna Upanishad*, 1.14; translated by Eknath Easwaran, founder of the Blue Mountain Center of Meditation, copyright 1987, 2007. Reprinted by permission of Nilgiri Press, P.O. Box 256, Tomales, CA 94971. www.bmcm.org.

The Jewish prayer translation is an excerpt from *Mishkan T'filah: A Reform Siddur*, copyright ©2007 by Central Conference of American Rabbis and Women of Reform Judaism, and is under the copyright protection of the Central Conference of American Rabbis and reprinted for use by permission of the CCAR. All rights reserved.

The gluten-free bread recipe on page 68 benefitted from two technical tips about gluten-free baking by the Editors at America's Test Kitchen. *The How Can It Be Gluten Free Cookbook*. (Brookline, MA: America's Test Kitchen, 2014), 173.

The Ayurvedic Institute. "Ghee." https://www.ayurveda.com/online_resource/ghee_recipe.html.

Bhavaprakasha 6.18.1; the translation is from *Ayurvedic Yogi.* "Ghee's Central Role in Ayurvedic Treatment." http://www.ayurvedicyogi.com/ghee%E2%80%99s-invaluable-place-in-ayurvedic-treatment/.

The recipe for almond milk was adapted from *Whole Food Recipes for Better Living* by Vitamix Corporation, (Cleveland, Ohio, 2004), 76. Reprinted with permission from Vitamix.

Chapter 6: Vegetable Soups

The epigraph is from Chitra Banerjee Divakaruni's novel *The Mistress of Spices*, (New York: Anchor Books, 1998), 7.

"Grace Before Food" from *The Celtic Spirit* by Caitlin Matthews. Copyright © 1999 by Caitlin Matthews. Reprinted by permission of HarperCollins Publishers.

The qualities of curry leaves were described by Dr. Vasant Lad in an interview with the author in 2003 and are printed with his permission.

Chapter 7: Legume-Based Soups

The epigraph is from Dr. Vasant Lad in an interview with the author. Printed by permission from The Ayurvedic Institute.

The translation of this Hindu prayer from the *Bhagavad Gita* 4.24, was taken from "Blessing Our Food as Part of God," July 11, 2012, https://www.ramdass.org/blessing-our-food-part-of-god/. Reprinted courtesy of Love Serve Remember Foundation, RamDass.org.

Lad, Usha and Dr. Vasant. *Ayurvedic Cooking for Self-Healing*, 47.

McGee, Harold. *On Food and Cooking: The Science and Lore of the Kitchen.* (New York, NY: Scribner, 2004), 489, 493.

Tyler Herbst, Sharon. *The New Food Lover's Companion: Comprehensive Definitions of Nearly 6000 Food, Drink, and Culinary Terms*, 3rd ed. (Hauppauge, NY: Barron's Educational Series, 2001), 345.

Chapter 8: Entrées

The epigraph is by Bethany Jean Clement, a *Seattle Times* food writer. These lines are the conclusion of an article titled "Why you should eat all the asparagus right now," originally published in the newspaper's May 10, 2016, edition. Reprinted with permission from *The Seattle Times*.

The Native American prayer is from an unpublished memoir by Jack Wagner and is printed with permission from Jack Gladstone, a member of the Blackfeet Nation in Northwest Montana and a direct descendant of the legendary chief Red Crow.

Regarding the Ayurvedic perspective on mushrooms: Dr. Smita Naram, *Secrets of Natural Health*, 29.

Chapter 9: Side Dishes

The epigraph is an excerpt from "The Vegetables" from *The Subject Tonight Is Love: 60 Wild and Sweet Poems of Hafiz* by Daniel Ladinsky, copyright 1996, and used with permission.

The Muslim prayer is reprinted with permission from the website *The Modern Religion*, "Everyday Duas in Arabic with Transliteration and Translation," http://www.themodernreligion.com/basic/pray/duas.html.

Consumer Reports. "Arsenic in Your Food." November 2012, http://consumerreports.org/cro/magazine/2012/11/arsenic-in-your-food/index.htm.

McGee, Harold. *On Food and Cooking*, 472.

US Food & Drug Administration. "Arsenic in Rice and Rice Products." August 4, 2014, http:www.fda.gov/Food/FoodborneIllnessContaminants/Metals/ucm319948.htm.

Chapter 10: Salads

The epigraph from Swami Muktananda is found in *Resonate with Stillness: Daily Contemplations*, (South Fallsburg, NY: SYDA Foundation, 1995), February 3. Reprinted by permission from the SYDA Foundation.

"The Five Contemplations" is a prayer commonly repeated by Zen Buddhists before eating. This version was rendered by Zen priest Andrew JiYu Weiss from prayers in the Zen traditions of Vietnam and Japan.

Chapter 11: Desserts

The epigraph is from email correspondence between Rabbi Zalman Schachter-Shalomi and the author, March 19, 2014. Printed with his permission.

The Christian prayer is from *The Book of Common Prayer*, (New York: The Church Hymnal Corporation, 1979), p. 835.

Pollan, Michael. *Food Rules: An Eater's Manual*. (New York: Penguin Group, 2009), 131.

WebMD. "Xanthan Gum." http://www.webmd.com/vitamins-and-supplements/xanthan-gum-uses-and-risks.

Glossary

Lad, Usha and Dr. Vasant Lad, *Ayurvedic Cooking for Self-Healing*, 239, 240, 242

Glossary

GLOSSARY OF INDIAN TERMS

As you study Ayurveda, you may be engaging with a new language, as the ancient Ayurvedic texts were all written in Sanskrit, the sacred language of India. In this glossary you will find the terms from Sanskrit and other Indian languages used in Sacred & Delicious.

AGNI: The biological power of digestion and metabolism that provides energy for bodily functions

AHIMSA: Nonviolence; a tenet of classical yoga

AMA (OR AAM): Toxins in the body produced by poor metabolism and non-food substances such as chemicals added to food when it is grown or processed

AYURVEDA: Literally, "knowledge of life;" also the traditional medical system of India

CHAPATI: A round unleavened soft flatbread, similar to a tortilla, traditionally made with wheat

CURRY (DERIVED FROM THE TAMIL *KARI*): A mixture of spices; a spicy sauce or a dish made from that sauce

DAL (OR DHAL, DAHL): a form of legume, especially mung, *chana* (split chickpeas) and *toor* (split pigeon peas); a soup made of any of these legumes

DHARMA: An individual's sacred duty or life purpose

DOSHA: An organizing principle that maintains the integrity of the physical body and is based on the traditional elements found in nature (earth, air, water, fire, and space)

JAGGERY: An unrefined sugar made from sugar cane

KAPHA: One of the three bodily *doshas,* made up of the earth and water elements

KHIR: A sweet pudding

MASALA: A mixture of dry, ground spices

OJAS: The subtle essence gleaned from pure foods that sustains the body and increases its vigor, immunity, and luster

PANCHAKARMA: A process involving five actions used to purify the physical body

PITTA: One of the three bodily *doshas,* made up of the fire and water elements

PRASAD: Blessed food; any gift from the Divine

PRANA: The life force that distinguishes what is living from what is dead; the breath

PRANAM: To bow before another with humility, gratitude, or devotion

RAJAS: An energy that is over-stimulating to the body, mind, and emotions

ROTI: A general name for Indian flatbreads

SATTVA: An energy that is pure and calming to the body, mind, and emotions

TAMAS: An energy that dulls the senses and creates lethargy and, in the extreme, negative tendencies such as violence

TARKA (OR TADKA, CHAUNK, THALIMPU): Herbs and spices that have been sizzled in hot oil to release their essential oils and full fragrance before being added to food

TRIDOSHIC: An English word form that refers to food or medicinal herbs that are balancing for all three *doshas* or constitutions

SPANDA: A divine pulsation

VAIDYA: An Ayurvedic physician

VATA: One of the three bodily *doshas,* made up of air and space

VIPAK: The post-digestive effect of a food after it has been assimilated in the body, either sweet, sour, or pungent

Index

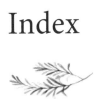

Author Biography

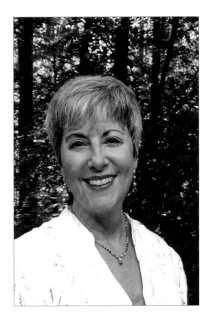

*L*isa Joy Mitchell, a busy public relations consultant, was drawn to study Ayurvedic cooking in 1998, when chronic health problems began taking center stage in her fast-paced life. On her road to wellness, Mitchell changed her diet and began an informal study with Ayurvedic physicians Dr. Vasant Lad and Ed Danaher in the United States and Dr. Smita Naram in India.

Mitchell is now a wellness mentor and cooking instructor based in Raleigh, North Carolina. She often works in partnership with her husband, Tom Mitchell, a chiropractic physician who practices Ayurvedic pulse assessment and herbal medicine. During the past decade, Mitchell has cooked for hundreds of participants in Ayurvedic clinics and meditation courses. You can find Lisa's blog and information about upcoming events at www.sacredanddelicious.com.

Selected Titles from She Writes Press

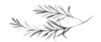

She Writes Press is an independent publishing company founded to serve women writers everywhere. Visit us at www.shewritespress.com.

Raw by Bella Mahaya Carter. $16.95, 978-1-63152-345-8. In an effort to holistically cure her chronic stomach problems, Bella Mahaya Carter adopted a 100 percent raw, vegan diet—a first step on a quest that ultimately dragged her, kicking and screaming, into spiritual adulthood.

Hedgebrook Cookbook: Celebrating Radical Hospitality by Denise Barr & Julie Rosten. $24.95, 978-1-938314-22-3. Delectable recipes and inspiring writing, straight from Hedgebrook's farm-house table to yours.

Away from the Kitchen: Untold Stories, Private Menus, Guarded Recipes, and Insider Tips by Dawn Blume Hawkes. $24.95, 978-1-938314-36-0. A food book for those who want it all: the menus, the recipes, and the behind-the-scenes scoop on some of America's favorite chefs.

Recipes for Redemption: A Companion Cookbook to A Cup of Redemption by Carole Bumpus. $19.95, 978-1-63152-824-8. A uniquely character-centered cookbook that offers delicious recipes—and savory stories—straight from the pages of A Cup of Redemption.

Note to Self: A Seven-Step Path to Gratitude and Growth by Laurie Buchanan. $16.95, 978-1-63152-113-3. Transforming intention into action, Note to Self equips you to shed your baggage, bridging the gap between where you are and where you want to be—body, mind, and spirit—and empowering you to step into joy-filled living now!

Think Better. Live Better. 5 Steps to Create the Life You Deserve by Francine Huss. $16.95, 978-1-938314-66-7. With the help of this guide, readers will learn to cultivate more creative thoughts, realign their mindset, and gain a new perspective on life.